SEIZED BY UNCERTAINTY

Seized by Uncertainty

The Markets, Media, and Special Interests
That Shaped Canada's Response
to COVID-19

KEVIN QUIGLEY, KAITLYNNE LOWE,
SARAH MOORE, AND BRIANNA WOLFE

McGill-Queen's University Press
Montreal & Kingston • London • Chicago

ISBN 978-0-2280-2289-3 (paper)
ISBN 978-0-2280-2332-6 (ePDF)
ISBN 978-0-2280-2333-3 (ePUB)

Legal deposit fourth quarter 2024
Bibliothèque nationale du Québec

Printed in Canada on acid-free paper that is 100% ancient forest free
(100% post-consumer recycled), processed chlorine free

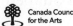

Funded by the   Financé par le
Government   gouvernement   Canada   Canada Council   Conseil des arts
of Canada   du Canada   for the Arts   du Canada

We acknowledge the support of the Canada Council for the Arts.
Nous remercions le Conseil des arts du Canada de son soutien.

McGill-Queen's University Press in Montreal is on land which long served
as a site of meeting and exchange amongst Indigenous Peoples, including the
Haudenosaunee and Anishinabeg nations. In Kingston it is situated on the territory
of the Haudenosaunee and Anishinaabek. We acknowledge and thank the diverse
Indigenous Peoples whose footsteps have marked these territories on which peoples
of the world now gather.

Library and Archives Canada Cataloguing in Publication

Title: Seized by uncertainty : the markets, media, and special interests that shaped
Canada's response to COVID-19 / Kevin Quigley, Kaitlynne Lowe, Sarah Moore, and
Brianna Wolfe.
Names: Quigley, Kevin, 1971– author. | Lowe, Kaitlynne, author. | Moore, Sarah
(Author of Seized by uncertainty), author. | Wolfe, Brianna, author.
Description: Includes bibliographical references and index.
Identifiers: Canadiana (print) 20240417585 | Canadiana (ebook) 20240417658
| ISBN 9780228022893 (paper) | ISBN 9780228023333 (ePUB) | ISBN
9780228023326 (ePDF)
Subjects: LCSH: COVID-19 Pandemic, 2020-—Government policy—Canada. | LCSH:
COVID-19 (Disease)—Government policy—Canada.
Classification: LCC RA644.C67 Q54 2024 | DDC 362.1962/414400971—dc23

This book was typeset in 10/13 Sabon by Sayre Street Books.

For those left behind

Contents

Tables and Figures

TABLES

FIGURES

Acknowledgments

We would like to thank the Social Sciences and Humanities Research Council of Canada for supporting our work on emergency management through a partnership development grant. We also wish to thank the Atlantic Canada Opportunities Agency for support through the Atlantic Canada Research Initiative Fund (ACRI) and the Province of Nova Scotia for support through the Change Lab Action Research Initiative (CLARI). ACRI and CLARI supported our work on tourism and the pandemic. CLARI also supported our work on home care and long-term care. This research would not have occurred without the generous and timely support of these organizations.

The MacEachen Institute for Public Policy and Governance (MI) at Dalhousie University in Halifax, Nova Scotia, served as a physical and virtual hub for our research. Scholars, students, advocates, and professionals with diverse backgrounds and expertise met at the MI over a three-year period to exchange views on the impact of the pandemic. While the authors are the exclusive owners of all errors in the manuscript, we would like to thank the many expert guests who attended our panels and round tables on the pandemic and offered such thoughtful and informed perspectives on the topic. The ideas generated at these events stimulated our thinking and served as a constant check on our research. We also owe a debt of gratitude to the original donors who enabled the MI to serve as a place for forward-looking policy debates and research.

Darrell Dexter, an honorary distinguished fellow of the MacEachen Institute, co-chaired many round tables with Scholarly Director Kevin Quigley. Darrell also attended exploratory discussions about the impact of the pandemic on long-term care, work that was supported by MI research assistant Mary MacGowan. Research assistant Hala Nader conducted much of the media analysis in the book and co-wrote chapter 10. Research assistant Noel Guscott conducted much of the research on lobbying, shared the lead on bureau-shaping analysis, and co-authored chapter 11.

MI program manager Jocelyne Rankin and copy editor Janet Lord have supported the work of the institute for years and played key roles in the research and writing process of the book. Jocelyne organized round tables and panels, contributed to writing grant applications, and designed and managed various budgets and project plans. Importantly, she made sure everyone was paid on time. Her deft planning ensured that the work met a predictable and ambitious timeline and included ample opportunity for academic rigour and input. We started the research at the beginning of the pandemic and drafted and necessarily redrafted material as events followed an unpredictable trajectory. Janet joined the team in the very early stages of this work and reviewed every word that is included in the book and, thanks to her sharp eye, many that are not.

We would like to thank everyone at McGill-Queen's University Press, and especially senior editor Emily Andrew, who supported us throughout the publication process in a variety of important ways, including securing thoughtful and robust reviews in a timely manner. The two anonymous reviewers provided two rounds of detailed and substantive comments that immeasurably improved the quality of the book. We hope they are satisfied with the result.

The authors have a number of professional responsibilities in their lives. These competing demands inevitably led to the authors sacrificing weekends and evenings to this work, which often shortchanged those in their personal lives. We are grateful to those who tolerated our misplaced priorities.

In Canada, 37,722 people are estimated to have died of COVID-19 between 1 January 2020 and 2 April 2022. The exact case count will never be known. At a lecture at the Society for Risk Analysis about twenty years ago, American risk psychologist Paul Slovic pointed out that we could not seem to process death and human suffering on such a large scale. This, he argued, was one reason that genocide continued to occur. While using objective data is crucial to understanding the magnitude of a problem, it is also important to remember that each death represents a lost life, as well as grief for those who knew the person.

Professor James Barker was a founding fellow at the MacEachen Institute and a renowned academic in leadership studies. Jim contributed to our round-table discussions on lessons learned from the pandemic, first on the subject of risk communication, and subsequently on management in complex contexts. Steven Estey was a highly respected human rights advocate who joined our round table to discuss the impact of the pandemic on those with disabilities. These leading thinkers, both in their sixties, passed away in the last year of our writing the book. They had considerable impact in their fields and challenged us to do better. We hope this book can help us understand better the role of government in such a complex context and the importance in the broadest sense of not leaving people behind, knowing that we do, and we did.

Abbreviations

9/11	11 September 2001 terrorist attacks
ACS	Association for Canadian Studies
AG	Auditor General of Canada
BI	business interruption
CAF	Canadian Armed Forces
CBSA	Canada Border Services Agency
CDC	Centers for Disease Control and Prevention
CERB	Canada Emergency Response Benefit
CERS	Canada Emergency Rent Subsidy
CESB	Canada Emergency Student Benefit
CEWS	Canada Emergency Wage Subsidy
CFIB	Canadian Federation of Independent Business
CHT	Canada Health Transfer
CIHI	Canadian Institute for Health Information
CMO	chief medical officer
CPHA	Canadian Public Health Association
CRA	Canada Revenue Agency
crsb	Canada Recovery Sickness Benefit
CRT	critical race theory
DC	Destination Canada
DMOS	destination-marketing organizations
EI	Employment Insurance
ESDC	Employment and Social Development Canada
G7	Group of Seven
GDP	gross domestic product
GPHIN	Global Public Health Intelligence Network
HRO	high-reliability organizations
IBC	Insurance Bureau of Canada
ICU	intensive care unit

IGH	interest group hypothesis
ILO	International Labour Organization
IPC	infection prevention and control
ITAC	Indigenous Tourism Association of Canada
LTC	long-term care
MERS	Middle East respiratory syndrome
MFH	market failure hypothesis
MHCC	Mental Health Commission of Canada
MPs	Members of Parliament
NACI	National Advisory Committee on Immunization
NAT	normal accidents theory
NESS	National Emergency Strategic Stockpile
NGO	non-governmental organization
NYT	New York Times
OCL	Office of the Commissioner of Lobbying of Canada
OECD	Organisation for Economic Co-operation and Development
ORH	opinion-responsive hypothesis
OWS	Operation Warp Speed
P&C	property and casualty (insurance)
PC	Progressive Conservative
PHAC	Public Health Agency of Canada
PHO	Public Health Ontario
PPE	personal protective equipment
PS	Public Safety Canada
PSW	personal support worker
QALYs	quality-adjusted life years
RAP	rational actor paradigm
SARF	social amplification of risk framework
SARS	severe acute respiratory syndrome
SDGs	sustainable development goals
SIN	social insurance number
SMES	small and medium-sized enterprises
TFW	temporary foreign worker
TIAC	Tourism Industry Association of Canada
UNWTO	United Nations World Tourism Organization
VSL	value of a statistical life
WFH	work from home
WHO	World Health Organization
WHTI	Western Hemisphere Travel Initiative
WTTC	World Travel & Tourism Council

SEIZED BY UNCERTAINTY

Introduction

By 31 March 2022 it seemed the worst of the crisis was behind us. COVID-19 case counts, hospitalizations, intensive-care-unit (ICU) visits, and deaths were dropping in most parts of the country, and vaccinations and diagnostic tests were in mass distribution. A month earlier, Canada's chief public health officer, Theresa Tam, had stated that as we braced for new waves, we needed "longer-term, sustained approaches and capacity-building so we're not in a crisis mode all the time as we fight this virus" (Tasker 2022a, para. 4). Who would have known it would be such a long journey?

Between 1 January 2020 and 2 April 2022 over 3.5 million Canadians were known to have contracted COVID-19, representing approximately 10 per cent of the population, and 37,722 were reported to have died from it.[1] The disease seized the vulnerable first. More than 840 outbreaks in the first wave occurred in long-term care (LTC) facilities across the country, accounting for over 80 per cent of COVID-19–related deaths in Canada by the end of May 2020 (CIHI 2020c, 1). Public attention was captured by families sitting vigil on the grounds of LTC homes, offering support to residents through the window. In time, the virus would kill infants, such was the reach and impact of the disease. Images from Italy, where the disease had appeared in February 2020, showed a health-care system in collapse. There were simply not enough ICU beds for the number of sick; doctors were "cry[ing] inside" as they made decisions with limited guidance about who would receive life-saving ICU treatment and who would not (*Mercury* 2020).

What was described in Canada as a low risk in February was, by 9 April, projected to infect anywhere from 22,580 to 31,850 Canadians and kill 500 to 700 in the coming weeks (PHAC 2020b). As it turned out, the estimates were low; by 15 April over 1,000 had died. In Quebec, hardest hit in the first wave, the case count doubled almost every other day. At its peak, eight of every 100 people who contracted the disease in Canada died (Government of Canada 2022j). In May 2020, researchers estimated that the demand for ICU beds would exceed thirteen times the number available (Shoukat et al. 2020, 494).

Governments were completely consumed by the issue. The prime minister and premiers accompanied by their chief medical officers (CMOs) gave daily press briefings. It was a powerful combination of science and democracy. After decades of the neoliberal criticism that governments were incompetent and untrustworthy, and new public management reforms had outsourced, downsized, and demoralized the public service, governments flexed their muscles and showed what they could do. They connected with global networks to learn about the disease; established massive testing and tracing operations across the country; closed borders, schools, public and recreational spaces, and businesses to limit the spread of the disease; set the rules for quarantines and enforced them; and secured millions of items of personal protective equipment (PPE) in a ferociously competitive global market, described by Finance Minister Chrystia Freeland as "the Wild West" (Reynolds 2020, para. 12). Slow bureaucratic procurement policies were dropped. Governments leveraged industry expertise and capacity to ensure that supply chains delivered critical supplies in order to maintain national stability. They partnered with other Western countries and incentivized the development of an effective vaccine in record time and distributed it with unprecedented speed.

In days, governments enabled millions of people to stay home to prevent onward transmission of the virus; they did this partly through legal and administrative changes and largely through economic programs to support the huge number of unemployed and the faltering businesses closed due to public health directives. "We are all in this together," Prime Minister Justin Trudeau said (Wherry 2020). In the end, the federal government borrowed an estimated $700 billion (Cochrane and Hartley 2022) to fund its pandemic response, an amount only governments with good credit can access so quickly.[2] A total of $81.6 billion was paid to 8.9 million unemployed through the Canada Emergency Response Benefit (CERB) program and regular Employment Insurance (EI) program between 15 March and 3 October 2020. By October 2020 the Government of Canada had allocated $80.8 billion to support 3.6 million applications from businesses through the Canada Emergency Wage Subsidy (CEWS) program, and $2.94 billion had been paid to 708,440 students through the Canada Emergency Student Benefit (CESB) (Government of Canada 2020a).

On the fringes there were anti-vaxxers and people protesting government overreach, but on balance governments rarely fell afoul of public opinion. During the first three waves of the pandemic, all governments that faced election were re-elected with increased numbers of seats.

Public health and health-care providers across the country were called upon and met the moment. They worked tirelessly, many without holidays or days off or even breaks, at personal risk to themselves and their families as the disease spread throughout health facilities; they coped with limited PPE and an ever-dwindling number of ICU beds. They were often exhausted and traumatized, working in life-and-death circumstances in a system at the brink, and these conditions went on for months. No matter how hard they worked, they were rarely ahead of the curve. People around the globe who were quarantined in their residences paid tribute to them nightly, from flickering the lights to banging pots and pans to singing operas from their balconies.

By March 2022 Canada had one of the lowest death rates from COVID-19 and one of the highest vaccination rates in the world (Ritchie et al. 2022b).

That is one narrative of the pandemic and government response. Pull back the curtain, and there is a much more involved story to tell.

Notwithstanding the death and hospitalization counts, the threat was effectively invisible, uncertain, and pervasive at the early stages. These characteristics lent themselves to a highly anxious reaction. Public-health directives saved lives but, as time would tell, the threat varied considerably due to several factors. While it is estimated that nearly 17 per cent of Canadians had had COVID-19 by 1 April 2022, with an additional 8 per cent suspecting they had had COVID-19, 90 per cent of Canadians had never formally tested positive for COVID-19 as of 2 April 2022.[3] Of those who tested positive by 21 July 2022, nearly 80 per cent are estimated to have had mild infections, and only 4.5 per cent required hospitalization (168,168 cases); of those, 16.5 per cent (27,747 patients) ended up in the ICU. People sixty years and older accounted for nearly 92 per cent of all COVID-19 deaths in Canada by 22 July 2022, with 60 per cent occurring among people over the age of eighty (Government of Canada 2022i). In the first six months, 90 per cent of those who died had co-morbidities, the most common being Alzheimer's and dementia (O'Brien et al. 2020; see also National Center for Health Statistics 2022; Government of Canada 2022i). The aged, the immunocompromised, and those in congregate facilities and densely populated environments were at highest risk. At one point 90 per cent of COVID-19 cases in Ontario occurred in just 10 per cent of its postal codes. By 2 April 2022, 14,382 people had died of the virus in Quebec, whereas eighteen had died in Prince Edward Island (Government of Canada 2022i).

Decisions to prioritize COVID-19 victims in the health-care system had consequences. For every person who died of COVID-19 in 2020, over three died from heart disease and five from cancerous tumours. A study conducted in the United Kingdom (UK) found that 45 per cent of those with possible cancer symptoms did not contact their doctor during the UK's first wave of the pandemic (March–August 2020), and approximately 40,000 fewer people than normal started cancer treatment (*Lancet* 2021). By spring 2021, models in Ontario indicated that the province had a surgical backlog of 250,000 procedures (CityNews Toronto 2021). Between the start of the pandemic and December 2021, an average of 35,000 fewer surgeries were performed across the country each month compared to previous years (CIHI 2021b). The biggest declines were in cataract surgeries and hip and knee replacements; sight restoration, less-essential heart surgeries, and diagnostic imaging also experienced significant delays (Canadian Medical Association 2020).

In any event, total death count is not the only way to think about mortality. An alternative way to measure the impact of the disease is years of life expectancy lost. Despite the popular press comparing the COVID-19 death count to that of the first and second world wars (Flanagan 2021; Waxman and Wilson 2021), in fact, the wars were each twenty times worse than COVID-19; soldiers died on average in their mid-twenties (National WWII Museum, n.d.; Brownell 2018). The number of years of expected life lost to road deaths each year is 75 per cent of the approximate years of life lost during the first year of COVID-19, 2020 (Transport Canada 2020a, 2020b). While we may not like road deaths, we regulate the risks and tolerate the deaths. What, then, triggered such a strong reaction to COVID-19?

Contrary to the prime minister's claim that we were all in this together, the disease and the associated government interventions affected people differently. With concern over high death counts, overwhelmed hospitals, and insufficient ICU capacity, governments frequently enacted similar strict public health measures across the board, which had an uneven impact on communities. Certain sectors, including finance and insurance, educational services, and scientific and technical services, were better able to have employees work from home and limit their risk exposure. In total, about 40 per cent of the workforce did so.

Likewise, some people were better off financially as the pandemic progressed. The average Canadian saved an additional $5,800 in 2020

(Schembri 2021) because there was so little to do. This figure masks considerable variation across income groups, of course; those with wealth and assets did better than those without. Some people redirected their savings to home renovations (Peesker 2020), and the sale of expensive recreational items jumped. Some speculated on the stock market, which increased 75 per cent in the year following the March 2020 collapse (Sraders 2021). By June 2021, home prices had risen by 16 per cent in key markets, the largest annual increase in Canadian history (BNN Bloomberg 2021).

The digital economy did well, too. Zoom's stock price rose by over 400 per cent. Netflix gained more than twenty-five million subscriptions and $70 billion in market capitalization, placing it above NBC, Universal Studios, and Disney (Pandey 2020). Big-box retail, like Walmart and Home Depot, could sell many items while maintaining social distancing and saw quarterly revenue increases and stock price increases range from 5 to 30 per cent (Yahoo Finance 2020e, 2020l). This was at times to the detriment of small businesses that could not meet government health directives and were forced to close or curtail business. Grocery chains, like Loblaws and Sobeys, saw increases in revenue, profits, and share value throughout the pandemic, particularly in March 2020, when sales were 29.2 per cent higher than in March 2019 (Statista 2021). Not all businesses were successful at maintaining normal operations, but some received considerable support from government. Air Canada received $5.9 billion in support, on top of $554 million from CEWS (Air Canada 2021a; Fife and Willis 2021). The insurance industry, arguably the sector that manages market risks, declared that many policies, such as business interruption (BI), were not valid due to the conditions of the pandemic. Ironically, during this crisis the property and casualty (P&C) insurance industry's net income rose by over 50 per cent from 2019 (Gambrill 2021).

As in many crises, the vulnerable were at higher risk and paid a heavy price. The mortality rate for COVID-19 was 1.7 times higher for those in the lowest-income areas compared with those in the highest-income areas. Neighbourhoods with higher proportions of racialized minorities experienced COVID-19 mortality rates that were twice as high as those in neighbourhoods with low proportions of racialized minorities. In 2020, people who identified as Arab, Middle Eastern, West Asian, Latin American, Southeast Asian, or Black were six to nine times more likely to test positive for COVID-19 than White populations (McKenzie 2020). As of November 2020, more people had died in Montreal Nord, a low-income area with a large population of African and Caribbean people, than had died in all of British Columbia (McKenzie 2020). In August 2020 the unemployment rate among those who identified as Arab or Black was twice as high as among those who did not identify as a minority (Statistics Canada 2020j). Despite these differences, only one in two Canadians believed during the pandemic that government should do more to address racial injustice.

Those in low-paying service jobs were more at risk, including those in food, manufacturing, and health care. The ability to work from home is strongly correlated with education level and age; only 20.0 per cent of workers under the age of twenty-five, and 12.7 per cent of those with less than a high school diploma, were able to work from home. By law, employers had to create a safe work environment. PPE had to be found and the safety measures enforced – and sometimes they were not, leading to major outbreaks at workplaces such as a Cargill meat-processing plant in Alberta and an Amazon warehouse in Ontario. Paid sick leave existed for some but not others; this raised questions of fairness and created perverse incentives for one to keep working when sick, which increased the risk of onward transmission. Small businesses were hit hard: in 2020, monthly business closures increased by 19 per cent, a net loss of about 2,300 businesses a month (Statistics Canada 2022a, 2022o). The unemployment rate in the tourism sector, where over 99 per cent of businesses are small, hit 30 per cent at one point. Although the tourism sector employs 10 per cent of the world's population, including in Canada, much of the work is low paid and casual and offers no benefits. A disproportionate number of immigrants, racialized minorities, and young people work in tourism (Tourism HR Canada, n.d.b). People's mental health deteriorated to the lowest levels ever recorded. Forty per cent of Canadians overall and 61 per cent of those unemployed said that their mental health deteriorated from March to December 2020 (Canadian Mental Health Association, n.d.). The pandemic led to the lowest levels of life satisfaction in Canada since the federal government began measuring it in 2003. UK data revealed that women aged sixteen to thirty-four, and thirty-five to sixty-four, groups at comparatively low risk of becoming seriously ill from the virus, saw the steepest decline in mental health (Helliwell et al. 2021, 115).

Media amplified the story in a selective and at times exploitative manner; it was characterized as a "media eclipse" (Lalancette and Lamy 2020). *The New York Times* published twice as many articles about COVID-19 as about 9/11, and four times more than about the financial crisis (2007–09). In Canada, while there was neglect and outright failure in some LTC cases, 78 per cent of people with family members in LTC said that the facilities did the best they could under the circumstances, a point rarely reported (Angus Reid Institute 2021a). After the first four months the media fell into a consistent pattern of high-volume coverage whether the death count was increasing or decreasing. In contrast to the depiction of the LTC facilities, the media regularly demonized younger people for breaking health directives by partying in large numbers and flouting citations. The story was oversimplified. One study found that younger adults had to implement more behavioural changes than older individuals did to comply with COVID-19 restrictions (Klaiber et al. 2021), even though they were at a much lower risk of developing severe illness due to the virus. The resulting layoffs also affected the young more: over 42 per cent of citizens who applied for CERB were under thirty-five years of age, as were 57 per cent of those applying for EI benefits between September 2020 and August 2021 (Government of Canada 2021h). Young people are more likely to live alone and use schools, campuses, bars, clubs, restaurants, sports teams, and arts clubs as social outlets and as ways of establishing relationships; all these venues were closed or curtailed for extended periods. People delayed getting married and having children. Young parents had to home-school their kids. Despite the media coverage of after-hours' parties, young people were only marginally more likely to break the rules than older Canadians were (Canadian Hub for Applied and Social Research 2021). The political priorities of younger people – environment, housing, social justice, and economy – were also sidelined to health issues. Mental-health conditions disproportionately affected young adults and were overlooked for months (Czeisler et al. 2020).

Public health agencies and the federal government landed clearly on the side of vaccines as a way out of the pandemic, as did most Canadians: by 3 April 2022, 83.3 per cent had received at least one vaccination, 80.0 per cent at least two, and 46.4 per cent at least one booster dose, and it was undeniably effective. Once double-vaccinated, people were thirty-six times less likely to be hospitalized and thirty-three times less likely to be in the ICU (PHAC 2021l, 7; Netherlands 2021). Nevertheless, there is a long history of anti-vaccination feeling in Canada; it did not start with COVID-19. Some people were reluctant to be vaccinated – the vaccine-hesitant at times were 28 per cent of the population – and had to be persuaded by the use of several strategies (B. Anderson 2021). Targeted efforts generated results. Anti-vaxxers, in contrast, were a small but determined minority that could not be persuaded. Both groups were often poorer and less educated than most and were marginalized in a variety of ways. It is ironic that many of the people who paid the most in terms of wealth and health throughout the pandemic were often least likely to get vaccinated. To the vast majority, these groups were uninformed, if not delusional. They were often treated as pariahs or fools or with incredulity by the government and mainstream media for failing to be vaccinated. They were an easy punching bag and presented political opportunities but also operational and ethical dilemmas, particularly when they started to fill the ICUs. The anti-vaxxers received considerable media coverage in February 2022 when they blocked bridges, border crossings, and the streets of Ottawa, but once it was clear that there were economic and political costs to pay, the power of the state descended on them, and they were removed. The hesitant to the adamant were compelled to be vaccinated or be excluded from many ordinary facets of life.

The containment strategy was pursued to save lives, partly because of the limited number of ICU beds. Canada had 12.9 ICU beds per 100,000 people, slightly above the Organisation for Economic Co-operation and Development (OECD) average (OECD 2020a). Shortage of ICU beds in Canada has been noted for years (CIHI 2016). In any event, whatever the ICU capacity, it would be tested during a serious pandemic; it would be unreasonable to pay the full cost for expensive ICU beds on an ongoing basis for "what-if" scenarios. At the same time, a crisis is not necessarily the best time to have a thoughtful, informed, and deliberative discussion about how to prioritize the sick. Triage policies in Canada vary but are generally based on which patients have the best chance of survival. If they have equal chance of survival, priority is given to the patient judged to have the most years of life ahead of them (University of Toronto Joint Centre for Bioethics Pandemic Influenza Working Group 2005, 16). There is no judgment on why a patient requires care; a principle of bioethics is that patients are not judged or treated differently based on a past behaviour that may have contributed to their condition. This principle applies equally to the unvaccinated, the chain smoker, the coal miner, and the skydiver.[4]

Institutions were ill equipped to make decisions about how to address various risk trade-offs and accommodate different degrees of risk tolerance with little time, inadequate resources, and intense media and political scrutiny. There are also questions about institutions' ability to learn and adapt. Despite the number of deaths in LTC in the first wave, for instance, more died in LTC in the second wave than in the first (CIHI 2021c). Vulnerabilities of racialized minorities during a pandemic are well documented, including in H1N1 influenza post-mortems nearly ten years earlier (PHAC 2010, 27–8; O'Sullivan and Bourgoin 2010, 15–16, 20).

The system needs to be prepared and more adaptive in the face of uncertainty. Following the outbreak of severe acute respiratory syndrome (SARS) in 2003, the government was roundly criticized by three separate commissions for having an inadequate infrastructure to prepare for, and coordinate a response to, national health emergencies. Public Health Agency of Canada (PHAC) was created partly because of government's poor performance during SARS. It was mandated to ready Canada for a pandemic, but problems persist. PHAC is increasingly drawn to health promotion over emergency and pandemic response; budgets have drifted that way since the inception of the agency. Clear gaps in Canada's pandemic response and preparedness were still evident in the early response to COVID-19, when action from January to March 2020 was characterized as "decentralized, uncoordinated, and slow" (Hansen and Cyr 2020). Audits have since found that pandemic plans prepared by the federal government were not regularly updated or tested, long-standing issues with health surveillance information had gone unresolved, and past recommendations on data-sharing agreements and privacy had not been implemented. The emergency stockpile was somewhat depleted. Accountability was opaque. Beyond the overlap of federal and provincial or territorial jurisdictions, politicians regularly said they were following the advice of the CMO and the science; the CMOs emphasized that their job was to advise, not to decide. CMOs took turns being heroes, then pariahs; two left amid significant criticism (S. Banerjee 2022a; Arthur 2021; CBC News 2021g, 2021j; L. Harvey 2020).

In sum, the government's response to COVID-19 was impressive but flawed. The information it had was incomplete and at times inaccurate, partly due to the nature of the threat and partly due to an unprepared system. The government's reach was vast, but its emphasis was narrow. Its response involved significant trade-offs, resulting in cascading effects across families, communities, businesses, and households; some were intended but many were not. By the time trucks were blocking Canada-US border crossings and the streets of Ottawa in February 2022, protesting government COVID-19 policies, politicians from the governing party as well as from opposition parties were calling for a cost-benefit analysis to assess more thoroughly the government and public health interventions. The call was rhetorical speech play; such analysis would be virtually impossible. It would require a consistent and logically sound model to reflect and align individual, institutional, and community-based knowledge and preference structure. While government response gained considerable support from the majority throughout the episode, COVID-19 was at times subject to competing and irreconcilable psychological, social, and institutional forces that converged in the face of uncertainty. A rational accounting could not explain it, let alone justify it. While the response at times shows the ability of the state to get things done, the picture is not always a reassuring one. It was an expensive, bureaucratic, precautionary response with unclear accountability; it lacked nuance, agility, and democratic oversight. Despite several early warnings – from weeks to years before the outbreak of COVID-19 – government was ill equipped to address and communicate trade-offs, different risk perceptions, and degrees of risk tolerance. In the face of an invisible and potentially devastating threat, the government opted largely for containment and stability, using specific interpretations of fairness and efficiency, which served the interests of some more than others.

THE PURPOSE AND FRAMEWORK OF THE BOOK

This book is written in the tradition of public administration and draws significantly on the social science of risk and risk-governance literature. The role of institutions figures prominently in the analysis. The book takes seriously the notion that risk regulation is a function of context. While the state of knowledge about the risk was uncertain, particularly at the beginning of the pandemic, information had to be sought, received, and processed in a particular social, economic, and legal setting and government institutions had to act within that setting.

We employ the Hood, Rothstein, and Baldwin (2001) risk regulation regimes framework to help us structure our analysis. The framework explores risk regulation according to competing rationales. They define *regime* as "the complex of institutional geography, rules, practice and animating ideas that are associated with the regulation of a particular risk or hazard" (2001, 9). Hood, Rothstein, and Baldwin read across various policy contexts while drawing together a variety of institutional perspectives to understand what shapes risk regulation.

To be clear at the outset, there is no single framework that can explain a case as complex as COVID-19 and how government responded to it. The Hood, Rothstein, and Baldwin framework, however, brings some needed discipline to the analysis of such a case. The term *context*, for example, was used throughout the pandemic often without a clear definition (Lemmens and Krakowitz-Broker 2020; Nixon 2021). Likewise, in the academic world, *context* is not always defined clearly or consistently (Bertin, Nera, and Delouvée 2020; Scardina et al. 2021; Dietz et al. 2020). Hood, Rothstein, and Baldwin give us a definition of *context* with specific lenses to examine features of regulatory response. The application of these concepts allows us to examine what had impact and in which ways, such as the application of health and safety laws, but also to note the things that did not influence outcomes, such as the role of business-continuity insurance, which was described as virtually useless for this kind of problem.

Hood, Rothstein, and Baldwin derive three separate (but overlapping) hypotheses to explore the contextual pressures that shape and explain regime response. The first hypothesis, the market failure hypothesis (MFH), considers the government's intervention as necessary given the technical nature of the risk and the inability of the market to manage the risk effectively without such intervention. This hypothesis examines the role of the law and insurance as well as information and opt-out costs. The second hypothesis, the opinion-responsive hypothesis (ORH), examines the popular context to assess the extent to which risk regulation is a response to the preferences of civil society. This hypothesis examines media coverage and polling data. The third hypothesis, the interest group hypothesis (IGH), examines the role of organized groups in shaping the way a risk is regulated in the industry. This hypothesis examines the concentration of power and how it is wielded to gain preferential treatment from governments. The framework is multidisciplinary; it incorporates economics and the law (market failure), social psychology (opinion-responsive), political science (interests), and sociology and anthropology (institutions) into its analysis.

Hood, Rothstein, and Baldwin use these three hypotheses to determine the extent to which each rationale explains the risk regulation content. Regulation content refers to the policy settings, the configuration of state and other organizations directly engaged in regulating the risk, and the attitudes, beliefs, and operating conventions of the regulators (Hood, Rothstein, and Baldwin 2001, 21). Each of the three critical elements of regime content is characterized further through the three elements of a cybernetic control system – information gathering, standard setting, and behaviour modification (figure 0.1). In this sense, control means the ability to keep the state of a system within some preferred subset of all its possible states. If any of the three components is absent, a system is not under control in a cybernetic sense (Hood, Rothstein, and Baldwin 2001, 23–5).

In this book we will first describe and analyze the information gathering, standard setting, and behaviour modification at play during the pandemic, essentially populating the right-hand side of figure 0.1.

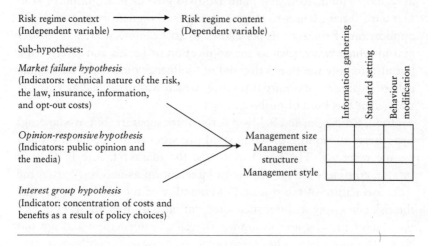

Figure 0.1 | Risk regulation regimes: understanding regime responses
Source: Hood, Rothstein, and Baldwin 2001.

Second, we will explore the context that influences the control mechanism through three specific lenses, captured by the left-hand side of the figure.

HOW WE STUDIED COVID-19, AND THE TIMELINES OF THE RESEARCH

We started to document the pandemic from the outset, recognizing that it was a significant event that would play out over time and that the threat was well beyond a medical and psychological phenomenon; it was a legal, economic, sociological, and geopolitical event, fraught with ethical dilemmas.

We recognize that people will research and write about COVID-19 for years. Some aspects will fall away while others will have lasting impact. Indeed, the pandemic may change profoundly how we organize ourselves: a more pervasive move to online commerce and work-at-home practices; a stronger focus on mental health as part of our overall well-being; clearer articulation of risk trade-offs in public health; a review of the ethical foundations of our health system; and a seismic shift in how we organize and deliver health care and LTC in the future.

This will not be the last word on COVID-19. We felt, however, that it would be valuable to document it as it was occurring, particularly the early stages, so that, as our interpretation of events changed over time, we would have the benefit of having been there at the start and documenting what we saw as it emerged.

We examine the period of January 2020 to March 2022, which generally aligns with the start of the pandemic to the point at which Canada's chief medical officer declared that Canadians would have to learn to live with the risk and that governments could no longer exist in a state of perpetual crisis, as noted at the outset of the book. Dr Tam noted this in February 2022. Our analysis generally ends in March 2022, which marks the end of a fiscal year for many organizations and funded programs. Occasionally our data extend slightly beyond March 2022, when, for instance, it represents publicly available data as close to 31 March 2022 as we could obtain, or when a particularly significant observation occurred after March 2022 that reveals important insights into the January 2020 to March 2022 period. The source and time frame of the data we use are indicated throughout the book.

We started documenting the case in March 2020 and concluded the process in July 2023. We depended largely on academic literature on the social science of risk and risk governance, as well as academic and professional opinions. Professional and academic opinions were often conveyed through the media, which created a challenge because we were also analyzing the media. As the reader will come to see, however, there was so much media coverage that it was possible to analyze the coverage at meso- and macro-levels and at the same time access expert opinions that were available in individual articles. Professional and academic opinions presented other challenges. In the early stages many experts speculated on various causes and outcomes that turned out to be inaccurate. This possibility required that we keep a watchful eye on audits and studies that were issued in the latter stages of our study to determine if the forecasts of excerpts were borne out by empirical studies.

Data collection was supplemented by several virtual and in-person events hosted by Dalhousie University's MacEachen Institute for Public Policy and Governance (MI), of which all the authors of this book were employees at the time of writing. We hosted nine panel events and four round tables and published six briefing notes in the first two years of the pandemic. We worked closely with seniors' advocates on home-care policies and with many groups in the tourism sector on their recovery plans. In fall 2022 the MI hosted a graduate class that included ten round tables, which nineteen experts attended to discuss various aspects of the pandemic and the lessons identified throughout the process. Topics ranged from health issues, such as risk communications, epidemiological modelling, emergency-room overload, and pandemic ethics; to economic issues, such as the pandemic's impact on tourism; to the impact on specific groups, such as people with disabilities, the elderly, and immigrants. Finally, we collaborated with Dalhousie University's Faculty of Medicine as part of its Catalyzing Systems Change initiative. This partnership resulted in two separate public panels in 2022 about the pandemic, one on social justice and one on ethics. Unless otherwise noted, all observations, conclusions, and mistakes belong to the authors of this book. Nevertheless, these events and meetings contributed to our thinking and our research and in some cases acted as an important check against our findings.

Finally, we make three brief definitional notes and one methodological one. First, we explain our use of the word *government*. Canada is a federation. There is a federal government, ten provincial governments, three territories, First Nations and Indigenous governments, and several municipal governments. When a specific government is responsible for an action, we name the government. At times, we refer to federal/provincial/territorial governments when circumstances had an impact on these orders of government, or they were working towards addressing an issue. At times, we refer to *government* (singular) when we are referring to the role that government plays in society and are less concerned about the specific jurisdiction that has responsibility.

Secondly, as we note in more detail in chapter 2, we draw on the work of German sociologist Ortwin Renn to refer to four types of risk throughout the book – simple, complex, uncertain, and ambiguous – to refine our analysis further. Risk is a function of *probability* and *consequence*. Both concepts were volatile and subject to various debates throughout the pandemic. A generic reference to risk lacks important nuance. We are most concerned with uncertain risk (characterized by an absence of predictive data), ambiguous risk (characterized by contested perspectives on the justification, severity, or wider measures of a threat), and complex risk (characterized by difficulty identifying links between a multitude of potential causal agents and specific observed effects).

Thirdly, we use the term *containment* to refer to the government strategy to stop the spread of COVID-19. We also refer to government's strategy to "slow" disease transmission. Most disease-transmission experts will note that complete containment of such a disease is a temporary strategy; ultimately, governments and public health agencies sought to slow disease transmission (Institute of Medicine (US) Forum on Microbial Threats 2007; WHO 2020e; Government of Canada 2020c; PHAC 2020k). We acknowledge the validity of both strategies, and that it is not always clear at which point one stops and the other begins. In the book we often use the term *containment* but acknowledge that it can also include the slowing of disease transmission.

Finally, we add a note about the data we use in this study, particularly the number of COVID-19 cases and deaths. Data sets in this study regarding COVID-19 cases, fatalities, and hospitalizations rely on data collected by September 2022. The availability of COVID-19 data has far surpassed past pandemics; more data have been available about the pandemic in real-time than about previous pandemics and disease outbreaks. The volume and variety of data, and the speed with which the data have been released, have had an impact on quality checks for research (Stoto et al. 2022). Variations in national data sets can partly be attributed to differences in definitions, reporting processes, and practices for data collection and management. COVID-19 case and death counts rely on collaboration between local, regional, national, and global public health agencies. These data have also been updated over time, and at times retroactively; as a result, there are differences between COVID-19 data reported in 2020, 2021, and 2022 and data currently available about those years. Definitions for metrics, rules for classifying a death as COVID-19–related, and the processes used to collect data and report these events vary across jurisdictions and change over time (Stoto et al. 2022). In short, while the COVID-19 data in this book will be close in total to published data on government health websites following the publication of this book, the data will certainly not be a perfect match.

THE PLAN OF THE BOOK

The book is divided into five sections: (1) introduction to the case and the social science of risk literature; (2) the government's response to the pandemic, using a cybernetic understanding of control, examining information gathering, standard setting, and behaviour modification; (3) case studies on LTC and tourism; (4) pressures and explanations, including market failures, public opinion, and the role of concentrated interests; and (5) a conclusion.

The introduction and chapters 1 and 2 introduce the case and situate it in the social science of risk and risk-governance literature. In chapter 1 we provide an overview of how COVID-19 first appeared in late 2019 and early 2020. We recall early actions taken by the Chinese government, the World Health Organization (WHO), and the United States (US) government including the Centers for Disease Control and Prevention (CDC), which allows us to introduce how Canada first learned of and responded to COVID-19. We conclude by summarizing key quantitative data about the Canadian experience, including case, ICU, and death counts between January 2020 and March 2022. Once we have established this basic storyline, chapter 2 situates COVID-19 in the risk literature, a study that dates to the Scientific Revolution but has grown exponentially over the last forty years. The chapter summarizes the rational actor paradigm and the dominant approach. It contrasts this approach with contributions from other disciplines, including psychology, sociology, and anthropology. All disciplines make important contributions to our understanding of the COVID-19 case, but none provides a complete account. We conclude this chapter by underscoring the value of a regimes approach to studying a wide-scale phenomenon like COVID-19, recalling Beck's risk society and noting in which ways the Hood, Rothstein, and Baldwin (2001) framework extends Beck's analysis.

Chapters 3 to 6 describe critically the mechanisms that government put in place to contain COVID-19 between March 2020 and March 2022. Chapter 3 examines selected information-gathering methods of the regime, including testing, contract tracing, and modelling. Chapter 4 examines standard setting, including health directives during the pandemic as well as the economic programs in place to support people and businesses during the episode and the governance that oversaw government decisions. Chapter 5 details how people's behaviour changed because of the disease and the related government directives. Government directives not only shaped the focus of the health sector but also triggered far-reaching changes in individual and organizational behaviour, which had significant and varying impacts on economic and social well-being in communities across the country. Vaccine development and distribution were unprecedented in their speed and reach; they represented a crucial part of the government's strategy and required broad-based acceptance and action by the public. We treat the vaccine and the related January and February 2022 protests against mandates separately in chapter 6.

Chapters 7 and 8 focus on two case studies. Chapter 7 examines perhaps the most noted failure on health grounds during the pandemic, LTC facilities. The chapter details how governments govern LTC facilities and the broader social and economic context in which that governance occurs. It then details the chronology of COVID-19 and LTC facilities; it includes a review of several audits and studies that detail the various shortfalls of facilities across the country and connects the failings with the broader context outlined in the chapter. Chapter 8 examines one of the most affected sectors on economic grounds during the pandemic, tourism. Like the LTC case, the chapter uses the Hood, Rothstein, and Baldwin framework to examine the context and governance of the sector and how that relates to the various vulnerabilities exposed in the sector throughout the pandemic.

Chapters 9 to 11 examine various contextual pressures that shaped government response. Chapter 9 tests Hood, Rothstein, and Baldwin's market failure hypothesis. The chapter examines the role of law and insurance and market dynamics during COVID-19, including a summary of the winners and losers in the market; it also examines information and opt-out costs as means to examine the extent to which market failures explain government response. Chapter 10 tests the opinion-responsive hypothesis. It examines media coverage and popular polling data and tries to determine the extent to which these popular contextual pressures aligned with government intervention. Chapter 11 tests the interest group hypothesis. It first uses Dunleavy's (1991) bureau-shaping model, which derives from public choice theory, to determine the extent to which government's response to the pandemic can be attributed to the preferences and behaviours of public health officials prior to the pandemic. It then uses Wilson's interest group typology to examine the role of lobbying during the pandemic and the relation between power and the concentration of benefits brought about by government policies.

The conclusion pulls the threads together; it summarizes key observations about the context and governance of COVID-19 in Canada. It concludes with comments about governments' ability to address low-probability, high-consequence events. The methods we employed for the study are captured in appendix 1.

PART ONE

Overview of COVID-19 and Situating It in the Risk Literature

In the following two chapters we provide an overview of the storyline of the COVID-19 pandemic and situate our research in the existing literature on risk governance, particularly as it applies to the COVID-19 case. In chapter 1 we detail how COVID-19 first appeared in late 2019 and early 2020, including actions taken by the Chinese government, the WHO, and the US government and CDC. This allows us to introduce how Canada first learned of and responded to COVID-19. We summarize key quantitative data about COVID-19 in Canada, including case, ICU, and death counts between January 2020 and 2 April 2022.

Next, chapter 2 situates COVID-19 in the social science of risk literature. This area of study dates to the Scientific Revolution but has grown significantly over the last forty years. We group the risk literature according to Renn's (1992, 2008a) four rationales. We then summarize the rational actor paradigm, the dominant approach, and contrast it with contributions from other disciplines, such as psychology, sociology, and anthropology. While these disciplines make important contributions to our understanding of COVID-19, none on their own provides a complete account.

As we note in the introduction, we refer to four types of risk throughout the book –simple, complex, uncertain, and ambiguous – to refine our analysis further. We are most concerned with uncertain risk (characterized by an absence of predictive data), ambiguous risk (characterized by contested perspectives on the justification, severity, or wider measures of a threat), and complex risk (characterized by difficulty identifying links between a multitude of potential causal agents and specific observed effects).

How It Started and Key
COVID-19–Related Health Outcomes

The chapter starts with a review of how the disease spread across Asian countries to the West, growing exponentially. It documents the way in which the Chinese government first communicated about the disease, and early reactions from the WHO and US government, including the CDC. Western governments were slow to react; they seemed unable to imagine what was to come and therefore to develop coherent strategies and mobilize resources. Despite Wuhan, a city of eleven million, being in lockdown by the end of January 2020, Western governments continued to describe COVID-19 as low risk and tinkered with small fixes and precautions.

By March 2020 there was a seismic shift as uncertainty turned to acceptance that what was to come would be disruptive if not devastating. There was a scramble for personal protective equipment (PPE), borders were closed, and the global economy ground to a halt. By the end of April, epidemiologists were forecasting deaths in Canada between 4,000 and 355,000 (PHAC 2020k). The strategy focused on trying to contain community spread as much as possible, recognizing that intensive care units (ICUs) would likely become overwhelmed, with 9,000 to 724,000 ICU cases forecast (PHAC 2020k). Despite the sombre tone of many press conferences in the first wave, future waves, such as the third, were actually worse when measured by deaths. Factors such as age, race, gender, ability, national origin, neighbourhood, and income were indicators of someone's vulnerability, with urban centres and more populous provinces being hit the hardest. By 2 April 2022 Canada had documented 3,503,141 cases of COVID-19, or about 10 per cent of the population, and 37,722 deaths, about 0.1 per cent of the population. Canada's pandemic response was a relative success compared to that of the US and Mexico (Béland et al. 2020). Countries like Australia, New Zealand, and South Korea were much more successful than most at containing the disease (Allin et al. 2022).

HOW IT STARTED

A novel coronavirus (2019-nCoV) was first reported to the WHO China Country Office as a pneumonia of unknown cause in Wuhan, Hubei Province, China, on 31 December 2019 (WHO 2020d, 1). On 3 January 2020 the WHO issued warnings via Twitter regarding the pneumonia cases reported in Wuhan (Staples 2020a). On 7 January 2020 China confirmed the new coronavirus. On 11 January the National Health Commission of China reported that the outbreak was associated with exposures in one open-air wet market in Wuhan. There have since been disputes over the origins of the virus, which we will discuss. China shared the genetic sequence of the virus on 10 January, which enabled other countries to develop diagnostic kits (WHO 2020d, 1).

The first evidence of human-to-human transmission of the virus recorded by doctors was likely on 7 December 2019. A patient presented with the virus but denied visiting the seafood market. Human-to-human transmission was not officially confirmed until the end of January 2020 (Staples 2020a; Huang, Sun, and Sui 2020). On 30 December 2019 Dr Li Wenliang, who worked at Wuhan Central Hospital, sent a private message to a group of doctors warning them of an outbreak in Wuhan of a similar illness to severe acute respiratory syndrome (SARS) (Staples 2020a; Green 2020). Dr Li was summoned to the Public Security Bureau on 1 January 2020, along with seven others, and made to sign a statement that accused him of providing "false statements that disrupted public order" (Staples 2020a, para. 14; Green 2020). By 31 December 2019 Taiwanese officials were on alert and screened passengers from Wuhan. At this time the Wuhan Municipal Health Commission declared that there was not any "obvious human-to-human transmission and no medical staff infection" (Staples 2020a, para. 13). This was contrary to the beliefs of medical professionals; at least two doctors were believed to have the virus at this time (Staples 2020a; Geraghty 2020).

Simultaneously, YY, a Chinese live-streaming platform, and WeChat censored keywords related to COVID-19, including *Unknown Wuhan Pneumonia*, *Wuhan Seafood Market*, references to Li Wenliang, and criticisms of the government. This information was not widely known until after 3 March 2020 (Staples 2020a; Ruan, Knockel, and Crete-Nishihata 2020). Furthermore, on 3 January, Caixin Global reported

that the National Health Commission (NHC), the top health authority in China, had ordered institutions not to publish any information
regarding the virus and to destroy any samples or transfer them to designated institutions (Staples 2020a; G. Yu et al. 2020).

On 13 March 2020 *South China Morning Post* reported that, in
fact, the first case of COVID-19 in China likely had occurred in Hubei
Province as early as 17 November 2019 (Staples 2020a). To further
complicate COVID-19's origin story, there have been reports about a
laboratory leak of the COVID-19 virus in Wuhan, which has two laboratories that research coronaviruses. Initially these notions were dismissed
as conspiracy theories; however, investigations into the matter did not
yield sufficient evidence to disprove the theory, a finding supported by
the WHO (*Economist* 2021a, 2021b). The US and WHO continued to
investigate possible sources of COVID-19, but there is still no conclu-
sive answer about the market or the laboratory leak as origins of the
virus (BBC 2021; White House 2021; Pompeo 2021; WHO 2021e).

The virus spread rapidly throughout Asia, primarily through countries
that border China. As noted, Taiwan took action on 31 December 2019.
On 3 January 2020 South Korea increased airport screening and quarantine processes for travellers from Wuhan, and on 7 January, Japan
did the same. On 9 January the WHO issued travel guidelines encouraging restraint but advised against travel and trade restrictions on China;
it also advised that the virus did not transmit easily between people,
which turned out to be inaccurate. On 14 January the WHO advised via
Twitter that there was no clear evidence of human-to-human transmission and that no cases of health-care workers with the disease had been
recorded (Staples 2020a). At the same time, the head of the NHC held
a teleconference and stated that COVID-19 would likely develop into a
major public health event, but did not communicate this information to
the WHO or any nation outside China (Staples 2020a; Associated Press
2020). This information was not widely known until April 2020.

On 17 January 2020 the US began screening passengers from Wuhan
at three of the most common entry points to the country (Staples 2020a).

By 20 January there were 282 confirmed cases of COVID-19 reported
by four countries, all traced back to Wuhan: China (278 cases), Thailand
(two cases), Japan (one case), and the Republic of Korea (one case).
Six people had died from COVID-19 in Wuhan. At this time, Chinese
respiratory expert Zhong Nanshan publicly confirmed human-to-human transmission (Staples 2020a). On 22 January the WHO confirmed
human-to-human transmission for the first time (Staples 2020a; WHO
2020b).

On 21 January, Taiwan issued a level-three travel alert for travellers from Wuhan and a fourteen-day quarantine period, tracked via mobile phones; two days later Wuhan residents were banned from entry (Staples 2020a). Taiwan was the first country to use mobile phones to monitor quarantine compliance (Huang, Sun, and Sui 2020). On the next day Canada implemented the screening of travellers from Wuhan arriving in Montreal, Toronto, and Vancouver and voluntary self-isolation for fourteen days (Staples 2020a).

The WHO focused on coordination, including the gathering and sharing of information between countries. The incident management system was activated on 2 January across the three levels of the WHO – headquarters, regional office, and country offices (WHO 2020d, 3). The WHO also released guidance on diagnosing the virus and reducing transmission, as well as updated travel advice (3).

On 23 January China made the unprecedented announcement of lockdown for Wuhan, China's seventh-largest city with a population of eleven million (Staples 2020a). At this time the WHO assessed the general risk of COVID-19 to be "very high" in Wuhan, "high" at the regional level, and "moderate" globally. The WHO has since stated that the global warning should also have been "high" at this point (Staples 2020a, para. 43).

By 25 January over 1,300 cases had been confirmed globally, with the vast majority in China (WHO 2020e, 1). The virus had spread throughout Asia to Australia, France, and the US (4). At this time the WHO issued updated strategic responses to COVID-19 with the following objectives: (1) disrupt human-to-human transmission in China, (2) prevent exportation of cases to other countries, and (3) prevent further transmission from exported cases. It recommended a combination of public health measures, such as testing, rapid diagnosis, contact tracing, infection prevention and control (IPC) measures for travellers, and raising awareness (5). The WHO also shared principles from previous coronavirus outbreaks, including Middle East respiratory syndrome (MERS) and SARS, which acted as a starting point to understand the virus. The understanding was that the spread of COVID-19, like other viruses, occurred between humans through droplets, contact, and fomites (e.g., contaminated objects).[1] The recommendation was to promote handwashing, reduce contact with ill people, avoid unprotected contact with animals (i.e., farm and wild), and enhance IPC practices in hospitals (4–5). We would learn much later that the risk of getting COVID-19 through touching contaminated objects and surfaces was likely overestimated (Goldman 2020).

Symptoms of the virus were like a cold or flu (e.g., fever, cough, pneumonia). In some cases, symptoms took up to two weeks to present, which is believed to be the longest incubation period for this disease (Government of Canada 2022j). Some people with the virus never displayed symptoms (i.e., asymptomatic), which had an impact on virus spread because many people did not know they had the virus (Government of Canada 2022j). Misinformation and confusion about asymptomatic transmission was a key issue for the WHO. As late as 8 June 2020 WHO representatives stated that asymptomatic COVID-19 cases were believed to be rare, but they clarified on the next day that asymptomatic transmission was an unknown factor (WHO 2020k, 2020l).

The first confirmed case of COVID-19 in Canada was reported on 25 January in Toronto, Ontario. The patient arrived in Toronto after travelling from Wuhan (CBC News 2020h). At this time the WHO advised countries to support surveillance efforts by reporting cases to it (Government of Canada 2022j). On 28 January it launched a digital platform to allow member states to contribute anonymized data to inform public health clinical responses (WHO 2020f, 1).

On 30 January 2020 the WHO Emergency Committee declared COVID-19 to be a public health emergency of international concern and provided measures to control the outbreak (WHO 2020g, 1). This did not result in the strong responses necessary from governments around the world (Independent Panel for Pandemic Preparedness and Response 2021). By 31 January nearly 10,000 cases of COVID-19 had been confirmed in five of the six WHO regions, including Western Pacific, Southeast Asia, the Americas, Europe, and Eastern Mediterranean (WHO 2020g, 4).

On 3 February the WHO unveiled a dashboard to share information about confirmed cases globally and the situation in each region (WHO 2020h). It also developed the "2019-nCoV kit," a diagnostic tool (1). The virus continued to spread to new countries across Europe, including Russia, Spain, Sweden, and the UK (4).

On 7 February Dr Li Wenliang, who warned other doctors early on about the risks of the virus, died of COVID-19 in Wuhan Central Hospital at the age of thirty-three (Staples 2020b; Xiao et al. 2022). He was posthumously exonerated, and Wuhan police formally apologized to his family on 19 March 2020.

On 11 February the WHO issued new guidance on travel restrictions for people and commercial trade, stating that they could help in the early stages to contain an outbreak. It advocated for active surveillance, early detection, isolation and case management, and contact tracing (Staples 2020b; WHO 2020a). On 12 February the United Nations (UN) activated a crisis management team, led by the WHO.

The cruise ship *Diamond Princess* departed Japan on 20 January 2020 and gained international attention as a high-risk situation. Between 7 and 23 February it accounted for the largest cluster of COVID-19 cases outside mainland China (Moriarty et al. 2020). On 2 February there were reports that a passenger from Hong Kong had tested positive for COVID-19, and the captain was ordered to have all 3,700 passengers and crew tested for the virus in Japan; many passengers were over sixty years old (Moriarty et al. 2020; Rocklöv, Sjödin, and Wilder-Smith 2020). By the end of the episode 712 cases had been confirmed and fourteen people had died. On 13 March the Cruise Lines International Association announced a thirty-day voluntary suspension of cruise operations in the US. By 17 March, confirmed COVID-19 cases were identified across twenty-five more cruise-ship voyages, and the CDC issued a level-three travel warning calling for a deferral of cruise-ship travel worldwide (Moriarty et al. 2020).

On 11 February the International Committee on Taxonomy of Viruses named the virus "severe acute respiratory syndrome corona-virus 2 (SARS-COV-2)," and the WHO International Classification of Diseases named the disease "COVID-19" (WHO 2020c).

By 29 February the sixth region of the WHO, Africa, had confirmed cases (WHO 2020l). Worldwide, over 85,000 confirmed cases had been reported, and nearly 3,000 people had died.

The WHO declared COVID-19 a pandemic on 11 March 2020, which spurred many governments around the world to unprecedented action. There were 118,000 cases across 114 countries (Independent Panel for Pandemic Preparedness and Response 2021, 16).

Early Responses from the WHO and Selected Criticisms

Reviews of the WHO's actions have been mixed. The WHO took on a large role with education about vaccines, it developed standards and guidance, and it helped facilitate equitable vaccine distribution with international partners through COVAX, which we will discuss in more detail in chapter 6. There have also been significant criticisms. COVID-19 has called attention to many long-standing governance issues with the WHO, especially regarding perceptions of undue influence by China and the US, decision-making powers and processes, and accountability measures. The WHO's reliance on information from the

Chinese government meant that the WHO was not acting on complete information, especially regarding the high risk of human-to-human transmission.

The WHO Independent Panel for Pandemic Preparedness and Response released a report assessing the actions taken by the WHO. It identified that, following SARS, the International Health Regulations (IHR) came into force, which were legally binding duties for member states and the WHO regarding information sharing, cooperation to contain a disease, and requirements to meet before the WHO director general could act on emergencies and which prevented the WHO from acting independently. Following H1N1, there were many recommendations made to improve pandemic response and strengthen the WHO's coordination, emergency response work, and funding; however, most of these recommendations were not implemented. Pandemic responses have not been a priority for many countries (Independent Panel for Pandemic Preparedness and Response 2021, 16).

The panel referred to February 2020 as a lost month (Independent Panel for Pandemic Preparedness and Response 2021, 16). It highlighted issues concerning the WHO's declaration of a public health emergency of international concern on 30 January 2020, for example indicating it could have been made at least a week earlier. Even when the declaration was made, there was a lack of understanding about what it meant, the urgency, and the severity of action that governments should have taken. This led to pressure on the WHO to declare a pandemic. At the time, the IHR did not use the term *pandemic*. Before this, the WHO primarily used the term to refer to pandemic influenza. Once the situation was categorized as a global pandemic, governments strengthened their responses (Independent Panel for Pandemic Preparedness and Response 2021).

The WHO has been praised for its ability to coordinate experts and disseminate robust information about COVID-19 quickly, especially early on, but has been criticized for how it characterized the risk. It characterized the global risk of the virus as moderate at the end of January and has since stated it should have been high. WHO guidance should have also assumed human-to-human transmission until evidence contradicted it, given what is known about infectious respiratory diseases (Independent Panel for Pandemic Preparedness and Response 2021).

The WHO depends on information gathering and sharing by its member states. Information revealed in March and April showed that the earliest cases of COVID-19 were identified in November 2019, not at the end of December, and demonstrated censorship of health researchers and institutions in China. This meant that the response to the pandemic was not only delayed but also grounded in misinformation. There was also conflicting guidance from the WHO regarding travel restrictions, the effectiveness of masks for the general public, and the risks of virus transmission from people who were asymptomatic (see chapter 4).

The WHO's ability to enforce regulations has been called into question; it can coordinate experts, create education campaigns, and provide guidance but ultimately relies on action from its member states. The organization is also largely dependent on funding from its member states and therefore is subject to their influence and priorities (Geraghty 2020; Weaver 2020). Researchers estimate that action taken a week or two earlier could have reduced cases in the first wave by 50–80 per cent in large urban centres such as New York City (Bokat-Lindell 2020).

EARLY RESPONSE FROM THE TRUMP ADMINISTRATION AND CENTERS FOR DISEASE CONTROL AND PREVENTION

At the World Economic Forum on 22 January 2020 President Trump assured reporters that he was not concerned about the novel coronavirus (Alper 2020; Belvedere 2020). By the end of January he had created a twelve-member coronavirus task force managed by the National Security Council, and he declared in his State of the Union address on 4 February that his administration would take the necessary steps to protect citizens (M. Cohen, Subramaniam, and Hickey 2020).

On 25 February, before leaving India to return to the US, President Trump told a press conference that the situation was under control in the US and that only a few cases had been reported (C-SPAN 2020a). On that same day Dr Nancy Messonnier, director of the National Center for Immunization and Respiratory Diseases at the CDC, announced that the situation in the US was about to change quickly and severely (Shear, Fink, and Weiland 2020). Officials say that President Trump was very upset by the announcement and concerned about potential closures causing panic and disruption to financial markets (Shear, Fink, and Weiland 2020).

On the following day, 26 February, President Trump held a press conference and announced Vice-President Pence as leader of the task force (C-SPAN 2020b). The president stated that the situation in the US was improving and that symptoms of the illness were often minor. Restrictions focused on travel, such as bans on inbound foreign nationals who had visited China within two weeks, and public health officials advised washing hands and staying home when sick (C-SPAN 2020b; Crowley 2020). Although the issue of low testing rates was raised, the president responded that they were testing everyone they needed to be tested (C-SPAN 2020b).

The Centers for Disease Control and Prevention

In late January CDC director Robert Redfield told state public health directors that "the virus is not spreading in the US at this time and CDC believes the immediate health risk from 2019-nCoV to the general American public is low" (Ortega et al. 2020, para. 15). By this time the virus had in fact arrived in the US and the problem was worse than they thought.

Before the pandemic the CDC had suffered years of declining funding, contributing to insufficient preparation (Parker and Terhune 2021; Kaplan 2021). Concerns were raised that the agency's infrastructure had been neglected for decades (Rabin 2022). The CDC had also been criticized for being too insular and academic (LaFraniere and Weiland 2022).

While not the only reason for issues and delays faced by the CDC, there was a high degree of politicization over its actions (Interlandi 2021; LaFraniere and Weiland 2022). The Trump administration was criticized for interfering with the CDC's operations and censoring internal experts (Parker and Terhune 2021; Kaplan 2021; Willman 2020; Interlandi 2021). Disagreements between federal and state political leaders and public health experts led to inconsistent public health messaging, enforcement of directives, and timing of public health restrictions (Kaplan 2021; Interlandi 2021).

The CDC made key mistakes particularly regarding surveillance and testing (Rabin 2022; LaFraniere and Weiland 2022; Interlandi 2021). It was criticized for underestimating the threat of the virus and overestimating its ability to design, manufacture, and distribute a test quickly. The WHO released a protocol (i.e., recipe or instructions) to create tests on 13 January, but the CDC took forty-six more days to develop its test (Willman 2020; Kaplan 2021). It is not unusual for the CDC to develop its own test and to control approval processes to enable labs to conduct testing; however, only five labs were approved by the CDC to test for COVID-19 early on (Fink and Baker 2020). Quality-control measures failed, and compromised kits were sent to many state- and local-level public health labs, which is significant because the CDC was their only source (Kaplan 2021; HHS Office of Inspector General 2020; Willman 2020; Ortega et al. 2020).

COVID-19 IN CANADA:
JANUARY TO EARLY MARCH 2020

The Canadian federal government worked to learn about the virus; initially much of its information came from other countries. As of 19 January 2020, Health Canada believed there was no clear evidence to suggest that the virus was easily transmitted between humans (Staples 2020a; Tasker 2020a). On 23 January Canada attended a teleconference with health officials from China, Japan, South Korea, and Thailand. Taiwan was excluded at China's insistence (Staples 2020a).

The Public Health Agency of Canada (PHAC) was caught off guard; the erosion of the Global Public Health Intelligence Network (GPHIN), an early-warning system, and a shift in focus to domestic projects and away from international surveillance contributed to the agency's weak stance. GPHIN had been used during past outbreaks, such as SARS, H1N1, MERS, and Ebola, and supplied approximately 20 per cent of the WHO's epidemiological intelligence (G. Robertson 2021b; Allin et al. 2022). The Auditor General (AG) noted that Canada was unprepared for COVID-19 partly due to incomplete information and flawed risk assessments (G. Robertson 2021a).

The Government of Canada announced on 2 February it would repatriate, or return, Canadians located in Wuhan and the broader Hubei province to Canada (Global Affairs Canada 2020a). The federal government spent $7 million to repatriate nearly 400 Canadians and accompanying family members. Passengers were screened before boarding, during the flight, and upon arrival in Canada and quarantined for fourteen days at the Canadian Forces Base in Trenton, Ontario (Global Affairs Canada 2020a). Two flights were organized and returned by 11 February (Global Affairs Canada 2020b). At this time the government encouraged all Canadians residing in China on a non-essential basis to return to Canada while commercial means were still available (Global Affairs Canada 2020b).

As noted, the first confirmed case of COVID-19 in Canada was reported on 25 January in Toronto, Ontario (patient first admitted on 23 January) (Government of Canada 2022j; Perkel 2021). As of 31 January 2020 there were four confirmed cases in Canada, in Ontario and British Columbia. At this time many members of the Opposition parties were concerned about screening at airports and voluntary self-isolation, emphasizing the "laxity" of the measure in comparison to those of other jurisdictions, such as the US and Taiwan (Staples 2020b). The first reported cases had a direct travel connection to China, but on

20 February Canada confirmed the first case related to travel outside mainland China (Government of Canada 2022j; Staples 2020b).

On 4 February Canada's Special Advisory Committee on COVID-19 recommended voluntary self-isolation for passengers from Hubei province, but travellers from Wuhan arriving on government-provided planes were mandated a fourteen-day quarantine period, which was stricter than that for other commercial air travellers (Staples 2020b; Lilley 2020). On 9 February Canada introduced screening requirements at ten airports across six provinces. At this time voluntary self-isolation was asked only of people with symptoms.

The position of the PHAC as of 26 February was to keep borders open. The federal government was considering social-distancing measures, closing schools, and cancelling mass events, but emphasized that these measures were merely being considered (Staples 2020b). On 27 February twenty-three Chinese-Canadian doctors signed an open letter calling for a fourteen-day quarantine to be imposed on all travellers from mainland China (Zheng 2020).

On 29 February 2020 there were fifteen cases of COVID-19 confirmed in Canada, all in Ontario and British Columbia. The first death due to COVID-19 occurred on 9 March in British Columbia in an LTC facility (Government of Canada 2022j).

On 11 March the WHO declared a global pandemic. By 15 March all provinces had confirmed cases of COVID-19, totalling approximately 250.

Monitoring and limiting international travel, developing capacity to test for the virus, and acquiring PPE were priorities for the federal, provincial, and territorial governments. Canada was able to develop tests from the virus's genetic information that China shared on 10 January (BC Centre for Disease Control 2020a, 2020b).

Major outbreaks across Canada in early March have been predominantly connected to the US, although a significant number of cases in Quebec have been traced to France. At this time much of the rhetoric regarding travel advisories referred to China; however, few cases in Canada at this time were due to travel from China (Desson et al. 2020). Initially measures to limit international travellers entering Canada exempted the US, but this decision had significant consequences given the high proportion of cases in Canada connected to the US. Less than a week following the implementation of international travel restrictions, Canada closed the border with the US to non-essential travel (Desson et al. 2020).

During this time there was also a scramble to procure PPE. The National Emergency Strategic Stockpile (NESS) has been in place since

1952 and is managed by the Canadian government to support provinces and territories during emergencies (Government of Canada 2019c). Provinces and territories have the responsibility to maintain their own stockpiles. Supplies, including ventilators, protective gear, pharmaceuticals (e.g., antibiotics), and equipment and supplies (e.g., blankets) are meant to supplement provincial and territorial emergency stockpiles (Government of Canada 2019c). Selected cities have federally managed warehouses, which in theory can deploy supplies within twenty-four hours of a request (Government of Canada 2019c). Funding for the NESS since 2012–13 was $3 million each year, down from a previous budget of $5.5 million. For comparison, Alberta budgets $9 million for its provincial emergency stockpile (M. Walsh 2020). Problems with the federal management of the NESS include "inaccurate" records and poor tracking of the age and expiry date of items (Tasker 2021, para. 9; Leo 2020a).

Despite recommendations following the 2003 SARS outbreak for governments to stockpile PPE and secure reliable supply chains, Canada was unprepared for the COVID-19 outbreak (M. Walsh, Robertson, and Tomlinson 2020). A 2006 report noted that the federal government should have a sixteen-week supply of equipment for a pandemic including masks, gloves, and face shields, but prior to COVID-19 there had been no mandated targets to acquire significant levels of PPE. A PHAC spokesperson stated in 2020 that the stockpile "historically only carried small amounts" of PPE because each province and territory generally sourced its own equipment directly from suppliers (M. Walsh 2020, para. 6). There was also a lack of knowledge at the federal level about provincial stockpiles early in the pandemic.

Federal decision makers had to choose between using PPE supplies to curb outbreaks domestically or using them abroad. Between 4 and 15 February 2020 Canada sent sixteen tons of PPE to China (Ling and Barton 2020). People managing the NESS warned on 13 February 2020 that there was insufficient PPE in the stockpile for the impending pandemic (Tasker 2020c). Shortages meant that the NESS could not meet most provincial demands for PPE until orders arrived in April 2020 (Tasker 2021). Health-care workers had to ration and reuse PPE; by September 2020, 54 per cent of doctors said they were still experiencing challenges to acquire PPE. Some said the stockpile failed during COVID-19 (Tasker 2021). The vice-president of PHAC said in April 2020 that the NESS was "monitored and stockpiled as it was mandated and funded to do" (Leo 2020, para. 25).

HOW COVID-19 PLAYED OUT IN CANADA: SELECTED DATA (1 JANUARY 2020 TO 2 APRIL 2022)

As of 2 April 2022 Canada had a reported total of 3,503,141 COVID-19 cases. We will likely never know the true number of COVID-19 cases as asymptomatic cases may never have been tested, some with symptoms may not have bothered to test, and surges in testing demand during the pandemic meant that many could not get tested at times even if they tried. The Omicron variant caused the largest surge in cases towards the end of 2021 and into 2022. Ontario and Quebec reported most of the COVID-19 cases.

People sixty years and older accounted for nearly 92 per cent of all COVID-19 deaths in Canada by 22 July 2022, with 60 per cent occurring among people over the age of eighty (Government of Canada 2022k). In the first six months 90 per cent of those who died had co-morbidities, the most common being Alzheimer's disease and dementia (O'Brien et al. 2020). Data from the CDC show that approximately 95 per cent of COVID-19 deaths in the US between 2020 and 2022 involved co-morbidities, including influenza and pneumonia, hypertension, diabetes, Alzheimer's, and sepsis (National Center for Health Statistics 2022).

Periods of rapid increase in COVID-19 cases are described as waves, and each wave of COVID-19 has some defining features and challenges, although jurisdictions' experiences varied.

The first wave in Canada occurred between March and June 2020. The fatality rate in the first wave was higher than experts anticipated, as large-scale outbreaks across Canada's LTC facilities resulted in an 8 per cent fatality rate in May 2020. Sweeping lockdown measures were put in place across the country, and there was a global search for PPE. COVID-19 restrictions included closures of non-essential businesses, physical distancing, restricted visitors to LTC facilities and hospitals, remote learning for schools, work-at-home directives, testing and isolation protocols, and travel restrictions. Provinces and territories with fewer cases of COVID-19 eased public health restrictions in the late spring and early summer, primarily in May 2020.

The second wave of COVID-19 started in the fall of 2020, as cases began to rise quickly in September. Cases continued to rise in the winter of 2020 and into the new year. Although cases were rising, there was more variation between the severity of public health restrictions across jurisdictions than in the first wave. In late November and December 2020, public health measures were strengthened in many jurisdictions.

Many Canadians celebrated winter holidays under lockdown restrictions that mirrored those of March 2020. The fatality rate decreased in the second wave, as younger people were contracting COVID-19 and their symptoms were not as severe as those in older populations; however, the second wave had even larger outbreaks in LTC facilities than in the first wave (PHAC 2020p, 2020s).

The third wave can be characterized by increased cases of COVID-19 variants of concern. As COVID-19 spread throughout the world, mutations in the virus made it more transferable and deadly. The third wave came on the heels of the second wave in January 2021 in some jurisdictions, whereas others saw sharp increases in cases in March 2021. Canada began distributing its first doses of the COVID-19 vaccine in December 2020. While the COVID-19 variants such as Delta posed significant challenges, such as increased infection rates and more severe symptoms, the vaccine was a way to reduce spread and symptom severity.

The fourth wave is characterized by the Omicron variant, first reported in Canada at the end November 2021; it had three times the genetic mutations of prior variants and spread more easily, even among vaccinated people. It was estimated that one person with Omicron could infect four people. Generally, Omicron cases were milder and had a lower risk of death, especially among those vaccinated (CDC 2022b; Semeniuk 2021; *Globe and Mail* Editorial Board 2022b). COVID-19 cases and hospital stays peaked in January 2022, with the highest case numbers and hospitalizations recorded between March 2020 and 2 April 2022 (Statistics Canada 2022i). The virus continued to mutate; "stealth Omicron" was estimated to be 30 per cent more contagious and caused a third of the new Omicron cases by the end of February 2022 (Ungar 2022, para. 1). The true number of cases was likely much higher than reported due to the challenges of getting tested during the Omicron wave. Although this was an issue throughout the pandemic, it was especially evident during this wave, as testing demands were so high that people with symptoms were directed to assume they had COVID-19 and isolate accordingly if they could not get tested.

While Omicron showed that the virus could return and be lethal, experts believed it was becoming weaker and that Omicron represented another significant turning point (Madhi 2022; Madhi et al. 2022; Malone 2022a). Decision makers emphasized the need to learn to live with COVID-19 and return to a sense of normalcy (Shaman 2022). Canada's chief public health officer, Theresa Tam, emphasized that as we brace for new waves, we need "longer-term, sustained approaches and capacity-building so we're not in a crisis mode all the time as we fight this virus" (Tasker 2022a, para. 4). In February 2022 provinces formulated plans to lift restrictions in March and April, two years after the first lockdown orders had been put in place (Malone 2022a, 2022b). Most states of emergency and government COVID-19 restrictions were lifted in March and April 2022, including mask mandates and proof-of-vaccination requirements. (For further discussion on COVID-19 mandates, see chapter 4.)

Excess Mortality and Impacts on Life Expectancy at Birth

Excess mortality measures changes in the number of deaths after accounting for changes in population (e.g., aging) and is one way to understand impacts of the pandemic. There were 28,987 excess deaths in Canada between March 2020 and November 2021,[2] meaning there were 6 per cent more deaths than expected without the pandemic; 28,117 (97 per cent) of these deaths were attributable to COVID-19 (Statistics Canada 2022i). There was especially significant excess mortality with the Delta variant (9.1 per cent) between August and November 2021 (Statistics Canada 2022i). Ultimately between March 2020 and July 2022, 7.4 per cent excess mortality was observed across Canada (Statistics Canada 2022j).

Life expectancy at birth in Canada decreased by more than half a year (–0.6) in 2020, the largest annual decline since the vital statistics registration system was introduced in 1921 (Statistics Canada 2022b). The direct impact of COVID-19 was estimated at –0.4 years; however, –0.6 years considers all causes of death (Statistics Canada 2022b). Although the pandemic influenced decreases in some deaths (e.g., influenza, pneumonia, workplace accident, road fatality), this was offset by increases in deaths caused by drug overdoses. Across Canada the largest declines in life expectancy were in Quebec, Ontario, Manitoba, Saskatchewan, Alberta, and British Columbia (Statistics Canada 2022b). The decrease was greater for males (–0.7 years) than for females (–0.4 years). Mortality rates also increased for most age groups, with rates for people aged twenty-five to thirty-nine being the highest in over twenty years.

Despite this, life expectancy at birth in Canada remained among the highest globally in 2020. Countries such as Spain (–1.6 years), Italy (–1.2 years), and the US (–1.8 years), experienced greater declines (S. Murphy et al. 2021; Eurostat 2021, 2022). The life expectancy in Norway, Denmark, and Finland remained stable or slightly increased. Canada fared better than the US. In Canada 5 per cent of deaths reported in 2020 were due to COVID-19, compared to 11 per cent in the US. By the end of 2020 there were 5.6 per cent excess deaths in Canada, compared to 17.4 per cent in the US.

There were three periods of excess mortality in Canada between March 2020 and November 2021; table 1.1 summarizes key details of these periods. The greatest impact shifted from predominantly older populations at the beginning to younger people later on. This could be due to indirect effects of the pandemic, such as missed medical appointments, increased substance use, and increased deaths caused by accidental poisonings and overdoses, which disproportionately affected younger Canadians (Statistics Canada 2022i). Excess mortality increased in December 2021, continued to rise in January 2022, and peaked at the end of the month. Alberta had nearly 150 excess deaths per week by the end January 2022, representing 25 per cent more deaths than expected (Statistics Canada 2022i). Excess mortality decreased across Canada into March 2022. By the end of March many COVID-19 restrictions had ended across the country, but excess mortality steadily increased again throughout 2022 (Statistics Canada 2023b).

Figures 1.1, 1.2, and 1.3 show, over time, case count, average incidence of COVID-19 over a seven-day period, total deaths, and fatality rate.

Factors such as age, gender, race, disability, national origin, and income were indicators of severity of COVID-19. In the first wave the elderly were the most likely to get severe cases of COVID-19; however, as the pandemic continued, younger people were increasingly affected. Women were more likely than men to test positive for COVID-19, partly due to the high proportion of women in the health-care and personal-care workforce, specifically in direct-care roles (Desson et al. 2020). As stated previously, most cases in Canada early on came from the US and France. Men were more likely to develop severe complications or die from COVID-19. The mortality rate for COVID-19 was 1.7 times higher for those in the lowest-income neighbourhoods compared with those in the highest-income neighbourhoods (Statistics Canada 2022b). Racialized people were also some of the most likely to die from COVID-19, particularly older immigrant males.' Many racialized people, including new immigrants, are employed in essential services work such as health care and LTC, earn low incomes, and live in multi-generational households. COVID-19 has disproportionately affected socially and economically marginalized communities, further demonstrating the impacts of social and structural determinants of health during the pandemic (Xia et al. 2022, 195).[3]

Table 1.1 | Three periods of excess mortality in Canada
(March 2020–November 2021)

Period	Dates	Details
1	April to June 2020	14.8 per cent more deaths than expected. People over the age of eighty-five were affected the most; vast majority of deaths attributed directly to COVID-19 during this period. Excess deaths for people over eighty-five were 22.5 per cent (women) and 17.4 per cent (men). Excess deaths for people under forty-five were 8.6 per cent (women) and 11.8 per cent (men).
2	October 2020 to the end of January 2021	9.9 per cent more deaths than expected. People under forty-five were affected the most, but only 1.6 to 1.9 per cent of their deaths were attributable to COVID-19, showing indirect effects of the pandemic. Excess deaths were 11.7 per cent (women) and 19.7 per cent (men). Impacts of excess mortality declined for Canadians eighty-five and older with 10.4 per cent (women) and 13.1 per cent (men).
3	August to mid-November 2021	People under forty-five were affected the most; excess mortality for this age group was 17.6 per cent (women) and 24.4 per cent (men). Excess mortality among people eighty-five and older decreased further: 3.8 per cent (women) and 6.4 per cent (men).

Source: Statistics Canada 2022i.

Neighbourhoods with higher proportions of visible minorities experienced COVID-19 mortality rates that were twice as high as neighbourhoods with low proportions, and even higher in Black neighbourhoods. People who identified as Arab, Middle Eastern, West Asian, Latin American, Southeast Asian, or Black were six to nine times more likely to test positive for COVID-19 than White populations (McKenzie 2020). The median age of infection was lower in racialized neighbourhoods.

Experiences with COVID-19 also varied between racialized subgroups (Subedi, Greenberg, and Turcotte 2020). For example, neighbourhoods with at least 25 per cent Black people in Montreal

Figure 1.1 | Total reported cases of COVID-19 across Canada between January 2020 and 2 April 2022. There were 3,503,193 confirmed cases of COVID-19 reported during this time.

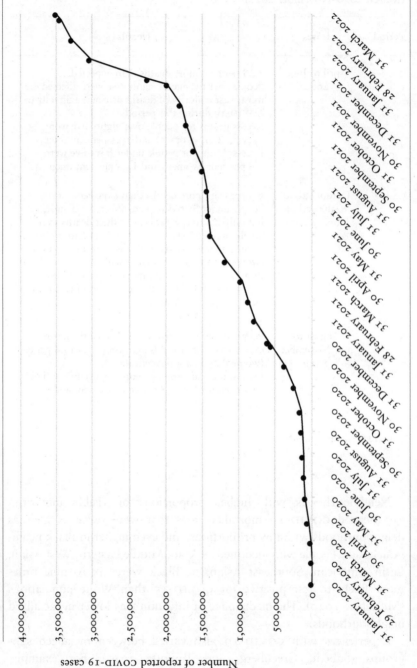

Source: Government of Canada 2022i.

Figure 1.2 | COVID-19 death rate over a seven-day period, January 2020–April 2022. The COVID-19 death rate peaked in three significant periods, April–June 2020, December 2020–March 2021, and January 2022–March 2022.

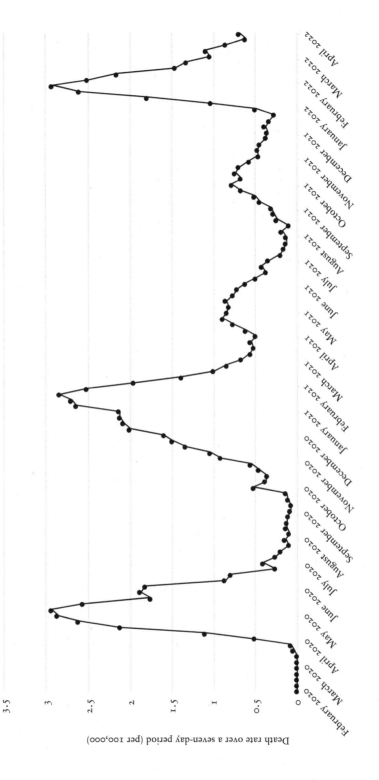

Death rate over a seven-day period (per 100,000)

Source: Government of Canada 2022i.

Figure 1.3 | Total reported COVID-19 deaths across Canada between January 2020 and 2 April 2022. There were 37,722 deaths due to COVID-19 in Canada by 2 April 2022.

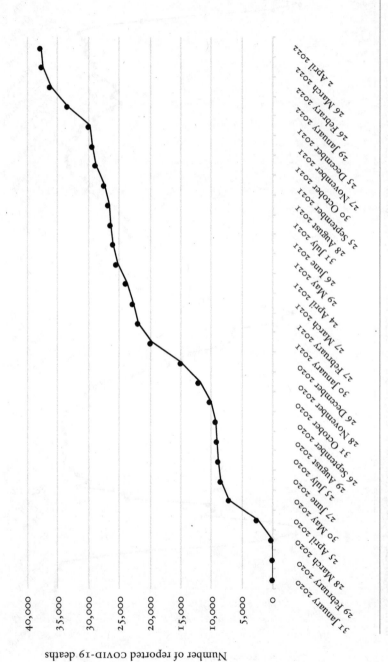

Source: Government of Canada 2022i.

reported a mortality rate four times higher than that of neighbourhoods with at least 25 per cent South Asian people living in Toronto (Subedi, Greenberg, and Turcotte 2020). As of November 2020 more people had died in Montreal Nord, a low-income area with a large population of African and Caribbean people, than had died in all of British Columbia (McKenzie 2020).

Impacts on Hospitals and Intensive Care Units

Many of the restrictions put in place were motivated by concern that the health system would become overwhelmed, particularly ICUs. Most people with COVID-19 had minor symptoms, but there were many who were hospitalized and admitted to the ICU. Data from the OECD have emphasized the limited hospital capacity of Canada compared to that of other OECD countries. In a ranking of hospital beds for acute care, Canada ranked near the bottom, at fourth from the last (1.97 per 1,000). Japan was at the top with 7.74 beds per 1,000, followed by Korea (7.08), Germany (5.95), and Austria (5.31) (OECD 2021). By 21 July 2022, 4.5 per cent of COVID-19 cases in Canada were hospitalized (168,168 cases), and 16.5 per cent of those (27,747 patients) were admitted to the ICU. ICU capacity was an immediate concern because of the situation in China and Italy, where hospitals were overloaded and there were ventilator shortages. Before the pandemic the average ICU capacity in OECD countries was 12 per 100,000 population, with Canada reporting a slightly higher number at 12.9 ICU beds per 100,000 (see table 1.2). While hospitals can convert a unit into an ICU, treatment for COVID-19 requires respiratory equipment (OECD 2020a). Capacity for an ICU patient is also more than just the hospital bed; it includes the necessary medical equipment and trained health-care workers.

A CIHI report noted that 33 per cent of ICU patients in Canada had required invasive ventilation in 2013–14, and there had been a need to increase ventilation capacity well before the pandemic (CIHI 2016). Surge capacity, or the ability of hospitals and health-care facilities to manage increased demand for ICU beds and ventilators, was also a key consideration.

A 2015 study estimated there were 3,170 ICU beds capable of invasive ventilation across Canada (Shoukat et al. 2020). The number of ICU beds in each province ranged from 0.63 to 1.85 per 10,000 population. Assuming an 80 per cent occupancy rate, ICU beds available for COVID-19 patients ranged from 0.13 to 0.37 per 10,000 population (Shoukat et al. 2020). In May 2020 researchers estimated that if up to

Table 1.2 | Of G7 countries, Canada ranked fourth for ICU capacity per 100,000 population before the pandemic

Country	Intensive care beds (per 100,000 population)
1 Germany (2017)	33.9
2 United States (2018)	25.8
3 France (2018)	16.3
4 Canada (2013–14)	12.9
OECD *average*	12.0
5 UK (England 2020 and	10.5
Ireland 2016 only)	5.0
6 Italy (2020)	8.6
7 Japan (2019)	5.2

Notes: While some of the beds and other resources in curative (or acute) care hospital units may be temporarily converted into flexible intensive care units, a key point, especially for COVID-19 treatment, is that intensive care beds need to be equipped with respiratory equipment.

There may be differences in the notion of intensive care that affect comparability of the data. Data refer to adults only in Belgium, Ireland, and Canada and to all ages in Germany, England, and Spain. Data in France include "*lits de réanimation adulte*" (except severe burns) and "*lits de soins intensifs*" (except neonatology) but exclude "*lits de surveillance continue adulte et enfants*" and "*lits de réanimation enfants.*" *Source:* OECD 2020c.

three people got COVID-19 from one identified case, and 40 per cent of people isolated themselves within twenty-four hours of the onset of symptoms, then the need for ICU care could exceed 2.6 times capacity (Shoukat et al. 2020). If the 80 per cent existing occupancy-rate estimate for ICUs were accurate, then the need would exceed 13 times the capacity (Shoukat et al. 2020).

Treatment at a hospital is expensive, and particularly for those in ICU, which invites difficult trade-offs about how much should be allocated for it. Hospital treatment for a COVID-19 patient averaged $23,000 in March 2021. ICU treatment was estimated to be around $50,000, nearly six times higher than ICU treatment for a heart-attack patient and four times higher than for an influenza patient.

Table 1.3 | Costs of COVID-19 care in hospital: $23,111 per patient, over three times the cost of the average non–COVID-19 hospital stay

Treatment	Cost ($)
Kidney transplant	27,093
COVID-19	23,111
Pneumonia	8,433
Heart attack	7,446
Hospital average (non–COVID-19)	6,349
Influenza	4,959

Source: CBC News 2021c.

CIHI estimated that the cost of COVID-19–related hospitalization in Canada, excluding Quebec, was approximately $3.5 billion between January 2020 and March 2022 (CIHI 2022b). Hospitalization costs tripled between November 2020 and March 2021 compared to earlier waves of the pandemic (CBC News 2021c). Total health expenditure in Canada increased by 12.8 per cent in 2020 due to pandemic responses; however, growth in health spending averaged 4 per cent per year between 2015 and 2019. COVID-19 response funding accounted for 7 per cent of total health spending in 2021, including federal, provincial, and territorial levels (CIHI 2021c).

Tracking hospitalization costs (table 1.3) by individual treatment can be misleading, as initial treatment costs of COVID-19 patients are much higher than average; however, cumulative costs for a decade of cardiovascular hospitalization due to unhealthy eating habits could cost $80,000.

The highest rates of hospitalization and ICU admission were among men over the age of sixty. Hospitalization was slightly more likely for males than for females, and males accounted for nearly 1.7 times more ICU cases than females. The highest rates of ICU admittance were in Quebec and Ontario (Statistics Canada 2021l). The highest number in one day occurred during the third wave in May 2021 with nearly 1,400 people in ICU in Canada due to COVID-19 (Government of Canada 2022k). Of the people hospitalized, 74 per cent were reported to have at least one underlying health condition as of May 2021 (PHAC 2020k).

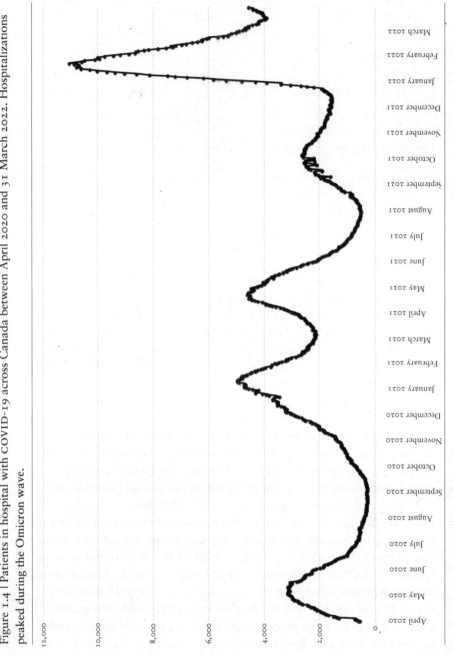

Figure 1.4 | Patients in hospital with COVID-19 across Canada between April 2020 and 31 March 2022. Hospitalizations peaked during the Omicron wave.

Source: Government of Canada 2022k.

Figure 1.5 | Patients in ICU and mechanically vented during COVID-19 across Canada between April 2020 and 31 March 2022. ICU admissions and ventilation peaked in May 2021 with the Delta variant.

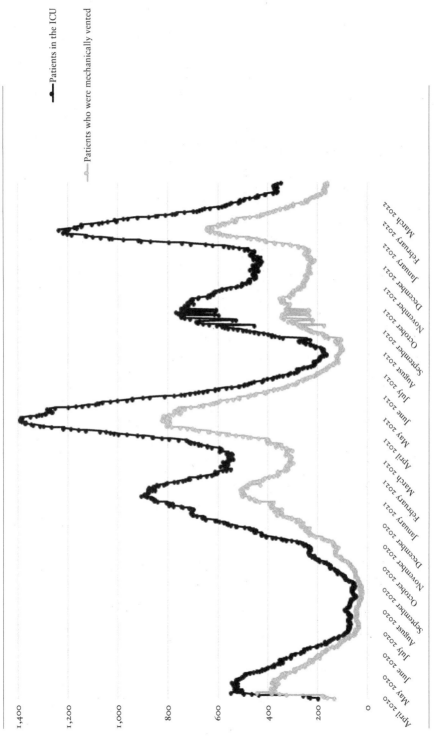

Source: Government of Canada 2022k.

The proportion of COVID-19 variants of concern climbed throughout 2021 (PHAC 2021g). ICU admissions increased between November 2020 and February 2021, and increased further throughout March and April 2021, as seen in figure 1.4 (PHAC 2021i). As the Omicron variant spread into 2022, there were more cases, but they were often less severe. Hospital stays were shorter than with the Delta variant, and slightly fewer patients needed to be mechanically vented. Figure 1.5 shows the number of patients admitted to ICU and mechanically vented during COVID-19 across Canada between April 2020 and 31 March 2022.

CONCLUSION

Canada is part of a global community in which there is regular trade and travel. This integration revealed vulnerabilities. At times China suppressed information, which increased the risk to the international community. Canada's largest trading partner and neighbour, the US, was slow to react; that Canada ramped up its effort largely after the US did suggests a vulnerability in Canada's dependence on the US response. While it is a crucial repository for global information about the pandemic, the WHO showed itself to be slow to appreciate the magnitude of the risk and ineffective at persuading powerful members to follow standards. In many cases, when confronted with uncertainty, governments described COVID-19 as low-risk; they were wrong, and their indecisiveness had serious consequences.

Public health was caught off guard. The slow reaction of Western governments when Wuhan, a city of eleven million, was under lockdown demonstrates their inability to react quickly in a crisis that demands speed in gathering information, setting standards, and changing behaviour. Its information gathering, testing capacity, and PPE stock were limited. The limited number of ICU beds available at any one time shows the importance of adaptive capacity. The concentration of population in urban centres, especially disadvantaged groups who worked in low-paying essential jobs and who were particularly vulnerable, was not appreciated early enough; this is where community spread at times was most virulent. Despite the vulnerability of their residents, LTC centres were also not adequately prepared. Although public health was not ready for the first wave, by many measures, the second and third waves were worse than the first in terms of hospitalizations and case numbers.

The purpose of this chapter has been to summarize how COVID-19 started and spread. We set out key COVID-19 data points. Our next step is to review how Canadian governments sought to understand

and control the disease, using the three lenses of cybernetics: information gathering, standard setting, and behaviour modification. Before we review governments' responses to control COVID-19, however, we will first situate COVID-19 in the social science of risk literature. This review will allow us to introduce key assumptions, terms, tools, and methods that must be explained before we analyze the case.

Situating COVID-19 in the Risk Literature: Four Rationales for Risk

COVID-19 exposes several epistemological challenges in risk research, analysis, and governance. When we are confronted with risks, what we think we know, how we know it, and what to do about it are contested. Scholars attribute our action in the face of uncertainty to several sources: rational analysis, biases, perspectives and feelings, lived experiences, institutional arrangements, and community identities and values, as well as the distribution of power in society. Although the origins of the study of risk, as we often refer to it, date back to the Scientific Revolution, the study has grown exponentially since the 1980s, marked in particular by the publication of Beck's (1986) *Risikogesellschaft* (*Risk Society*; first translated into English in 1992), reflecting progress and debates in and across several disciplines, including psychology, sociology, and anthropology.

This chapter groups the key risk literature according to four rationales and gives examples of how each provides important insights into our understanding of and reaction to the pandemic. It draws significantly on C. Jaeger et al. (2001) and expands on Quigley (2008) and Quigley, Bisset, and Mills (2017). The four rationales are distinguished by the extent to which risk is understood as objective or subjective and interpreted at an individual or institutional-community level. Importantly, the literature reviewed in this chapter will allow us, over the course of the book, to draw on a wide range of literature from the last few decades to explore the case. While the literature is rich and diverse, the organizing concepts of objective versus subjective, and individual versus institution or community, demonstrate that many observations about the pandemic and what do about it were premised on different focal points for analysis. When taken together, these result in inconsistent and incompatible claims; this epistemological confusion underscores

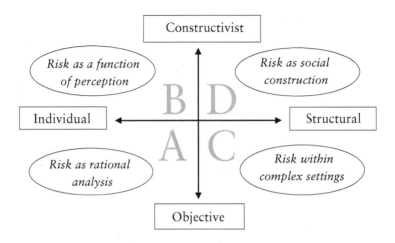

Figure 2.1 | Risk rationality diagram: four rationales for risk
Renn (2008) uses the term *realistic* as an organizing concept rather than the term *objective*. *Source:* Adapted from Renn 2008a.

part of the challenge of articulating what constituted an appropriate response to the threat. The chapter concludes by highlighting why a regimes approach offers an opportunity to bring these at times divergent concepts together for a more holistic understanding of the pandemic and governments' responses.

RISK AS RATIONAL ANALYSIS (BOX A IN FIGURE 2.1)

The rational actor paradigm (RAP) approach to risk is underpinned by Western notions of rationalism. It upholds reason as the key source of knowledge, and understanding is pursued through intellect and logic. In the RAP tradition of risk, knowledge is largely dependent on abstract mathematical reasoning; the methods can be both deductive and inductive, and abstract or empirical. There is optimism that complex problems can be reduced to simpler forms. It implies, if not directly supports, the notion of universal truth, and that truth can be obtained through reasoning and expressed in numbers to obtain abstract universals. It assumes the view of an individual, not a collective, and is utilitarian.

The Western study of probability, central to the concept of risk, started during the Scientific Revolution and included studies of games of

Table 2.1 | Public Health Agency of Canada's COVID-19 predictions, 2020

Percentage of population with COVID-19	All cases	Hospitalized	ICU	Deaths
1.0%	376,000	29,000	9,000	4,000
2.5%	940,000	73,000	23,000	11,000
5.0%	1,879,000	146,000	46,000	22,000
10.0%	3,759,000	292,000	92,000	44,000
25.0%	9,397,000	730,000	229,000	111,000
50.0%	18,795,000	1,461,000	459,000	222,000
70.0%	26,312,000	2,045,000	642,000	311,000
80.0%	30,071,000	2,337,000	734,000	355,000

PHAC estimated between 376,000 and 30,071,000 cases of COVID-19 in Canada.
Source: PHAC 2020a.

chance by Cardano, Pascal, and Fermat and continued with Bernoulli's law of large numbers, Gauss's discovery of the normal distribution, and Laplace's discovery of the central limit theorem. These studies laid the groundwork for the modern study of statistics. The study of probability and statistics allows us to structure problems of uncertainty and provides predictive capacity. In risk analysis, models and calculations are necessarily simplified representations of reality with the aim of capturing the key features of the problem. In this view, risk is defined as probability multiplied by consequence (Starr 1969; Lowrance 1976). There is also a sense of agency. Technical risk analyses are intended to reveal causal agents associated with unwanted effects; it is assumed that we can act on this information. Until the early 1980s this understanding of risk was largely uncontested (Adams 1995, 8).

Formal risk modelling is a growing practice and fits comfortably within RAP. Modellers identify entities and interdependencies; the models can include data on probability, vulnerability, consequence, and time. Table 2.1 exemplifies the outputs of government models throughout the pandemic to understand and communicate the threat of the disease (PHAC 2020a).

Models that represent the infection rate of COVID-19 were founded on various assumptions, including assumptions about people's behaviour as well as the infection, hospitalization, and death rates (Adam 2020). Uncertainty is a constant challenge to modelling; the parameters include several estimates, such as latency period, proportion of asymptomatic cases, duration of infectivity, and distribution (Ogden et al. 2020, 201). More detailed discussion about models can be found in chapter 3.

RAP and Risk in Comparative Perspective

Rational analysis allows us to compare risk using common measures. One way to understand the consequences of the pandemic is to consider the number of people who died from COVID-19. Table 2.2 shows where Canada fits in comparison to other countries when considering deaths from COVID-19 in absolute terms and on a per capita basis. Table 2.3 shows the number of reported deaths caused by COVID-19 from its inception to 2 April 2022 (37,722) and where it fits in a ranking of causes of death in 2019 (Statistics Canada 2020l).

The tables can help us situate COVID-19 in relation to other phenomena; still, they are oversimplifications of a more complex story. Reporting processes varied by jurisdiction, including how COVID-19 fatalities and co-morbidities were reported, which undermines any death-count comparisons. In fact, it is not that easy to categorize someone as dying strictly from COVID-19. Most people who died of COVID-19 died from the virus plus additional causes, such as heart disease, chronic obstructive pulmonary disease, asthma, and/or diabetes. Ninety per cent of COVID-19–related deaths that occurred between March and July 2020 in Canada occurred among individuals with pre-existing chronic conditions (Government of Canada 2021g).

As noted in the previous chapter, there were 28,987 excess deaths in Canada between March 2020 and November 2021,[1] meaning there were 6 per cent more deaths than expected without the pandemic; 28,117 (97 per cent) of these deaths were attributable to COVID-19 (Statistics Canada 2022i). (For further discussion on COVID-19–related deaths, see chapter 1.) Mortality rates also increased for most age groups, with rates for people aged twenty-five to thirty-nine being at the highest in over twenty years.At the beginning of the pandemic, excess deaths were largely among seniors and primarily due to COVID-19. Between March and June 2020, excess deaths for people over eighty-five were 22.5 per cent (women) and 17.4 per cent (men). This trend changed as the pandemic progressed, and there began to be more excess deaths among younger Canadians. Between October 2020 and mid-November 2021, Canadians under forty-five were the most affected by excess mortality

Table 2.2 | Reported COVID-19 deaths per capita in selected countries, 22 January 2020 to 2 April 2022

Country	Total population (2019)	Total deaths due to COVID-19	Total deaths due to COVID-19 per capita (x 1,000)
Brazil	211,049,519	660,371	3.13
United States	328,239,523	984,312	3.00
United Kingdom	66,796,800	192,543	2.88
Italy	59,729,081	159,666	2.67
Mexico	127,575,529	323,212	2.53
Spain	47,332,614	102,541	2.17
France	67,287,241	142,544	2.12
South Africa	58,558,267	100,032	1.71
Germany	83,092,962	129,987	1.56
Canada	37,589,262	37,722	1.00
India	1,366,000,000	521,345	0.38
Australia	25,522,169	6,383	0.25
Japan	126,264,931	9,216	0.07
China	1,408,000,000	120, 827*	0.086
Taiwan	23,773,876	853	0.04
New Zealand	4,979,300	28	0.006

* Data on COVID-19 deaths and cases from China have been unreliable. Deaths due to COVID-19 in China are estimated to be 390,000, with a range of 77,000 to 945,000 based on global fatality rates as of 16 January 2023 (Bloomberg 2023). As of 20 September 2023, 121,679 cumulative deaths due to COVID-19 in China were reported to the WHO (WHO 2023).

Canada had a low death count relative to other countries. *Sources:* United States Census Bureau 2019; Statistics Canada 2019a; Office for National Statistics 2021; World Bank 2018, 2020a–i; National Institute of Statistics and Economic Studies 2021; National Statistics Institute 2021; Macrotrends, n.d.; Australian Bureau of Statistics 2019; Ritchie et al. 2022a.

(19.7 per cent for men and 11.7 per cent for women), yet COVID-19 caused only 1.6 to 1.9 per cent of these deaths as of the end of January 2021, meaning these deaths were from other causes such as an overdose. Between August and mid-November 2021, excess mortality among

Table 2.3 | Leading causes of death in Canada, 2019–20

Cause of death	Total fatalities in 2019	Rank of cause of death in 2019	Total fatalities in 2020	Rank of cause of death in 2020
Malignant neoplasms (i.e., tumours)	80,372	1	81,242	1
Heart diseases	53,364	2	54,430	2
Accidents (unintentional injuries)	15,527	3	16,818	3
COVID-19	N/A	N/A	15,890	4
Cerebrovascular diseases	13,717	4	13,761	5
Chronic lower respiratory diseases	12,902	5	11,844	6
Diabetes mellitus	6,987	6	7,654	7
Influenza and pneumonia	6,945	7	6,037	8
Alzheimer's disease	6,181	8	5,788	9
Intentional self-harm (suicide)	4,581	9	4,152	11
Nephritis and nephrosis	3,770	10	4,065	12
Chronic liver disease and cirrhosis	3,708	11	4,199	10

COVID-19 was the fourth leading cause of death in Canada in 2020.
Source: Statistics Canada 2020l.

people eighty-five and older decreased to 6.4 per cent (men) and 3.8 per cent (women). January 2022 to 5 March 2022 was the deadliest nine-week period during the pandemic at the time. The majority of provinces were affected, in contrast to other periods in which the most populated provinces were primarily affected. There were 8,959 excess deaths, or 16.2 per cent more deaths than expected, with 78 per cent attributed to COVID-19 (6,985 deaths), but other factors, such as the record number of accidental poisonings (including overdoses) reported in 2021 were contributing factors. Throughout the rest of March 2022 the number of deaths fell within the range of what would be expected had there been no pandemic; however, another period of excess mortality started in mid-April 2022. At one point in the pandemic it was common to compare the death rate from COVID-19 to that of the first and second world wars, particularly in popular media coverage (Waxman and Wilson 2021; Flanagan 2021). This comparison is made more complicated by the fact that the average age at death of someone during COVID-19 was much higher than the average age of death of a soldier during war; soldiers typically died in their mid-twenties. Therefore, if we estimate years of life lost, the consequences of those world wars were over twenty times more severe than the consequences of COVID-19. (See appendix 2 for data and calculations.)

The novelty of the event can also be an important consideration. One of the most significant risks we take almost every day is to drive a car. Each year about 2,000 Canadians die on the roads. COVID-19 killed many more people in Canada than car accidents did at the time of the pandemic. Deaths by car accidents and by COVID-19 are quite different in several ways. For our purposes here, we underscore that deaths by car accidents are not new; road safety is regulated, but road deaths occur regularly and are tolerated to a degree. COVID-19 in contrast was new, poorly understood, and with high dread characteristics, which we will explore in more detail in the "Risk as a Function of Individual Perception" section. For the purposes of rational analysis we might compare road deaths over a ten-year period (dating back to the last pandemic, H1N1) to the number of deaths attributed to COVID-19 between January 2020 and March 2022 to have a sense of how pandemic deaths compare to road deaths. If we consider years of life lost, we can estimate that we lost an average of 188,610 years of life due to COVID-19 (March 2020–2 April 2022) and 642,810 years of life due to vehicle-related fatalities (2009–19). In other words, over the past decade, car accidents have been about 3.4 times more deadly than COVID-19. In fact, years lost due to COVID-19 roughly equal the number of years lost by car deaths every two years and nine months. (See appendix 3 for data and calculations.)

When the Omicron variant peaked at Christmas 2021, and experts recommended people drive rather than fly to family gatherings across the country (see, for example, Compton and Sampson 2020), they were asking people to shift their risks from contracting Omicron on a flight to driving long distances in the winter, which can also be dangerous, but these trade-offs were rarely noted. There was a similar occurrence after 9/11 when many Americans chose to drive rather than fly; in the months that followed, there was a sharp increase in road deaths (J. Ball 2011; Blalock, Kadiyali, and Simon 2009).

Economic Tools

There are economic tools that help us reason through health and cost trade-offs that are largely consistent with RAP. Cost-effectiveness analysis and cost-utility analysis are commonly used to evaluate health interventions and can be used to analyze trade-offs for an individual as well as at community, regional, and national levels. Cost-effectiveness analysis is used regularly in the fields of medicine and public health. It estimates how much an intervention may cost per unit of health gained compared to other options (CDC 2021).

Cost-utility analysis can also be used to compare costs and effects of alternative interventions. It measures health effects in quantity (life years) and quality of life and combines them into a single measure, quality-adjusted life years (QALYs). This estimates how an intervention can extend people's lives (life-year gains) and improve the quality of life compared to alternative options (UK Health Security Agency 2020). It can be challenging to capture effects such as impacts on mental health, as well as other non-health effects. Measures for quality of life can also be more subjective than other clinical measures (UK Health Security Agency 2020). These types of cost-benefit-analysis tools can be used to inform and assess a variety of interventions, some more explicitly than others. Throughout COVID-19 they were used to assess decisions about maintaining surge capacity in hospitals, designing vaccine trials and policies, implementing virtual health care, and approving new products and technologies (Frank, Concannon, and Patel 2020; Berry et al. 2020; Emanuel et al. 2020).

The value of a statistical life (VSL) calculation is a tool that decision makers use to assess the costs and benefits of specific standards and interventions, and the calculation is often published by US government officials when assessing proposed policies. If each premature death due to COVID-19 in the US is valued at $7 million, as Cutler and Summers (2020) suggest for example, the economic cost of these premature deaths would be approximately $4.4 trillion over the course of a year

(2020–21). What constitutes a legitimate cost and how one measures it are difficult to determine. In October 2020, if one includes in the calculation the value of lives lost due to COVID-19, to long-term health complications, and to mental-health issues resulting from the pandemic, researchers estimated the cost to US gross domestic product (GDP) to be $16 trillion for one year; the financial crisis (2007–09) is estimated to be only one-quarter of this cost. COVID-19 is thought to be more costly than all the wars fought by the US since 9/11 (Afghanistan, Iraq, and Syria) and comparable to damages from fifty years of climate change (Cutler and Summers 2020). Even from within the tenets of RAP, there are many challenges associated with the use of VSL (see, for example, Quigley 2018). There is no universally accepted single value for statistical life. There are also many ways to calculate the VSL, for example by factoring in age (Cutler and Summers 2020; Treasury Board Secretariat 2022; L. Robinson 2020). A wide range of values for a statistical life are used across government departments in the US, for example, anywhere from $7 million to $12 million (Cutler and Summers 2020; Office of the Assistant Secretary for Planning and Evaluation 2017; US Department of Transportation 2021), and all have various normative implications.

The RAP approach to understanding risk has been criticized on several grounds. First, what people perceive as unwanted effects or consequences differ according to their values and preferences, and they may change over time and in different circumstances; a challenge in supporting any solution to a decision problem is the ranking of options, which will not reflect everyone's preferences. Relatedly, people have a hard time comparing risks; they would rather know what is being done to manage a risk than to hear that the risk they are facing is not as serious as a more common one. Second, models based on RAP typically require data, yet it is difficult to obtain reliable data for these models. To start, modellers assume people can express themselves accurately in numerical terms. Moreover, the interaction between human activities and consequences is more complex, and perhaps subtle, than the average probabilities captured by most risk analyses. When data are unavailable for these models, which is often the case when we explore rare events, such as pandemics, acts of terrorism, and rare natural disasters, they are often estimated; estimations have errors associated with them. What is more, models are often built on past experiences or data from other jurisdictions. These models will fail to predict new or rare events because the assumptions do not necessarily hold. Third, the institutional structures for managing and controlling risks are prone to organizational failure, which may increase actual risks (C. Jaeger et al. 2001, 86).

From a normative standpoint, RAP embeds key assumptions. To start, RAP assumes that we can understand complex technological systems and that a reductionist approach is the best way to understand them. Motivation, organization, politics, context, and culture are ignored (C. Jaeger et al. 2001, 91). Moreover, people also do not normally like to have their lives expressed in dollar values, even if the insurance industry does it as a matter of course. It is telling, for example, that during the pandemic governments rarely employed or presented any rational economic analysis to justify interventions. Governments referred almost strictly to containment, "flattening the curve," and protecting the healthcare system and ICUs from being overwhelmed. An RAP approach also upholds the privileged position of the one who designed the model (i.e., the expert); it values expert views over lay views. Finally, risk minimization and even resilience are not necessarily the only ends in mind; equity, fairness, and flexibility are also plausible and potentially desirable goals, but they are frequently overlooked (86).

RISK AS A FUNCTION OF INDIVIDUAL PERCEPTION (BOX B IN FIGURE 2.1)

Risk as individual perception helps us understand how people felt about the risks associated with COVID-19 and the various challenges that public health faced in communicating risk to people in light of these feelings. As one editorialist in the *New York Times* noted, a pandemic is over medically when death and incidence rates plummet and socially when people's fear of the pandemic wanes (Kolata 2021). When it comes to risk psychology, emotion is important. Understanding risk perception also helps us to understand and predict people's behaviour and to improve communication between technical experts and lay people (Burns 2012) as a means to shape that behaviour. The psychometric paradigm – theory and technique of mental measurement – draws on the work of cognitive psychologists such as Slovic, Fischhoff, and Lichtenstein (1982) to conceptualize risks as personal expressions of individual fears or expectations. In short, individuals respond to their perceptions whether or not those perceptions reflect reality. The study of risk perception has grown in popularity over recent decades, partly due to the study of psychology and the associated pre-eminence we put on individual perspectives and testimonies.

The psychology of risk literature identifies several biases in people's ability to draw inferences in the face of uncertainty. Risk perception can be influenced by personal control (Langer 1975), familiarity (Tversky and Kahneman 1973), exit options (Starr 1969), equitable sharing of benefits and risks (Finucane et al. 2000), and the potential to blame an institution or person (Douglas and Wildavsky 1982). Risk perception can also be influenced by how a person feels about something, such as a particular technology or a disease (Alhakami and Slovic 1994; Assailly 2009). People also show confirmation bias (Wason 1960), which suggests they seek information to confirm, not to challenge, how they feel.

Risk perceptions are often faulty when we consider consequence and probability (Slovic, Fischhoff, and Lichtenstein 1982). Risk cannot be directly observed. Rather, people construct risk perceptions based on their understanding of hazards in everyday life, often making judgments about risk by using incomplete or erroneous information. They also rely on biases or heuristics to comprehend complexity. Heuristics are cognitive tools people use to analyze risk and complexity (Slovic, Fischhoff, and Lichtenstein 1982; Spencer 2016). In some ways, heuristics are helpful because they allow people to render simplistic understandings of complicated subjects. However, they can also oversimplify or distort our understanding. Heuristics have two primary dimensions: the unknown factor and the dread factor. Unknown risks include those that are new, unobservable, not known to science or to those exposed, and have a delayed effect. High-dread risks include those understood to be uncontrollable, inequitable in their reach, potentially catastrophic, of high risk to the future, not easily reduced, inclusive of involuntary exposure, and able to affect people personally (Slovic, Fischhoff, and Lichtenstein 1982). These characteristics figure prominently during a pandemic. One of the most common heuristics is availability. Under the influence of the availability heuristic, people tend to believe that an event is more likely to occur when they can imagine or recall it easily; people underestimate risks they cannot imagine or recall. This can lead to probability neglect, when we focus on outcomes but overlook likelihood (for examples see Slovic, Fischhoff, and Lichtenstein 1982; Folkes 1988; Betsch and Pohl 2002; Tversky and Kahneman 1973; Maldonato and Dell'Orco 2011; Sjöberg 2000; Pachur, Hertwig, and Steinmann 2012). From a risk psychologist's point of view, the availability heuristic helps us understand why we were slow to respond to COVID-19 in the first place. We had never experienced such a large-scale pandemic; we could not imagine it and therefore we could not respond to it.

A psychometric approach to risk provides more insight into the effect of media than a rational approach does. The media tend to report the dramatic over the common, but more dangerous (Soumerai, Ross-Degnan, and Kahn 1992), and tend not only to sensationalize generally

(Johnson and Covello 1987) but also to sensationalize the most negative aspects of events (Wahlberg and Sjöberg 2000; Young, Norman, and Humphreys 2008; Young et al. 2013).

The degree of trust in institutions and authorities is an important factor in considering how people receive and process information (Earle 2007; Siegrist and Bearth 2021). The term *trust* is used in a variety of distinct and not always compatible ways in organizational research (Rousseau et al. 1998; R. Kramer 1999). Barbalet (2009) argues that trust is often confused with consideration of legitimacy or loyalty. R. Kramer (1999) describes several ways to think about trust: history-based trust, category-based trust, and roles-based trust, for example. Hardin (2006) argues that the key is trustworthiness – the context that allows trust to develop. Peters, Covello, and McCallum (1997) identified three dimensions that people tend to look for in others to develop trust: knowledge and expertise; care and concern; and openness and honesty (cited in Eiser and White 2005). Medical doctors, for example, tend to rank well in all three categories, which is why they tend to be highly trusted (Ipsos and Royal College of Physicians 2009). These concepts can be applied equally at the organizational level (Gillespie and Dietz 2009). The concept of open communication, in particular, appears repeatedly in research on developing organizational trust (M. Clarke and Payne 1997) and encompasses free data-sharing, inclusive decision making, and collaborative work (Firth-Cozens 2004; Jeffcott et al. 2006). Trust is easy to lose because negative information that can diminish people's feelings of trust is more attention grabbing, more powerful, and often more readily available than positive information (Eiser and White 2005).

Psychologists and social psychologists have proposed frameworks to explain risk challenges, including the social amplification of risk framework (SARF) (Kasperson et al. 1988) and the mental models approach (Morgan et al. 2001). SARF explains how risks are amplified or attenuated by scientists, media, cultural groups, and interpersonal networks. The mental models approach examines how to align the thinking of lay people with expert views by addressing knowledge gaps.

There are many psychological biases that work against public health initiatives. The relationship between people's anxiety levels and their willingness to engage in preventive or containment measures is well documented (for example, see Tausczik et al. 2011; Hilton and Smith 2010; J. Jones and Salathé 2009). Governments' recommendations about health care are more likely to be followed by those who perceive the risk to be significant. Unfortunately the relationship between people's anxiety and the probability of them dying or becoming debilitated by a threat is quite weak (J. Jones and Salathé 2009). From a probability point of view, people often feel anxious about the wrong things. Medical advice may also conflict with personal, cultural, or religious beliefs. (For a recent example see the Ebola case in 2014–15 as described in Manguvo and Mafuvadze [2015] and Landen [2014].) Additionally, people do not identify with "statistical lives" and meso- and macro-level analyses; they are moved by human stories. Finally, the successes of public health initiatives suffer from a dilution of benefit, whereby the perceived benefit is diminished because in time the public no longer observes the consequences of the disease (Poland and Jacobson 2001), and at times questions the benefits of intervention, which is referred to as the paradox of preparation when considering things like pandemics and natural disasters (Kottke 2020).

It is also difficult to prove conclusively that disease prevention is successful. When it is successful, it is quietly successful over time. Disease-prevention rewards are delayed and not accrued necessarily to the payer. Professional advice can be inconsistent, and permanent, long-term (and unpopular) behaviour change may be required.

Risk psychology brought several important issues to the fore during COVID-19, which we will explore throughout the manuscript and particularly in the opinion-responsive hypothesis (ORH) discussion (chapter 10). Here, by way of example, we will simply point out the contrast between expert and lay views of risk. Experts may develop models that identify who is at greatest risk of the disease, but this may not correspond with who feels most anxious about the disease and behaves accordingly (Trifiletti et al. 2021). When we think about risk strictly in rational terms, we might look at ICU patients and death rates, for example. Older people were more likely to become sick with the disease. Men were more likely to die than women. Yet mortality rates do not correspond with mental health. UK data reveal that women reported the most significant impacts to their mental health across all age groups; those aged sixteen to thirty-four, and thirty-five to sixty-four, saw the steepest decline in mental health (Helliwell et al. 2021).

Like RAP, risk psychology has limitations. It suffers from the same micro-orientation as RAP does. It assumes that an individual will act on subjective estimates of consequences and probabilities. It is not clear if an individual will pursue a strategy to verify or validate perception before acting on it (C. Jaeger et al. 2001). Moreover, lay judgments of risk are seen as multi-dimensional, but a strong distinction between the subjective "popular" level and the objective "expert" level is maintained

(Taylor-Gooby 2006, 7). People can also be subject to manipulation through various techniques, which raises questions about ethics. Methodologically, psychometrics has also been criticized for gathering data through questionnaires, in which the issues are already predefined (6–7), which may reveal bias towards certain issues.

RISK WITHIN COMPLEX SETTINGS (BOX C IN FIGURE 2.1)

Understanding how governments responded to the pandemic in an organizational context is crucial because public policy and management occur in organizational contexts and are therefore subject to the constraints and opportunities of organizational dynamics. There are two main schools of thought on the safety and reliability of complex technological and social systems: (1) high-reliability organizations (HRO); and (2) normal accidents theory (NAT). The tenets of the HRO literature, common in business schools and operational research, suggest that complex risks can be safely controlled by organizations if the correct design and management techniques are followed, such as strong and persuasive leadership, commitment and adherence to a safety culture (including learning from mistakes), creating redundancies, and increasing transparency with respect to accountability and operations (La Porte and Consolini 1991; La Porte 1996; Weick and Roberts 1993; Weick and Sutcliffe 2001). In contrast, the NAT literature, which is an extension of chaos theory, holds that failures are inevitable in organizations that are socially and technically complex. NAT advocates argue that the discipline required of HRO is unrealistic. Systems fail because of their inherent fallibility and the non-responsive nature of bureaucratic organizations. Efforts to increase accountability result in the shifting of blame. Indeed, safety is only one priority, which competes with many others (Sagan 1993; Vaughan 1996; Perrow 1999; Taleb 2007).

More recently, the search for security is understood as a dynamic process that balances mechanisms of control with processes of information search, exchange, and feedback in complex multi-organizational settings. This dynamic process, which evolves over time, is guided by public organizations and seeks participation from private organizations, not-for-profits, and informed citizens (Comfort 2002; Aviram and Tor 2004; Aviram 2005; Auerswald et al. 2006; De Bruijne and Van Eeten 2007; Egan 2007; M. Howlett 2019). The risk debate has now expanded from avoiding failure to coping with failure in a variety of complex organizational settings (D. Palmer and Maher 2010;

Aldrich 2013; Casler 2014; Sheps and Cardiff 2011; Huck, Monstadt, and Driessen 2020; Normandin and Therrien 2016).

Increasingly, there is a movement towards a systems approach within medicine. In this view, complex health problems can only be addressed by understanding basic science, clinical science, and the system in which they operate (Skochelak and Hawkins 2017; Ovens and Petrie 2021), including the interdependence that exists among organizations (Therrien, Normandin, and Denis 2017). "Health systems science is defined as the study of how health care is delivered, how health care professionals work together to deliver that care, and how the health system can improve patient care and health care delivery" (Skochelak and Hawkins 2017, 6). Systems science offers insights into the nature of the whole system that often cannot be gained by studying the component parts in isolation (Mabry et al. 2008). Health systems science "includes knowledge and skills related to value-based care, quality improvement, social determinants of health, population health, informatics, and systems thinking" (Gonzalo, Chang, and Wolpaw 2019, 501).

From a complex systems perspective, RAP is misleading because it tends to assume regression to a mean; in fact, events like pandemics and climate disasters are becoming more extreme, and the mean is no longer a useful guide (Flyvbjerg 2020). The CDC's Pandemic Influenza Plan and National Strategy in 2005 (CDC 2022a; US Department of Health and Human Services 2005; Homeland Security Council 2005) is a touchstone document for public agencies around the world and provides structure and guidance in a complex context. The plan identifies the key actions to take during a pandemic: international surveillance, determining the feasibility to contain an outbreak, obtaining and analyzing samples of the virus, isolating exposed patients and their contacts, enhancing ways to track the spread of the virus in real time, implementing public health measures such as physical distancing and gathering limits, monitoring and assessing response mechanisms, and developing vaccines and treatments (US Department of Health and Human Services 2005). While it is presented as a step-by-step process, the complex nature of disease transmission means that many of these steps may occur out of order or simultaneously.

Throughout the pandemic, there was certainly no shortage of remarkable institutional feats that support the optimism of HRO advocates. There was an incredible amount of minute-by-minute information exchange around the globe; testing was set up in a matter of weeks; vaccines were developed and distributed in record time; and large organizations learned to adapt to changing circumstances under intense scrutiny.

There were also failures, which would not surprise an NAT advocate. Uncertainty led to errors. Officials underestimated the fatality rate in the first wave because of extensive transmission in LTC and seniors' facilities (Ogden et al. 2020, 202); LTC facilities, however, experienced higher fatality rates in the second wave than in the first, which also raises questions about our capacity to learn and adapt during the process. The failures in LTC are discussed in more detail in chapter 7. Taking a step back and considering the response from a longer time horizon, we see some other important organizational failings. The federal, provincial, and territorial governments have had a regularly updated pandemic plan since 1988 but have failed to make progress in a number of important areas, as various reports and audits over several decades have shown (National Advisory Committee on SARS and Public Health 2003; Expert Panel on SARS and Infectious Disease Control [Walker] 2003; A. Campbell 2004; Macdougall et al. 2014). These organizations' failings are discussed in more detail in chapter 11.

HRO and NAT are like a nagging couple; they have irreconcilable differences, and neither will go away. They make different assumptions about systems and people. HRO is much more optimistic about both. In practice, both schools are useful: HRO represents best practice in systems management; NAT is a constant reminder of people's hubris and organizational inertia and the high price we pay for both.

RISK AS SOCIAL CONSTRUCTION (BOX D IN FIGURE 2.1)

Risk as a Function of Organizational Culture and World Views

Cultural theory is useful for interpreting how different organizational types respond to risk (Douglas 1982, 1992; Hood 1998). It contrasts with complexity studies as outlined earlier because the focal point for analysis is not the complexity of the problem and the setting but rather the way people with different world views experience, interpret, and respond to risks, and how those different world views are shaped by organizational settings. Cultural theorists see risk as a danger or threat to a value system that is embedded in institutional arrangements, not as a calculable probability. Douglas's grid-group theory measures regulation (grid) and social integration (group) to determine value systems and the preferred institutional arrangements flowing from them, leading to the characterization of four cultural types: hierarchists, individualists, egalitarians, and fatalists. Each type has a preferred governance arrangement and particular blind spots and vulnerabilities.

To the hierarchist (high grid, high group), good governance means a stable environment that supports collective interest and fair process through rule-driven hierarchical organizations. Any departure from this rule-bound hierarchy represents risk for the hierarchist. To the individualist (low grid, low group), good governance means minimal rules and interference with free-market processes. Individualists understand risk to be government regulation of the economy or the management of public services. To the egalitarian (low grid, high group), good governance means local, communitarian, and participative organizations. For egalitarians, authority resides with the collectivity; herd immunity achieved through collective solidarity fits comfortably within egalitarianism.[2] Fatalists (high grid, low group) doubt straightforward cause-effect relationships; to them, good governance means management that assumes surprises and is adept at adaptive capacity.

Each of these types represents a world view. Throughout the pandemic, cultural theory helped us detect the different world views at play when confronting uncertainty. The dominant approach was that of the hierarchist: expert-led, supported, and regulated by large public bureaucracies. This view was often in tension with the individualist's market-oriented view, which held that the governments' interventions were too heavy handed and that the health restrictions were disproportionate to the risk. We saw expressions of the individualist when businesses argued to roll back regulations between waves; we saw more extreme expressions of this type during the Freedom Convoy protests. Egalitarianism was manifest in several social-justice arguments, which included calls for collective strategies and contended that the government's response privileged some over others. The randomness with which the disease spread and the constant demand for adaptation represented fatalism. Despite its limitations when tested empirically (for examples see Dake 1991; Brenot, Bonnefous, and Marris 1998; Sjöberg 1998), cultural theory's capacity to show the recurring debates and irreconcilable difference in these world views has been described as a revolutionary advance in the study of risk (Royal Society 1992).[3]

Critical Theory, Ethics, and Critical Race Theory

For critical theorists, the tools and methods derived from RAP lead to administrative structures that are insensitive to true human needs; the approach reduces humans to mere objects to be manipulated. If society is not sufficiently vigilant, power can be concentrated in the hands of a small group of specialists in social and political elite apparatuses (C. Jaeger et al. 2001). Critical theory takes seriously that individuals living together must intentionally discuss preferences, interests, norms, and values in a rational way and reach uncoercive consensus among competing views. It can be understood as institutional and objective but, given its connection to critical race theory (CRT), we will include it in institutional and subjective.

Critical theory is particularly important in three ways for our examination of COVID-19. First, it highlights that risk models are an abstraction. They de-emphasize the actual people involved; they are developed by experts, often far from the lived experience of the most affected communities. Relatedly, public health disease prevention can be in tension with normal clinical practice. Clinical practice centres on patient autonomy, while public health disease prevention starts at the population level and then translates to the individual. Rather than dwell on the pathology of an individual's disease, disease prevention focuses on the risk in the population as a whole.

Secondly, critical theory underscores the importance of ethics in risk decision making. As a result of the SARS outbreak in 2003, the University of Toronto Joint Centre for Bioethics (2005) produced a report detailing ethical considerations in pandemics. The report argues that influenza pandemic plans must be founded on widely recognized values. Both decision makers and the public need to be engaged in ethical discussions to ensure that plans reflect what is widely accepted as fair and good for public health. In a pandemic there are key ethical issues: health workers' duty to provide care during a communicable disease outbreak; the restriction of liberty in the interest of public health (e.g., quarantine); priority setting (e.g., allocation of scarce resources); and global governance implications (e.g., travel advisories). The report also includes substantive values to guide ethical decision making for a pandemic influenza outbreak:[4] individual liberty; protection of the public from harm; proportionality; privacy; duty to provide care; reciprocity (e.g., society must support those who face a disproportionate burden, such as health-care workers); equity; trust; solidarity; stewardship. It also outlines procedural values: reasonableness; openness and transparency; inclusivity; responsiveness; and accountability.

Ethical questions occurred throughout the pandemic but became particularly salient when officials had to distribute limited PPE and prioritize who had access to medical treatment and services, such as ICU beds. The issue of access to ICU beds and the resources required to support them received considerable attention after vaccines became available and those who chose not to be vaccinated were occupying a high number of ICU beds.

The speed with which decisions had to be made in some cases prevented prolonged periods of reflection and public engagement. The federal government issued an ethics framework during COVID-19 (Government of Canada 2022n). In fact, many ethicists contributed to discussions about the allocation of limited resources throughout COVID-19. Emanuel et al. (2020), for example, made six recommendations with respect to the allocation of limited resources: benefits should be maximized, focusing particularly on saving lives and improving recovery; critical interventions should go first to front-line workers and those who keep critical infrastructure operating; for patients with similar prognoses, equality should be invoked through random allocation of resources, as opposed to first-come, first-served processes; prioritization guidelines should differ by intervention type and change to reflect advances in scientific evidence, focusing in particular on maximizing benefits; people who participate in safety research on vaccines and therapeutics should receive some priority for COVID-19 treatment; and there should be no preferential treatment for patients with COVID-19 compared to patients suffering from other illnesses.

Recommendations such as these were helpful in establishing signposts for decision makers. Most governments received ethics advice from advisory boards. Still, goals had to be set, such as minimizing death, and trade-offs had to be weighed, such as how to allocate limited resources within the health-care system as a whole and how to balance COVID-19 health restrictions with other economic and social considerations. As noted by M. Smith (2022), an ethicist who sat on the Ontario government's COVID-19 vaccine-distribution task force, claims such as "follow the science" can be damaging because they obscure the role that values and ethics play in decision making. In Smith's words, science can tell us what is happening and help us forecast, but science "cannot tell us what to do." Those are ethical, political, and broader social decisions. Decisions may have been guided at times by ethical principles, such as solidarity and social justice, but there was always a degree of ambiguity in these decisions, and the accountability could be opaque. Some of these decisions were made at individual hospitals while others were made by political decision makers in provincial or territorial cabinets.-

Thirdly, critical theory serves as an intellectual foundation for CRT, which emerged from civil rights scholars such as Derek Bell, Kimberlé Crenshaw, and Richard Delgado. CRT underscores that race is socially constructed; it examines the intersection of race and institutional arrangements and the resulting laws and policies that perpetuate racist behaviours and outcomes.

Racialized people were some of the most likely to die from COVID-19 (Xia at al. 2022). Neighbourhoods with higher proportions of racialized minorities experienced COVID-19 mortality rates that were twice as high as those in neighbourhoods with low proportions of racialized minorities (McKenzie 2020). That racialized minorities so disproportionately lived in lower-income neighbourhoods, in crowded housing that led to rapid disease transmission, is already an indication of systemic bias (McKenzie 2020). Beyond this initial observation, however, one notes that these different death rates were not identified in early models. In fact, most public health authorities did not collect race-based data. In some cases, community leaders themselves have voiced concerns about race-based data for fear that it would lead to further discrimination (Ahsan 2021; Varcoe et al. 2009).

CRT asserts that institutions manage risks for some and perpetuate it for others. It centres on racialized minorities who have access to experience and a perspective that is not available to non-racialized people. This has important governance implications. CRT can lead to better engagement between those responsible for a traditional power apparatus and racialized communities, but also to a transfer of power that enables them to interpret risk and to control their own response. The absence and importance of context-specific responses to pandemics in Indigenous communities had been noted in H1N1 post-mortems (National Collaborating Centre for Aboriginal Health 2016). Overcoming the racial gap in COVID-19 vaccine uptake, for instance, took deliberate effort and required engagement with community leadership (Burch and Schoenfeld Walker 2021; Wiafe and Smith 2021; Nuriddin, Mooney, and White 2020, 950; Canadian Public Health Association 2018, 3). Indeed, after targeted efforts, vaccine support among many First Nations, Inuit, and Métis people increased (Parkin et al. 2021). In Nova Scotia the premier and the CMO were criticized for singling out racialized communities for their failure to follow public health orders (*Nova Scotia Advocate* 2020; McSheffrey 2020). Certain communities established community-based committees and expected governments to engage with them and through them (PHAC 2021b) rather than criticizing the communities through the media.

An approach that validates community leadership, and, in so doing, the unique community experience, can be empowering for marginalized communities. It can also be limiting. It sets stricter limits on objectivity and emphasizes that the human experience is subjective, and therefore has an impact on people's ability to work collectively to solve problems (Farber and Sherry 1997); for some, life through a social constructivist lens is bleak (Christensen 2005). While a strong advocate for social justice, having seen first-hand the atrocities of the Second World War and the Holocaust, Habermas, who was one of the original architects of critical theory, wondered how successfully people could understand and articulate what was in their own interests (1971, 1984, 1987). This is a particularly important point when we consider the low vaccine participation rates among marginalized populations, which we discuss further in chapter 6.

A REGIMES APPROACH TO COVID-19

The social science of risk literature outlined in this chapter is at once enabling and constraining. Beyond its traditional rationalist roots in statistics, the literature has grown exponentially since the 1980s from numerous disciplines. These literatures use different focal points for analysis. While these different contributions help us analyze the COVID-19 pandemic, it is difficult to imagine a single risk framework that could accommodate such a multi-faceted challenge, let alone bring together such fundamentally different literatures into one coherent explanation. Notwithstanding this challenge, the risk regulation regimes framework provides us with several lenses through which to explore the pandemic.

Our application of the framework builds and extends on its original intention. Hood, Rothstein, and Baldwin (2001) developed the framework as a response to the broad claims about the "risk society" (Beck 1992). Beck defines risk as a systematic way of dealing with hazards and insecurities induced and introduced by modernization itself (21) and argues that modern science and technology have created a risk society in which the production of wealth has been overtaken by the production of risk (19–20). The creation and distribution of wealth has been replaced by the quest for safety. Progress has turned into self-destruction as an unintended consequence through the inexorable and incremental processes of modernization itself, as evidenced through the climate crisis and the proliferation of nuclear power, for example. Beck distinguishes modern risks from older dangers by their scale and invisibility and the need for experts to detect them, despite their limited ability to do so. Risks, as opposed to older dangers, are consequences, which relate to the threatening force of modernization and globalization. Risks brought on by modernization go beyond national borders (41–2), as we saw in the rapid global transmission of the virus. Even as risks become more global, transcending national borders, risks simultaneously become more intricate and personalized. People have their own views of risk based on their own experiences and rationales. Social, cultural, and political meanings are embedded in risk; there are different meanings for different people (24). The natural scientists' monopoly on rationality is broken, and gaps emerge between scientific and social rationality (30).

Hood, Rothstein, and Baldwin (2001) argue that a systems approach to risk problems – like Beck's risk society – is necessary but there is nuance to the way we respond to risk that general claims fail to capture. They use the risk regulation regimes framework to examine how governments' responses to risk vary by policy domain, and they examine and compare risks such as attacks by dangerous dogs outside the home, radon at home and at work, road safety, and pedophile offenders released from custody. They demonstrate that at times governments' control mechanisms are influenced by the logic of market failures, public opinion, or organized interests.

Our study contributes to debates about the risk society by considering a global risk like COVID-19, which transcended borders and economic classes and affected people in different ways, and about which individuals held different and deeply personal views. Like Hood, Rothstein, and Baldwin (2001) we are also interested in variation in responses to risk although in a slightly different way. We use the risk regulation regimes framework to describe not independent policy domains but rather the cascading consequences, intended and unintended, of governments' risk regulation approaches to a pandemic across interdependent policy domains.

The separate hypotheses provide us not only with an opportunity for a positive account of how governments responded but also a somewhat loosely defined normative one. In liberal-democratic societies most would expect governments to address market failures, however elusive an exact definition might be. It is also reasonable to think that governments respond to public opinion – again, a concept not easily captured. Organized interests also play an important role in a modern democratic society, particularly in terms of bringing forward problems and solutions to elected leaders. There is concern about privileged access among these groups and the benefits that come with it; there is also concern about those that are not organized and whether their concerns are addressed. Each hypothesis has its own normative appeal; the framework allows us to test the power and complexity of each one and, in doing so, explore the nuances of a risk society.

The framework leaves some things out. Hood, Rothstein, and Baldwin (2001) do not include path dependency explicitly in the framework but acknowledge the important role that path dependency plays in public administration as articulated by institutionalists (March and Olsen 1989; Brans and Rossbach 1997). There is some opportunity to examine path dependency in the framework. The authors' use of cybernetics coupled with size, structure, and style included in the framework allows us to describe various characteristics of the risk regulation regime, including its organizational culture, which leans towards stability. While the urgency of the pandemic did prompt atypical behaviours, such as fast-tracking purchasing decisions and vaccine development and distribution, generally the pandemic did not recreate public administration in Canada; instead, the pandemic was addressed through existing institutional and constitutional frameworks. Changes in design may come later in light of lessons from the pandemic – as the creation of the US Department of Homeland Security by merging twenty-two separate agencies following 9/11 allowed more coordinated intelligence-gathering and effective security measures against terrorism (Bush 2002) – but it is striking how few fundamental institutional changes occurred throughout COVID-19. In Canada the constitutional division of responsibilities will almost certainly constrain any ambitious redesign.

Hood, Rothstein, and Baldwin (2001) also do not include "ideas" as a contextual factor. They argue that ideas, such as the precautionary principle, and their impact cannot easily be separated from interests and the power of those advocating specific ideas. We agree, but the argument has limitations that should be noted. The risk literature at times holds up the concept of the precautionary principle as an ethical one (J.M. Macdonald 1995; ter Meulen 2005). While the limits of this claim are explored more fully in chapters 9 and 10, ethical considerations played an important role in governments' decision making. Like path dependency, ethics can be captured in the control mechanism: under government information gathering, as we saw when governments included ethicists on their advisory committees (Ontario COVID-19 Science Advisory Table 2022), and in the standards and behaviours that governments adopted, as we saw in the prioritization of vaccine distribution, for instance. Which contextual pressure to point to in order to explain ethics is more challenging.

Risk Refined: Four Risk Types

Given Hood, Rothstein, and Baldwin's (2001) interest in nuance beyond the general claims of the risk society, a singular reference to the concept of risk is also limited. Risk is a function of probability and consequence. These concepts were highly fluid and at times contested throughout the pandemic. A generic reference to risk lacks important nuance. In this book we refer to four classifications of risk: simple, complex, uncertain, and ambiguous. The classification of risk is "not related to the intrinsic characteristics of hazards or risks themselves but to the state and quality of knowledge available about both hazards and risks" (Renn 2008b, 18). The four types of risk allow us to consider how knowledge of the pandemic changed and interacted with the risk regulation regime.

With *simple risk*, predicted events are frequent and the causal chain is obvious (e.g., car accidents). Simple risks generate reliable data that help to inform our view of risk; we can be more confident about the extent to which the threat will materialize and the consequences of that threat.

Complex risks exist when there is difficulty identifying and quantifying causal links between a multitude of potential causal agents and specific observed effects (Renn 2008b, 19). There are two kinds of complex risks: epistemic, which result from imperfect knowledge, and aleatory, which result from randomness. Epistemic risks include those associated with the characteristics of a new virus as well as interconnected infrastructure and for which uncertainty can potentially be reduced through data collection and increased institutional capacity. Aleatory risks include randomness, such as disease transmission that occurs in social systems; we know that it will happen, but we cannot know when or to whom. Complex risks are examined largely based on expert opinion both within and outside public regulatory agencies and rely on formal probabilistic modelling.

For the most part, we consider COVID-19 an *uncertain risk*, particularly in the early stages. Uncertain risks exist when the factors influencing the issues are identified but the likelihood of any adverse effect or effects themselves cannot be precisely described. There is "a lack of clear scientific or technical basis for decision making" (Renn 2008b, 18–19). The absence of predictive data diminishes confidence in traditional objective measures of risk estimation, and therefore risk management becomes more reliant on "fuzzy" or subjective measures of risk estimation (18–19). Uncertain risks frequently generate surprises or realizations that risk modelling frameworks fail to anticipate or explain (e.g., rare natural disasters, terrorism, pandemics).

Ambiguous risks result from divergent or contested perspectives on the justification, severity, or wider meanings associated with a given threat (Renn 2008b, 19). With ambiguous risks, there are two types of ambiguity: interpretative ambiguity, which stems from different interpretations of the same results (e.g., effectiveness of vaccines); and normative ambiguity, which stems from different beliefs about which risks are tolerable (e.g., limiting personal freedoms through lockdowns to limit community spread). For ambiguous risks, we have the data, but we may not agree on what they mean and what to do about it.

CONCLUSION

RAP continues to be the dominant model for thinking and framing most risk questions. It is an expert-driven approach to risk analysis; the problem is often narrowly defined, and it reduces complexity to simplified models. The risk psychology literature underscores that people have different views and preferences, and they are not particularly rational from an expert's point of view. While this increases complexity, understanding these views is important because it helps us anticipate how people are likely to feel and respond to highly uncertain and high-dread risk events like a pandemic. Notwithstanding the various psychological biases among members of the lay public that confront public health initiatives, understanding these feelings can lead to a better-informed communications plan that will try to motivate desirable behaviour in the general population. Institutional studies reveal organizational successes and failures in addressing complex problems; the COVID-19 episode raises important questions about our capacity to learn and improve, and indeed whether our organizational cultures will allow us to learn lessons that undermine the dominant behaviours and hold people to account. The ethics literature, in particular, challenges us to think about the limits of science and sheds light on the values that underpin decisions and actions in the face of uncertainty.

These disciplines have contributed to our understanding of risk and its management. Each field brings its own assumptions, tools, and perspectives, contributing to a much richer understanding of risk. Using one approach is narrow; using all approaches is unwieldy. Each of these lenses can help us understand aspects of our response to COVID-19, but none will give a complete account.

Hood, Rothstein, and Baldwin's (2001) risk regulation regimes framework, which builds on Beck's risk society and shapes this book, tests for different explanations for governments' responses, be it market failure, public opinion, or the influence of organized interests. The framework provides us with the necessary flexibility to analyze such a complex case like COVID-19, drawing on a variety of concepts from several disciplines. Renn's four types of risk are a necessary enhancement to the study; it allows us to distinguish between different degrees of knowledge of risk problems, and the demands these different types of knowledge will make on the risk regulation regime.

This chapter serves as risk-theory primer for the reader before we start this analysis. Each of the rationales can help to examine the control mechanism (chapters 3 to 5) and contribute to our understanding of each of the hypotheses (chapters 9 to 11). Generally, RAP is commonly deployed to examine a bureaucratic control mechanism and the market-failure hypothesis, which includes concepts of insurance and the rule of law. The psychology of risk helps us examine the opinion responsive hypothesis; it gives us ways to analyze how the media construct and report risk stories and how people feel about risks, as expressed through polling data. Institutional studies help us understand the processes and nature of power that underpin the interest-group hypothesis and how different world views and values are expressed in different forms of governance. In short, the four rationales described in this chapter give us the vocabulary and concepts, as articulated in the traditional and emerging risk literature, to examine the contextual pressures that shaped governments' responses.

PART TWO

Regime Content: The Government's Control Mechanisms

Now that we have provided an overview of COVID-19 in Canada and the existing literature on risk governance that pertains to this study, we turn to the mechanisms that government put in place to contain the disease between March 2020 and 2 April 2022. We structure the following three chapters based on the three elements of cybernetics. In chapter 3 we examine selected information-gathering methods of the regime. This includes testing, contact tracing, and modelling. Next, chapter 4 looks at standard setting, including health directives, economic programs like Canada Emergency Response Benefit (CERB), and governance practices. Lastly, chapter 5 examines how people's behaviour changed as a result of COVID-19 and related government directives and standards. Some of these changes were intended; others, as we shall see, were not.

Chapter 6 starts with a review of the development, distribution, and take-up of the vaccine. This analysis is framed according to cybernetics and once again examines the information-gathering, standard-setting, and behaviour-modification elements in relation to the COVID-19 vaccines. We discuss the anti-vaccine mandate protests, which attracted attention in January and February 2022. In March 2022 many provincial and territorial governments announced that COVID-19 restrictions would end. This arguably represents one of the final stages before people began to accept and live with the threat of COVID-19.

3

Information Gathering:
Testing, Contact Tracing, and Modelling

In cybernetics, obtaining accurate information about a threat is the first step in addressing that threat. Information may be gathered actively or passively from outside or within a system (Hood, Rothstein, and Baldwin 2001, 22). There were challenges. Mechanisms and processes had to be put in place to understand the threat, which took time, relied on assumptions, and included many imperfections. Once data were collected, the problem could be characterized as complex, meaning the risk was affected by many variables interacting in diverse and unpredictable ways. More data helped epidemiologists to model and estimate the disease spread, but the models are highly reliant on expert opinion. What constitutes relevant information is biased by institutional education, practices, and values, which can create blind spots. The interdependence of systems across society makes it difficult to determine when one system stops and another starts; decisions to contain COVID-19 had cascading effects across several systems, including health and economic ones, which created additional consequences and uncertainty.

This chapter focuses on the three key information-gathering mechanisms that governments had put in place as of March 2020 to better understand the risk COVID-19 presented in Canada: testing, contact tracing, and modelling. We will review the methods, outcomes, and strengths and weaknesses of each.

TESTING

Public health officials relied on COVID-19 testing to learn who was infected with the virus and where and how quickly it was spreading. Testing enabled officials to identify and isolate COVID-19–positive people, trace their contacts, understand better the transmission of the virus, and inform public health responses (Government of Canada 2022p). The novelty of the virus meant that new tests and technologies had to be created and approved. The absence of testing capacity, and delays in conducting testing, in the early stages were among the most criticized aspects of the public health response.

Canada used three types of testing most often during the pandemic: molecular/PCR, point-of-care, and antibody. The first two detect the virus and diagnose COVID-19. Swabs are used to collect samples from the nose or throat. Point-of-care is a rapid test usually done in a hospital or a doctor's office; throughout the COVID-19 pandemic, designated testing clinics were used to limit virus spread in hospitals. This form of testing was primarily used in rural, remote, and isolated communities where results could be gathered without sending them to a lab for testing. Antibody testing, or serological testing, was used to determine if someone had been infected by the virus previously. Test accuracy varied depending on how long a person had been infected. As the pandemic progressed, home self-administered rapid tests were developed. False-negative (i.e., patient is positive, but test result is negative), false-positive (i.e., patient is negative but tests positive), and inconclusive results were possible and occurred (Government of Canada 2022p).

False-negative results have a particularly negative impact on pandemic control because cases categorized as uninfected can unintentionally transmit the virus. The accuracy of molecular tests was affected by the stage of the disease (i.e., how long a patient had been infected), the type of sampling, and the quality of the sample. The time window in which false-negative results are more likely to occur was also not clear. False-negative results were possible with both self-testing rapid test kits and PCR tests. The summary estimate of the false-negative rate from reverse transcription polymerase chain reaction (RT-PCR) tests was 12 per cent, with an estimated range of 2 to 58 per cent (Pecoraro et al. 2021).

PHAC released testing advice through the federal, provincial, and territorial COVID-19 Special Advisory Committee (Government of Canada 2022p). The committee intended to establish a national approach to testing that optimized the use of local resources by the provinces and territories based on regional needs.

The federal government provided funding to the provinces and territories to support testing and contact tracing and to approve testing devices. The national target was to have the capacity to test up to 200,000 people per day. The federal government allocated $4.28 billion from the Safe Restart Agreement to help provinces and territories expand testing and contact tracing capacity, as well as improve data management and information-sharing systems. Each province and territory determined its own guidelines for testing and contact tracing to meet its specific needs, including the criteria for who could be tested (e.g., asymptomatic individuals) (Government of Canada 2022q). This resulted in varied testing protocols and capacities across the country; it is estimated that as of December 2020 approximately 75 per cent of testing capacity was used nationally each day (Allin et al. 2022; Health Canada 2021, 9). The Canadian Public Health Association (CPHA) has since recommended a pan-Canadian framework for testing protocols, capacity, and laboratory-surge capacity, as well as stockpiling testing kit components through the NESS (CPHA 2021).

Delays in reliable testing data were partly due to the National Microbiology Lab being the only one that could officially confirm COVID-19 tests in Canada at the outset of the pandemic. This meant that all test samples had to go to the laboratory in Winnipeg, Manitoba, to confirm a case of COVID-19 (Allin et al. 2022). Both the virus and the tests to confirm it were new, and capacity needed to be scaled. As more tests were developed and each province and territory had at least one lab approved to confirm test results, they could expand internal testing capacity and hasten confirmation of test results. The ability to test for COVID-19 varied due to capacity limits, such as available staff and resources, and to the policy choices made in each jurisdiction. For example, Quebec worked quickly to expand testing capacity but only reached its provincial target (set in mid-April 2020) at the beginning of September 2020. Ontario increased capacity over time but was one of the last jurisdictions to report COVID-19 testing data in Canada and only met its provincial target at the end of November 2020 (National Institute of Public Health Quebec 2021; COVID-19 Canada Open Data Working Group 2021; MacLellan 2020; Allin et al. 2022; Desson et al. 2020).

Selected Similarities and Variations in
Testing Standards across Canada

Many provinces and territories took a similar approach to testing but there was some variation. Public health officials prioritized those most vulnerable to the virus such as seniors and people with pre-existing conditions; those living in congregate facilities like hospitals and long-term care facilities; health-care and other essential workers; close contacts of confirmed COVID-19 cases; travellers from areas with COVID-19 outbreaks; and people who displayed COVID-19 symptoms. The severity and number of symptoms people displayed determined whether public health officials would order a test, and these criteria varied across the country throughout the pandemic. As the known COVID-19 symptoms changed, provinces and territories updated their lists of symptoms accordingly. Often, eligibility requirements were changing so quickly, in real time, and were shared frequently with the public that there were disconnects between decision makers and front-line health-care workers. This meant that the health-care professionals responsible for administering tests, and later vaccines (see chapter 6), were learning about decisions to change eligibility criteria at the same time as the public was.

There were differences in approach to universal testing throughout the pandemic. Universal testing means that anyone who wanted a COVID-19 test could have one regardless of whether they were symptomatic. These tests were provided at no cost to the person being tested, particularly early in the pandemic. British Columbia, Alberta, Saskatchewan, and Nova Scotia implemented universal testing (BC Centre for Disease Control 2020a, 2020b; Fletcher 2021a; Government of Saskatchewan, n.d.; Government of Nova Scotia, n.d.). Alberta was the first province to expand testing to asymptomatic people, first in Calgary and then to areas with outbreaks. As of 29 May 2020, any person in Alberta could be tested for COVID-19 regardless of whether they displayed symptoms, and there was no limit to the number of times a person could be tested (CBC News 2020a). This was demanding on Alberta's health system. In late October 2020 the Government of Alberta chose to suspend asymptomatic COVID-19 testing to help reduce testing wait times and hasten the delivery of results (Government of Alberta 2020f; Piller 2020).

In contrast, Manitoba, the Northwest Territories, Nunavut, Quebec, New Brunswick, Newfoundland and Labrador, and Prince Edward Island (PEI) did not implement universal testing at this time.[1] There were exceptions for asymptomatic testing of health-care and essential workers, as well as people who may have been exposed to COVID-19. Public Health Ontario (PHO) did not recommend routine testing for asymptomatic persons, except for health-care workers, caregivers, first responders, essential workers, persons living in the same household, and those who were Indigenous (PHO 2020b, 2020c). Similarly, Yukon implemented asymptomatic testing for specific groups. In mid-December 2020, testing was expanded in Ontario to persons requiring a test for international travel. By early December, Yukon had expanded its test strategy to cover asymptomatic persons with a high risk of exposure. Asymptomatic testing in Quebec was limited to close contacts of COVID-19 cases or people exposed to the virus, with slightly expanded criteria for those living in Montreal (Government of Quebec, n.d.).

Expanding Testing Capacity

Once testing capacity had been established, it constantly had to be expanded and made more efficient. As of 16 March 2020, capacity in British Columbia was 2,000 tests per day, which more than tripled by the end of April to over 6,200 (BC Centre for Disease Control 2020b). Testing was most common in the largest cities: 42 per cent of all tests in Alberta in the first six months took place in Calgary, and 33 per cent in Edmonton (Government of Alberta, n.d.a). As cases spiked in Calgary, asymptomatic testing was implemented and expanded to other areas with outbreaks and, by the end of May 2020, was expanded to the entire province (Fletcher 2021a).

PHO expanded testing capacity by adding additional shifts at testing laboratories and implementing 24-7 testing at its lab in Toronto (PHO 2020a). A survey of provincial lab capacity was conducted in early March 2020 that resulted in capacity being expanded to additional hospital and private labs. As of 3 April 2020, Ontarians could book COVID-19 testing appointments, access results, and provide information about close contacts online (Ontario Ministry of Health and Long-Term Care 2020). New tools and testing methods were developed using automated processes. PHO invested in equipment that could run more tests at a time to increase capacity and reduce wait times for results (PHO 2020a).

In early April, New Brunswick received a donation from the Saint John Regional Hospital Foundation's COVID-19 emergency fund to upgrade testing and purchase equipment such as ventilators. With the new equipment, seven locations across the province were expected to have the capability to offer faster results of COVID-19 tests (Office of the Premier of New Brunswick 2020a).

Testing capacity in PEI was expanded on 1 April 2020 when the system GeneXpert was brought online. An additional system, BD MAX, was introduced on 10 April and increased local testing capacity significantly (Yarr 2020). Even with capacity expanded, PEI still needed to confirm COVID-19 positive results with labs in other provinces at this time.

In early April 2020 the Government of Newfoundland and Labrador changed testing strategy to focus on people who had symptoms, were vulnerable to the disease, or worked with vulnerable populations (D. Maher 2020). Hospital patients, residents at LTC facilities, health-care workers, and people over seventy-five years old were prioritized for COVID-19 testing (Newfoundland and Labrador Provincial Public Health Laboratory Network 2020). In early May 2020, testing criteria were expanded to include anyone presenting with two or more symptoms of COVID-19. Figure 3.1 outlines the average number of COVID-19 tests reported across Canada.

Rapid self-test kits became prevalent to monitor COVID-19 infections in households, particularly during the Omicron wave. Individuals could test themselves if they experienced symptoms or had been exposed to COVID-19. PCR tests would be used to confirm results. During the Omicron wave, self-testing was especially encouraged because the high demand for tests meant it was challenging to get an appointment, and at times tests were limited to high-priority populations (Freeze 2021; S. Banerjee 2022b). Public health advice to anyone with symptoms was to isolate as though they had COVID-19 until they could have a test or the recommended isolation period had elapsed since the onset of symptoms (S. Banerjee 2022b). Many people stopped being tested altogether, and testing rates declined (A. Miller 2022).

In sum, testing increased from about 178,000 tests in March 2020 to over two million per month by March 2022 (Ritchie et al. 2022a). By 12 July 2022 the federal government had distributed 27,489,079 COVID-19 rapid tests to workplaces, community groups, and non-profit organizations. It shipped an additional 573,476,183 to the provinces and territories, 66 per cent of which were distributed. Distribution rates varied across the country (Government of Canada 2022q). Most COVID-19 tests were provided at no cost to members of the public, but there were options to pay for COVID-19 tests, and the degree to which people paid out of pocket varied by jurisdiction, point of time in the pandemic, and situation for testing. For example, tests to meet travel requirements were paid out of pocket by the traveller.

Socio-economic factors, such as income and status as an ethnic minority, resulted in pronounced differences in the effects of the pandemic across Canada, but most Canadian health-care providers do not regularly collect sociodemographic data aside from age and gender (Desson et al. 2020; Allin et al. 2022; CPHA 2021). This gap limited the insights that public health officers could derive from the COVID-19 tests and models. This had also been an issue during the H1N1 pandemic. PHO published a report that emphasized the disparities in H1N1 transmission among Black, Indigenous, South Asian, Southeast Asian, and White Ontarians. People who identified as Southeast Asian were three times more likely to be infected, South Asian people were six times more likely to be infected, and Black Ontarians were ten times more likely to be infected with H1N1 than White Ontarians were (McKenzie 2020). In the first year of the COVID-19 pandemic, death rates from

Figure 3.1 | Number of daily COVID-19 tests, February 2020–March 2022. Average daily testing rates were less than 200,000 throughout the pandemic with testing rates peaking during the Omicron wave.

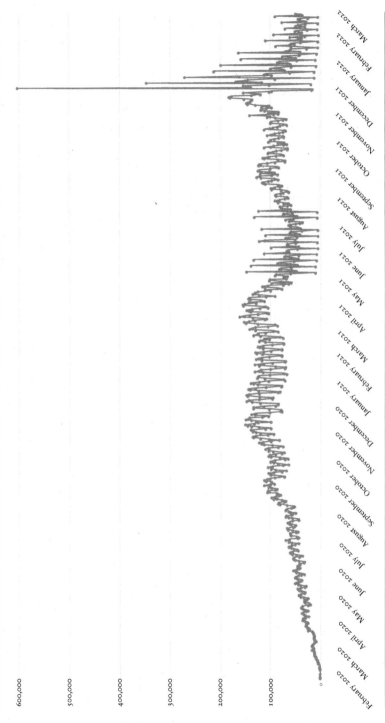

Source: Ritchie et al. 2022a.

COVID-19 were higher for people living in apartments and low-income neighbourhoods, recent immigrants, people who were a visible minority, and people who did not speak English or French as a primary language (Government of Canada 2022o). First Nations, Inuit, and Métis communities were also disproportionately affected by COVID-19. There are significant systemic inequities (e.g., housing, health care, infrastructure, and health outcomes) as well as vaccine hesitancy and distrust of governments and health authorities. As of the start of October 2021, COVID-19 rates were 3.3 times higher on reserves than among the general population (Mauracher 2021). There were many challenges in collecting and sharing data, as well as distrust of how governments would use the data, in addition to there being a lack of disaggregated data. The Assembly of First Nations National COVID-19 Task Force formed a COVID-19 data working group to support First Nations in their data and information governance and to address data challenges (Assembly of First Nations COVID-19 Data Working Group 2021). Collecting sociodemographic data of COVID-19 cases was a contentious issue throughout the pandemic due to the greater impact of COVID-19 observed in racialized communities. Manitoba was the first province to mandate race-based data collection as part of its COVID-19 response (McKenzie 2020). In Ontario this culminated in the decision to mandate health-care providers to collect race-based data in June 2020 (Government of Ontario 2020b). Collecting sociodemographic data across the country would have helped identify trends of negative impacts on marginalized communities in real time, as opposed to after the fact (Ng 2021). For example, much of what was learned about the significant negative impacts of COVID-19 on racialized communities came from comparing maps of confirmed COVID-19 cases with known information of racialized and low-income communities.

CONTACT TRACING

Contact tracing is a long-standing public health practice used to identify people who have likely been exposed to a virus. Once a person tests positive, efforts are made to reach close contacts to identify possible chains of transmission and other cases of, in this instance, COVID-19 (Christakis 2020; WHO 2021c). These close contacts are identified and directed to self-isolate and be tested. Contact tracing helped to identify sources of exposure, such as whether a case was travel-related, the result of attending a "superspreading" event, or community exposure, so that related public health interventions could be implemented accordingly

(WHO 2021C). Private businesses like restaurants were required to keep patrons' contact details for tracing purposes in case they were later found to have been exposed to COVID-19.

This process has been used for centuries to address epidemics and pandemics, including syphilis, bubonic plague, typhus, measles, and tuberculosis (Christakis 2020). Throughout the twentieth century, contact-tracing efforts were used to control infectious diseases such as smallpox, HIV, tuberculosis, influenza, and Ebola (Christakis 2020).

Countries' governance arrangements, laws, culture, infrastructure, available labour, and population demographics result in different approaches to contact tracing around the world. The level of access that governments had to personal data and the degree of centralization also influenced how public health officials conducted contact tracing (WHO 2021C). Singapore, Israel, China, Taiwan, and South Korea used telephone records, financial records such as credit-card information, and facial-recognition software to support surveillance and tracing efforts (Christakis 2020). In April 2020 the Singapore Health Department employed 5,000 contact tracers for a population of five million, meaning that one person per thousand was employed to conduct contact tracing (Christakis 2020).

Contact-tracing efforts in Canada were led by the provinces and territories, but the federal government provided $4.3 billion in support, as noted earlier (Government of Canada 2021k). Statistics Canada staff conducted contact-tracing interviews because of their experience and ability to interview in more than thirty-five languages (Statistics Canada 2021k). During 14–20 March 2021, Statistics Canada made between 5,985 and 9,461 calls a day (Statistics Canada 2021k).

At the start of the pandemic Alberta had the capacity to trace an average of six close contacts per COVID-19 case. By July 2020 the province could trace up to twenty close contacts for every case, which contributed to pressure on testing in Calgary (C. Tait 2020). At the end of September 2020 the Government of Ontario announced a $1 billion investment to expand testing and contact-management efforts (Herhalt 2020). During the summer of 2020 there were approximately 4,000 people conducting contact tracing in Ontario, but many jurisdictions struggled to keep pace with increasing case numbers. As a result, contact tracers in Toronto, for example, were able to reach only 55 per cent of new cases within a day of confirmation to begin contact-tracing efforts. At the end of September the province hired an additional 1,000 staff to support testing and contact-tracing efforts (Herhalt 2020), including 500 from Statistics Canada (Canadian Healthcare Technology 2020). In

early October, contact-tracing efforts had to be scaled back in Toronto
to focus on high-risk groups; however, the full program resumed by the
end of November (Cox and Keller 2021).

Like Ontario, many jurisdictions across Canada struggled to keep
pace with tracing contacts of cases as numbers rose throughout fall
and winter 2020. By the end of November 2020 the responsibility to
track secondary COVID-19 exposures mainly fell on the person who
tested positive (Cox and Keller 2021). This meant that someone who
received a positive COVID-19 test result would be responsible for notifying their household about the exposure and identifying close contacts.
Contact-tracing efforts in British Columbia at this time focused on
identifying sources of infection rather than alerting people who might
have been exposed (Cox and Keller 2021). For a time, Alberta had one
of the most robust contact-tracing programs, but as cases rose during
fall 2020, the province had to suspend contact-tracing efforts for all
except high-priority cases, which included health workers, residents of
LTC homes, and students and staff in schools. At this time, Alberta had
approximately 800 contact tracers and announced that an additional
400 would be hired to address the significant backlog of cases. In early
November nearly half of newly confirmed cases did not have a known
source of infection, and by the end of the month over 80 per cent did
not (Cox and Keller 2021). Saskatchewan also faced challenges in contact tracing, so much so that pauses in tracing for new COVID-19 cases
announced in November 2020 were, in part, to enable tracers to catch
up (Cox and Keller 2021).

The use of technology has been a distinguishing feature of the COVID-
19 pandemic. The private sector developed technology for contact
tracing, including smart-phone apps, that were implemented by various
governments. Governments across Canada, Australia, Asia, and Europe
implemented various forms of technology-based contact-tracing methods (Kleinman and Merkel 2020). While there are many benefits of
digital approaches to contact tracing, their use raised questions about
privacy, effectiveness, technical limitations, cost, degree of public uptake
(i.e., adoption), and voluntariness (Kleinman and Merkel 2020). Trade-
offs between effectiveness and privacy must also be weighed. In January
2022, Canada's privacy commissioner announced an ethics investigation into the PHAC's use of data from mobile phones (Bailey 2022).

Several countries in Asia, such as South Korea and China, used
involuntary forms of data collection, such as security-camera foot-
age, financial records, and cellphone records as noted, whereas North
America and Europe used more voluntary forms, such as mobile

applications where a user had to opt in (Kleinman and Merkel 2020). While the scale of this data collection was unique, using big data to inform public policy is part of a larger trend in policy-making (Longo and McNutt 2018). In the case of many Western countries, the success of contact tracing depends on people being forthcoming, accurate, and truthful about their contacts once they test positive for COVID-19; key information could be withheld or may not be fully accurate as human memory is fallible (Cox and Keller 2021).

Residents of tech-savvy countries were much more likely to download and use the technology. In Singapore the government app was downloaded by 20 per cent of the population in the first month after launch (Kleinman and Merkel 2020). In South Korea private developers created an app to alert users if they came within a 100-metre radius of someone who tested positive for COVID-19; it was downloaded over one million times within a few weeks (Huang, Sun, and Sui 2020). Another South Korean app, Corona Map, plotted the locations of diagnosed COVID-19 patients and became the second-most downloaded app in South Korea. Some apps were used to track people in quarantine to ensure compliance, such as in Taiwan and Hong Kong, whereas others were used primarily to aid governments' contact-tracing efforts.

In Canada the effectiveness of the federal COVID-19 app COVID Alert was limited as submitting data to the app was voluntary, and relatively few who tested positive uploaded their information to the site. The app did not track user-location data or collect personal information that could make someone identifiable (Government of Canada 2022h). British Columbia, Alberta, Nunavut, and Yukon each expressed concerns about the federal app (ISED 2021). Progress was slow. At the beginning of October 2020 the app was available in just four Canadian provinces, meaning only 45 per cent of the population could access it (ISED 2021; Hill and Pazzano 2020). It was the end of November 2020 before the app was available to most people in the country. By 11 February 2021 just over 6.2 million people had downloaded the app, but it is estimated that only 2 per cent of people who tested positive for COVID-19 had used it (Pinkerton 2021). To upload data about a positive test result, provincial and territorial public health units created a one-time key (OTK) and provided it to the COVID Alert user. This OTK could be entered in the app by the user to confirm that they had tested positive for COVID-19 and to alert other app users that they may have been exposed. Overall estimates suggest that fewer than 5 per cent of positive cases had obtained an OTK from their public health authority by the end of February 2021 (Government of Canada 2021j).

By the end of May 2022, use of the app had increased over the year across Canada, and 69 per cent of users given a unique OTK had entered it in the app to confirm their positive test result. There was variation between the provinces and territories in the rates that OTKs were entered in the app; Quebec had the highest (95 per cent), and Saskatchewan had the lowest (59 per cent) (Government of Canada 2022h).

CANADA'S APPROACH TO MODELLING

Models represent a simplified version of reality and can be used to inform decision making, provide insights into trade-offs, and motivate behaviour change. In January 2020, PHAC convened an expert modelling group that included over fifty federal, provincial, territorial, and university-based modellers and epidemiologists. Similar groups had been developed in other countries, and many shared information via the WHO modelling group (Ogden et al. 2020, 199).

Many types of models were developed and used throughout the pandemic. Canada used two main approaches based on (1) an agent-based model and (2) a deterministic compartment model. Both are SEIR-type models (susceptible-exposed-infected-recovered) that include the impacts of non-pharmaceutical interventions (Tang et al. 2020, 199). Once vaccinations had been introduced, models were updated to account for these new data. Initial versions of the deterministic model were adapted from Tang et al. (2020). In this study Tang et al. adopted a deterministic model to demonstrate the transmission dynamics of the virus and assess the impact of public health interventions on infection rates. In this approach the effects of physical distancing are modelled by using daily per capita contact rates that are informed by several data sources, such as cellphone data. The deterministic approach used homogenous mixing but was modified to include specific contact rates to account for variation within and between age groups (Ogden et al. 2020, 199, 202).

The agent-based model approach used specific details about communities, such as homes, communal meeting spaces, workplaces, schools, retail stores, and restaurants, and was used to estimate the impacts of closures in more detail and the various scenarios of community transmission. The agent-based approach included contact rates within and between age groups. In early models, data specific to the UK and other European countries were used instead of contact rates in Canada because similar studies had not yet been conducted in Canada (Ogden et al. 2020, 199, 202). Transmission rates and fatality rates used in the calculations for these models were also informed by data from China, the *Diamond Princess* cruise ship, and Italy and forecast that severe cases could quickly overwhelm Canada's health-care system. In some cases the group also adapted models used for H1N1 and other influenzas to model COVID-19 (Ogden et al. 2020, 200).

Canada primarily used forecasting models to make short-term estimations, and dynamic models to make more long-term estimations. Forecasting models used data to estimate how many new cases were expected within a short time, such as weeks (PHAC 2020b, 10). Dynamic models showed how the epidemic might unfold over the coming months by applying knowledge of the virus's behaviour and the potential impact of public health measures (e.g., social distancing, gathering limits, business closures) (PHAC 2020b, 10). The models themselves were a measure to change behaviour, as the forecasts were used to motivate the public to take the virus and restrictions seriously to avoid the projected worst-case scenarios. In addition to the PHAC models for all of Canada, provincial and territorial public health agencies released models for their jurisdictions.

Although COVID-19 was a global pandemic at this time, the term *epidemic* is used here because of specific geographical focus on a jurisdiction, in this case Canada. A key goal was to reduce the number of people whom a COVID-19 patient could infect to less than one, on average (PHAC 2020b, 4). Prior to the implementation of strong public health measures in mid-March 2020, each infected person in Canada infected 2.2 others on average. A series of models was used to generate several scenarios, including (1) no control, (2) weaker control (delay and reduce the peak of the epidemiological curve), and (3) stronger epidemic control (PHAC 2020b, 13). No-control efforts refer to governments taking no action, which would result in an estimated 70 to 80 per cent of the population becoming infected. Stronger epidemic-control models include a high degree of physical distancing, a high proportion of cases identified and isolated, and a high proportion of contacts traced and quarantined, resulting in 1 to 10 per cent of the population becoming infected (PHAC 2020b, 14). Weaker control models include a low degree of physical distancing, a low proportion of cases identified and isolated, and a low proportion of contacts traced and quarantined, resulting in 25 to 50 per cent of the population becoming infected (PHAC 2020b, 14).

COVID-19 outbreaks were not uniform across Canada. Key factors in this variation included demographics, such as population, population density, age, socio-economic status, living arrangements; when and how

COVID-19 first arrived in a jurisdiction; and the degree of community transmission, as well as variance in provincial and territorial laboratory testing capacity and confirmation methods (PHAC 2020b, 7).

On 9 April 2020, forecasts for the short-term epidemic trajectory predicted 22,580 to 31,850 cases and 500–700 deaths by 16 April (PHAC 2020b, 11). As of 16 April there were over 28,000 confirmed cases and over 1,000 deaths due to the virus across Canada (Government of Canada 2022j). The observed case-fatality rate was higher than that initially predicted largely due to extensive transmission in LTC and seniors' facilities (Ogden et al. 2020, 202).

On 3 April 2020, COVID-19 was projected to kill 3,000 to 15,000 in Ontario, even with public health measures in place. Projections at this time revealed that with no intervention there could be 300,000 cases and 6,000 deaths; current prevention measures could result in 80,000 cases and 1,600 deaths; and with extreme interventions there could be 12,500 cases and 200 deaths (*National Post* 2020). As of 30 April 2020, Ontario had over 16,000 confirmed cases and over 1,000 deaths due to COVID-19 (Government of Canada 2022j).

On 28 April 2020, PHAC produced a follow-up to its 9 April report. Information at the time showed that implemented measures, such as physical distancing, detection and isolation of cases, tracing and quarantine of contacts, and travel restrictions, had been partly effective in controlling COVID-19 epidemics across the country (PHAC 2020a, 2). Assumptions for these models included that 7.8 per cent of all cases were hospitalized, 2.4 per cent required ICU care, and 1.2 per cent resulted in death. The case-fatality rate did not take health-care capacity into account, which is to say that the case-fatality rate could have increased had health-care capacity been exceeded.

Modelling COVID-19 Posed Many Challenges

Models generally include many estimates and assumptions because there are limits to the data that modellers can collect as well as apply to different jurisdictions. Arguably, the most significant challenge for modellers was how little was known about the virus and how quickly information was changing. Models were continuously updated as new information was accepted by the medical community (Ogden et al. 2020, 198; Adam 2020). The models used many assumptions: average number of people that one infected person would contact each day; percentage of cases that would be identified and isolated; percentage of people who would be in contact with a COVID-19 case; and percentage of people who would be correctly traced and appropriately isolated (PHAC 2020b, 10). Many COVID-19 models also made assumptions about health directives, and that stay-at-home and social-distancing orders would continue (Bui et al. 2020).

Some key developments in knowledge about COVID-19 in the early stages were that the virus was highly transmissible by respiratory and possibly fecal-oral routes, it could be transmitted before symptoms appeared (pre-symptomatic transmission), and some cases might be entirely asymptomatic, which would mean that known symptoms never developed. The virus could cause severe illness in older people and some younger people, particularly those with pre-existing conditions, but how the virus could have an impact on children was uncertain (Ogden et al. 2020, 199).

Despite the rapid learning, there were many unknowns when modelling and, as a result, models were based on estimated input values. Experts did not know the exact or true rate of death for people who became infected, the transmission rate between individuals, the total number of people who had been infected, whether infected persons were immune to the virus, how long such immunity could last, or the true number of deaths due to COVID-19 (Bui et al. 2020; Grenier 2020b; Giattino 2020). Another limitation of the models was that the observed case-fatality rate was higher than initially predicted because of extensive transmission in LTC and seniors' facilities, as noted earlier. Outbreaks in these facilities were severe because contact rates were high and the population highly vulnerable. These death rates were not anticipated in earlier models; they also varied throughout the country (Ogden et al. 2020, 202).

Initial modelling estimates used age-specific severity estimates from international surveillance data about the virus and Canadian demographic information. These data were combined to model the number of total cases, the proportion of cases that might be mild or asymptomatic, the proportion that might require hospitalization or ICU treatment, and the number of deaths. More precise estimates on health-care needs could have been assessed at the community level in earlier models to account for the specific demographics, such as age and co-morbidities, of a given community (Ogden et al. 2020, 201).

The models used low-end and high-end projections to reflect a range of possibilities depending on the public's adherence to public health measures. The high-end estimates in the models were generally accurate throughout the pandemic although there were a few times when the models fell short. Throughout the fall of 2020, during the second wave, the models often underestimated the number of cases by several thousand. Projections for deaths were also underestimated, especially early on as noted, and with the emergence of new variants of COVID-19 (Forani 2020).

Models had to be constantly adjusted as new information was gathered and public health measures changed. Human behaviour, such as compliance with public health restrictions, is also challenging to anticipate, particularly in long-term projections. It has less impact on short-term projections because public health interventions often take two weeks to affect the epidemic curve (Forani 2020). The findings of the models and the alarming messages that go with them can also be used to motivate behaviour change and encourage compliance with public health orders. In this sense, somewhat ironically, if models have the desired effect, they will prompt behaviour change and ultimately overestimate case and death count. Table 3.1 compares short-term model projections to the known cases and deaths.

Indeed, there were times when projections overestimated cases and deaths. For example, models from September 2020 predicted 3,000 cases a day by mid-October, but the actual number was 2,300 to 2,500 (Forani 2020). It was estimated that by November cases could exceed 5,000 a day, but they averaged 3,000 a day in early November (Forani 2020). There were also times when models underestimated case and death count. PHAC estimated that there could be 155,795 cases by 2 October, but there were over 160,500 cases by that time (Tumilty 2021). At the end of October 2020 it was projected that daily cases could exceed 6,000 by early December if the level of contacts was maintained. In early December, 6,200 daily cases were recorded (Forani 2020). Variants of the COVID-19 virus also posed a challenge because their infection and fatality rates were difficult to determine (Blackwell 2021).

The worst-case scenarios that PHAC had anticipated did not come to pass (Tumilty 2021, para. 8). PHAC anticipated a large increase in cases in the new year (2021) from increased social interactions over the holidays. In November 2020 it warned of a worst-case scenario in which Canada could have 60,000 cases per day by early January 2021 if restrictions eased and people gathered in large numbers (Tumilty 2021), and up to 25,000 cases if there was no change in social interactions and restrictions. On 4 January there were 14,000 daily cases of COVID-19 reported (Tumilty 2021).

Modelling can be used to inform vaccine-distribution strategies and prioritize groups for vaccination (M. Galloway 2021). Decision makers had to determine whether to prioritize the most vulnerable or the most exposed, and models can help develop scenarios based on different parameters. According to some models, for example, essential workers should be prioritized for vaccines rather than all people over sixty-five years of age (CBC News 2021f).

Models were criticized throughout the pandemic because of the range of forecasts they provided, and how they changed over time and varied in their accuracy. Modelling is challenging; errors may come from the model's methodology, the inaccuracy of assumptions made to produce the model, or the inherent challenges in predicting accurately how individuals and governments will behave, such as loosening restrictions and complying with public health orders (Bui et al. 2020). Different types of expertise are also needed to develop more accurate models. Modelling specific communities and neighbourhoods requires knowledge of those communities and neighbourhoods. The ability to communicate to decision makers and lay people what the models mean and what to do about it was at times in short supply. To mitigate this, many modellers considered a variety of factors and a range of values for each input. As new variants emerged, the models needed to be recalibrated with new data. It is important to consider the outputs or scenarios of a wide range of models to compare findings and assess limitations to develop a more complete understanding of various forecasts.

CONCLUSION

The threat of COVID-19 changed dramatically over time. As late as February 2020, officials continued to describe COVID-19 as "low risk" in Canada. Later, it would be described as the biggest public health crisis of the century (Romo 2020; Staples 2020b). There were two immediate problems in understanding the threat. First, the capacity to gather information did not exist in the early stages. There was a necessary delay as public agencies across the country developed a test, expanded their testing capacity, and increased the speed with which they obtained and communicated results. From a logistics standpoint, this was a significant undertaking.

Secondly, the virus's reach was constantly changing; growth was exponential, and where and how it was growing were always in question. Gathering information depended on people getting tested, disclosing positive results, self-isolating, and, in some cases, notifying close contacts. Asymptomatic transmission made this even more challenging because people would not even know they had the disease and were passing it on to others. Public health officials were always playing

Table 3.1 | Public Health Agency of Canada's modelling projections, April 2020–January 2022

Report date	Model forecast	Actual outcome	How correct the models were
9 April 2020	22,580–31,850 cases and 500–700 deaths by 16 April	28,381 cases and 1,015 deaths by 15 April	Actual cases within model range, but actual deaths beyond model range
28 April 2020	53,196–66,835 cases and 3,277–3,883 deaths by 5 May	60,772 cases and 3,859 deaths by 5 May	Actual cases and deaths within model range
4 June 2020	97,990–107,454 cases and 7,700–9,400 deaths by 15 June	98,787 cases and 8,156 deaths by 15 June	Actual cases and deaths within model range
29 June 2020	103,940–108,130 cases and 8,545–8,865 deaths by 12 July	107,346 cases and 8,788 deaths by 12 July	Actual cases and deaths within model range
8 July 2020	106,015–111,260 cases and 8,560–8,900 deaths by 17 July	109,264 cases and 8,847 deaths by 17 July	Actual cases and deaths within model range
14 August 2020	121,650–127,740 cases and 8,980–9,115 deaths by 23 August	124,629 cases and 9,096 deaths by 23 August	Actual cases and deaths within model range
22 September 2020	150,780–155,795 cases and 9,220–9,300 deaths by 2 October	160,535 cases and 9,349 deaths by 2 October	Both total cases and deaths underestimated
9 October 2020	188,150–197,830 cases and 9,690–9,800 deaths by 17 October	194,106 cases and 9,757 deaths by 17 October	Actual cases and deaths within model range
30 October 2020	251,800–262,000 cases and 10,285–10,400 deaths by 8 November	260,055 cases and 10,525 deaths by 8 November	Total cases within range, but deaths underestimated
20 November 2020	366,500–378,600 cases and 11,870–12,120 deaths by 30 November	372,036 cases and 12,104 deaths by 30 November	Actual cases and deaths within model range
11 December 2020	531,300–577,000 cases and 14,410–14,920 deaths by 25 December	535,149 cases and 14,797 deaths by 25 December	Actual cases and deaths within model range
15 January 2021	752,400–796,630 cases and 18,570–19,630 deaths by 24 January	748,381 cases and 19,094 deaths by 24 January	Total cases overestimated, but actual deaths within range

Table 3.1 | continued

19 February 2021	841,650–878,850 cases and 21,510–22,420 deaths by 28 February	867,694 cases and 21,994 deaths by 28 February	Actual cases and deaths within model range
26 March 2021	973,080–1,005,020 cases and 22,875–23,315 deaths by 4 April	1,008,106 cases and 24,219 deaths by 4 April	Both total cases and deaths underestimated
23 April 2021	1,209,780–1,281,040 cases and 24,000–24,570 deaths by 2 May	1,235,696 cases and 24,300 deaths by 2 May	Actual cases and deaths within model range
28 May 2021	1,387,210–1,426,400 cases and 25,590–26,310 deaths by 10 June	1,398,292 cases and 25,873 deaths by 10 June	Actual cases and deaths within model range
25 June 2021	1,413,010–1,420,740 cases and 26,175–26,475 deaths by 4 July	1,416,732 cases and 26,090 deaths as of 3 July	Actual cases and deaths within model range
30 July 2021	1,432,555–1,441,610 cases and 26,570–26,700 deaths by 8 August	1,439,068 cases and 26,394 deaths as of 7 August	Actual cases within model range, actual deaths overestimated
3 September 2021	1,534,770–1,570,230 cases and 27,025–27,260 deaths by 12 September	1,542,954 cases and 26,917 deaths as of 11 September	Actual cases within model range, actual deaths overestimated
8 October 2021	1,672,370–1,713,060 cases and 28,370–29,030 deaths by 17 October	1,680,193 cases and 28,200 deaths as of 16 October	Actual cases within model range, actual deaths overestimated
5 November 2021	1,734,290–1,757,170 cases and 29,075–29,620 deaths by 14 November	1,747,987 cases and 29,037 deaths as of 13 November	Actual cases within model range, actual deaths overestimated
10 December 2021	1,845,770–1,873,780 cases and 29,845–30,285 deaths by 19 December	1,877,102 cases and 29,752 deaths as of 18 December	Actual cases underestimated, actual deaths overestimated
14 January 2022	2,917,370–3,562,450 cases by 25 January and 31,620–32,660 deaths by 23 January	2,913,322 cases and 32,120 deaths as of 22 January 3,031,544 cases and 33,238 deaths as of 29 January	Actual cases and deaths within the model range

PHAC modelling projections correct nearly 57 per cent of the time.
Source: PHAC 2020i–s, 2021e, 2021g–m; Government of Canada 2021l.

catch-up against a largely invisible enemy. Both challenges required the active participation of an informed and concerned public. Public health surveillance and information sharing between agencies and governments were also significant challenges. These issues had been raised following SARS in 2003, and COVID-19 scaled them to unprecedented levels, including deficiencies in surge capacity; timely scaling of and access to laboratory testing and results; data access and sharing among orders of government; coordination across institutions; and national electronic surveillance systems (Health Canada 2003; Allin et al. 2022).

Models were an important device by which to understand the risk but also to communicate the risk to decision makers and the lay public. It was a complex task. Models required data that at times could only be estimated, and assumptions about the transmissibility and severity of the virus varied as it mutated, meaning that the values of certain variables changed over time (e.g., infection rate) and could vary by jurisdiction. Many assumptions were made about the pathogen and human behaviour that were estimates based on expert education, experience, and in some cases data from other parts of the world. Many of the models provided reasonably accurate forecasts, and they were dire. Models that forecast short-term outcomes were largely accurate; of the twenty-three modelling reports noted, thirteen (or approximately 57 per cent) came within the estimated range for cases and deaths; seven fell out of range for one category and three fell out of range for both measures. Even when estimates were out of range, they were often close. Despite the ranges, assumptions, and sensitivities of the model, they were able to communicate forcefully the immediate danger and the need to change behaviour to have a chance of meeting the challenge in the coming weeks. These were among the most powerful moments of the pandemic; the immediate forecasts offered little hope in the short term.

The true case count will never be known. Given the novelty and magnitude of the challenge, models could only be so reliable. The range of estimates generated from models that made short-term projections often included the observed case and death counts within the range, and in some respects this is unsurprising. Models that generated estimates for the short term had wide ranges, and, in any event, interventions in the short term had limited impact; the trajectory was clear and difficult to alter. Modelling for the longer term was more difficult and ultimately less accurate. In some respects, longer-term projections are set up to fail. Health officials hope that people will change their behaviour in light of the projections and that the result will be a less severe outcome.

Managing information about COVID-19 in Canada was made more complex because of the division of responsibility for health care between the federal and provincial or territorial governments (Desson et al. 2020). The variation in provincial and territorial capacity and response to COVID-19 also influenced the success or failure of government operations. The federal government depended on data from provincial and territorial health authorities. It released statistics about COVID-19, including case numbers and deaths, but the quality of national-level data was significantly affected by reporting delays, particularly until late June 2020 (Desson et al. 2020). For example, on 25 May 2020, Canada had 85,679 confirmed COVID-19 cases, but the federal government only had complete data on 40,660 cases – less than half the total (Desson et al. 2020). Provincial and territorial data were much more reliable, although the provinces and territories differed in their abilities and willingness to manage and share data. There are many trade-offs associated with sharing data, especially health data where there are additional considerations of privacy and restrictions on its use. For example, Quebec was significantly affected by COVID-19 but only began publishing official data in May 2020 following pressure from academics. This was due in part to the l'Institut de la statistique du Québec's policy that prevented official determination of cause of death until two years after the death (Desson et al. 2020). The level of detail of the data also varied by province and territory. For example, collecting race-based data was not a common practice at the provincial and territorial level, though it clearly would have revealed important insights, as previously mentioned (see chapter 1).

The approach was underpinned by a rationalist paradigm as outlined in chapter 2 and exemplified the blind spots of such an approach: it was top-down and expert-driven. There was optimism that with technology and data, public health officials could control to a degree the disease spread and that existing pandemic practices could simply scale up to address the challenge.

Addressing such a risk by the rationalist method provides a means to an end, but the parameters of the exercise had to be set. The information was largely communicated through a health lens with a focus on one particular issue, the containment of COVID-19. There were flaws in the information gathering, including in detecting trends among demographic groups such as racialized people. There was also considerably less attention paid to other health issues, such as delayed diagnoses and treatment of serious illnesses, such as heart disease. As we would come to learn, governments' regulations and directives themselves would contribute to other health problems, such as increases in mental-health issues, substance use and overdoses, delays in cancer treatments, and changes to physical activity and healthy behaviours (see chapter 5). There is also the question of economic information. How was information considered about the overall cost of governments' interventions, such as unemployment, underemployment, business failures, and social costs? All these factors contribute to a degree of complexity that is susceptible to being overlooked in a narrowly focused rationalist approach. Indeed, these cascading effects contribute to uncertainty and ambiguity; the need for broader stakeholder engagement and more on-the-ground intelligence was evident.

4

Standard Setting: Health and Emergency Response, Economic Support, and Governance

While early characterizations of COVID-19 suggested the disease could be devasting, the episode also reveals the reach and power of the state. Governments made extraordinary declarations, the likes of which most had never seen in their lifetimes. In a matter of days the federal government closed national borders, enforced the Quarantine Act, and legislated massive economic programs to support businesses and those unable to work. Provincial and territorial governments enacted states of emergency that gave them sweeping powers to close businesses and schools and restrict movements. Governments decided what was essential and what was not. In the midst of this, democratic checks, like Parliament and legislative assemblies, altered their processes, often reducing opportunities for public scrutiny by elected members, for example during question periods.

According to cybernetics, standard setting involves establishing goals or guidelines. In government, standards often take the form of policy or directives. COVID-19 standards reached across every government department and jurisdiction; no one was left untouched by the standards enacted by governments. While there was some variation across jurisdictions, an aggressive and largely uniform approach was deemed to be the best way to contain the disease, particularly in the early stages. Yet changes in one policy area had cascading effects in other areas; there were trade-offs implicit in every decision. While the focus of governments was to contain the spread of the disease and ensure ICUs were not overwhelmed, policy-makers had to adjust programs and standards in various fields as a result of health directives. Suddenly every sector and policy area had some type of interdependence with health and health directives.

This chapter is divided into three sections. The first section, "Health and Emergency Response," reviews selected health guidelines, emergency powers, and the determination of essential services; it also considers salient topics such as school closures and travel advisories. The second section, "Economic Support," examines programs that the federal government enacted to ensure economic stability during periods of lockdown and restricted movement. It also considers the role the Bank of Canada played in the crisis to ensure capital was available and the economy could continue to function. The third section, "Governance," reviews changes to selected administrative legal processes and democratic accountability.

For the most part, the standards were blunt. They were enacted quickly, with an eye to ensuring that essential services could function and that the health system would not be overwhelmed. Some regulations were adjusted over time. The fairness and precision of these standards were less important than ensuring stability, quickly, in a crisis. The response exemplified the strengths and weaknesses of bureaucracies in such situations.

HEALTH AND EMERGENCY RESPONSE

Division of Health-Care Responsibilities between Federal and Provincial/Territorial Governments

Governments' responses to COVID-19 were underpinned by the formal division of responsibility for health care between the federal government and the provinces and territories. The federal government has a strategic role to set national standards, fund and facilitate information gathering and research, and regulate prescription drugs and medical devices (Allin, Marchildon, and Merkur 2021). The federal government generally plays a coordination and funding role, and the provinces and territories deliver the services (Fierlbeck 2010; Migone 2020; Allin, Marchildon, and Merkur 2021).

Canada has a predominantly publicly financed health system, with nearly 70 per cent of health expenditures being financed through tax revenues from federal, provincial, and territorial governments (Allin, Marchildon, and Merkur 2021). The system allows Canadian residents "reasonable access to medically necessary hospital and physician services without paying out-of-pocket" (Government of Canada 2016, para 3). Health-care roles and responsibilities are shared between federal and provincial or territorial governments. The federal government sets national standards for the health-care system through the Canada Health Act (1984), provides most of the funding for provincial and territorial health-care services, supports delivery of services to specific groups of people (e.g., First Nations, people living on reserves, Inuit, members of the Canadian Armed Forces, veterans, federal inmates, and some refugees), and approves medication and health-related devices (Government of Canada 2016, 2022c).

Provincial and territorial health-care insurance plans must meet the minimum standards outlined in the Canada Health Act to receive full payment under the Canada Health Transfer (CHT). The CHT represents the largest federal transfer to the provinces and territories (Government of Canada 2011a). The provinces and territories are responsible for administering their own tax-funded and universal hospital and medical care plans, as well as additional coverage for health services excluded from universal health care (e.g., prescription drugs, long-term care, home care). Provincial and territorial ministers of health are responsible for the legislation and regulations to administer universal coverage for hospital and physician services (Allin, Marchildon, and Merkur 2021). Provincial and territorial governments manage, organize, and deliver health-care services in their jurisdiction, meaning there is variation in how provinces and territories operate their health-care systems and public health offices.

In short, most health-care responsibilities throughout the pandemic lay with the provincial and territorial governments, which played a pivotal role in containing the disease while also trying to maintain other health-care services. The federal government played a crucial role in controlling borders, enforcing quarantine measures, providing economic support to the provinces and territories, and in some cases directly to citizens, to ensure stability during periods of dramatic restrictions. The federal government was also responsible for obtaining and approving vaccines. At times, Canada's federated health system is criticized for being highly fragmented (Emanuel 2020). While federalism can give provincial and territorial governments the flexibility to respond to the unique needs of each region, some argued that uncoordinated efforts on a national scale may have prevented the country from using all its resources and capacities effectively (Desson et al. 2020; Flood and Thomas 2020). For further discussion of the Canada Health Act, the division of responsibilities, and health care as a market failure, see chapter 9.

Emergency Powers Enacted to Maintain Health-System Capacity

The federal government was reluctant to declare a national state of emergency. Some argued that early on it might have been helpful to support testing and contact-tracing capacity in the provinces and territories. There were political risks with enacting a state of emergency, such as being seen as intrusive and damaging to intergovernmental relations (Flood and Thomas 2020; Fierlbeck and Hardcastle 2020, 46–7; Allin, Marchildon, and Merkur 2021). It is also not clear that it was necessary. All provinces and territories were dealing with similar issues; reallocation of resources among them was not necessarily the problem. Instead, existing legislation (e.g., the Quarantine Act) was used, and the COVID-19 Emergency Response Act was created.

As COVID-19 spread across Canada, many provincial and territorial governments declared states of emergency or public health emergencies, which granted them powers to make changes quickly to restrain actions and mobilize resources to where they were needed (Allin, Marchildon, and Merkur 2021). Quebec was the first province to declare a public health emergency on 13 March 2020 (Lawson et al. 2022). By 22 March, all provinces and Nunavut had declared a state of emergency or a public health emergency, and by 27 March Yukon and the Northwest Territories had declared states of emergency (Lawson et al. 2022). These imposed travel restrictions, gathering-size limits, closure of non-essential services and businesses, school closures, and physical-distancing requirements.

The federal government did enact far-reaching legislation. An Act respecting certain measures in response to COVID-19, enacted on 25 March 2020, amended other legislation to support the federal government's emergency response, for example, the Financial Administration Act and Canada Labour Code (Parliament of Canada 2020). In mid-April, regulatory amendments to the Contraventions Act came into force that enabled law-enforcement agencies to ticket individuals who did not comply with the federal Quarantine Act (Department of Justice Canada 2020).

No sooner had lockdowns occurred than there was pressure to communicate how long they would last. In April 2020, provinces and territories started to release plans to reopen their economies and relax public health restrictions. Saskatchewan was the first to unveil its recovery plan, on 23 April (Government of Saskatchewan 2020). By the end of May, most provinces had released plans to reopen, many of which used a phased approach.

COVID-19 infections continued to occur throughout the summer of 2020 as businesses reopened and physical-distancing measures relaxed across the country. By the fall, most provinces and territories were in the midst of a second wave of COVID-19. The majority limited travel and gathering sizes, including gatherings at households and indoor facilities, throughout the fall and into 2021. Closures within provinces and territories were not always uniform, as some jurisdictions adopted a zone-based approach, in which areas with outbreaks of COVID-19 were under tighter restrictions than areas with fewer cases. This was not a perfect solution as people in zones with tighter restrictions would travel to regions with fewer restrictions to go shopping or visit seasonal properties, for example. Additionally, the line between zones could seem driven more by jurisdiction than science. In some parts of Toronto, for example, one side of the street was under stricter orders than the other side. As the third and fourth waves persisted into 2021, provinces and territories that had relaxed regulations, such as masking and lockdowns, needed to re-enact them.

Determining Essential Services

The *National Strategy for Critical Infrastructure* defines critical infrastructure as "processes, systems, facilities, technologies, networks, assets, and services essential to the health, safety, security or economic well-being of Canadians and the effective functioning of government" (PS 2020b, para. 1). For the ten key sectors, Public Safety Canada (PS) identified the functions in table 4.1 as essential, but the examples shown are not exhaustive.

The ten critical sectors were articulated in the national strategy in 2007 and co-authored by the federal, provincial, and territorial governments. The details in this case, however, were developed in light of the pandemic. Municipal, provincial, territorial, or First Nations, Inuit, and Métis jurisdictions had the legislative authority to implement response actions in their jurisdictions, including determining which services were essential. Generally, many provinces and territories followed this list of sectors when designating essential services. There was some variation, however, when certain jurisdictions identified services for vulnerable populations as essential, as well as when there were debates about the designation of liquor and cannabis as essential retail products. Jurisdictions such as Saskatchewan and Manitoba had specific designations of essential services for both the province and the northern communities within the province.

School Closures and Effects on Education

Approximately 5.7 million children and youth attend primary and secondary school across Canada (Statistics Canada 2021i). Provinces and territories suspended in-person classes in school and child-care facilities, and educators worked to transition their programming to online

Table 4.1 | Public Safety Canada's list of essential functions

Essential function	Examples
Health	Workers providing health-care services (e.g., doctors and nurses), caregivers, social service workers, medical technicians, COVID-19 testing and clinical research, and medical supplies manufacturers (e.g., PPE)
Water	Operation of drinking water and waste-water facilities, including associated testing
Food	Grocery workers, restaurants with take-out and delivery capacity, agriculture workers, and other food producers, manufacturers, and distributors
Information and communication technologies	Operations of communications infrastructure, dispatchers, and repair and maintenance workers
Energy and utilities	Workers operating the generation or transmission of power (e.g., natural gas, electric, nuclear), and petroleum production and transportation
Transportation	Workers transporting both goods and people, trucking, shipping, and automotive maintenance
Finance	Consumer and business banking, and related financial services (e.g., call centres, automatic teller machines, bank branches)
Safety	Law enforcement, emergency management, search and rescue, laboratory technicians, and 911 call-centre employees
Government	Services that have an impact on the health, safety, security, or economic well-being of Canadians or the effective functioning of the Canadian government
Other services	Tradespersons (e.g., plumbers, electricians, exterminators), education, hotel workers, researchers, and professional services (e.g., real estate, law, accounting)

Source: PS 2020b.

and remote learning. Some provinces and territories noted the closure would be temporary, while others cancelled in-person classes for the remainder of the school year.

In many jurisdictions, child-care spots were made available for essential workers but access to them varied across the country. Capacity was expanded over time to accommodate not only children of health-care workers but also those of other essential workers, such as employees who supported critical infrastructure and the military (Government of Alberta 2020a; Government of British Columbia 2020c; Government of Manitoba 2020a; Government of Northwest Territories 2020a; Government of Alberta 2020b, 2020f).

Many schools resumed in-person classes in September 2020 with masks, sanitation practices, and social distancing. Some schools underwent renovations to improve ventilation. The school year would not be smooth and uninterrupted, as in-person classes were suspended during the second and third waves of the pandemic.

Post-secondary students and instructors also made the transition to online learning. Many post-secondary institutions implemented a hybrid model of online classes with some in-person classes in September 2020. This model continued for the 2021 academic year with cancellation of in-person classes in favour of remote learning when cases peaked. Universities were in a somewhat precarious position; many had large numbers of international students who had become significant sources of income. For example, the total tuition from international students in 2020 was $1.7 billion, which represented 68 per cent of all tuition revenue and was more than the provincial and territorial grants that the institutions received (Friesen 2021). University administrators worried that these numbers would drop dramatically because international students would have to navigate travel restrictions and quarantine rules. For example, those returning to Nova Scotia were required to pay out of pocket to quarantine at a hotel even if they had their own residence locally (Xu 2021). Financial assistance to help cover some of these costs was made available, for example through post-secondary institutions (Dalhousie University 2021). There were 28 per cent fewer international students in Canada in 2020 than in 2019 (A. Tucker 2021). By fall 2020, many universities had seen enrolments increase, especially of part-time students, and their total enrolments increased throughout the pandemic (Friesen 2020a, 2022). In some cases, students demanded tuition waivers and reductions because of decreased in-person services and experiences, but these demands were rarely met. In fact, many universities increased tuition (Friesen 2020b).

At the start of the pandemic many people – including policy-makers and parents – were concerned that schools could become hotspots for transmission (Lewis 2021). As the pandemic continued through 2021, experts had mixed views about the effectiveness of school closures. Some studies found them to be effective in reducing community transmission and mortality, but many found that other interventions, such as mask mandates, social-gathering limits, travel restrictions, and non-essential business closures were more effective (El Jaouhari et al. 2021, 516).

Teachers' unions across the country argued that teachers should be included in provincial and territorial vaccine-prioritization plans, similar to the inclusion of health-care and other essential workers. Their efforts were rebuffed. The main reasons were that there were generally low case rates in schools, and any high-risk adults, such as the immunocompromised, would have been included in vaccine prioritization anyway (Hager and Keller 2021; Kane 2021).

Travel Advisories and Restrictions

Border control, including closures and mandatory quarantine, is primarily a federal responsibility. The travel restrictions early on have been considered a contributing factor to the containment of COVID-19 during the first wave in Canada. At the same time, some experts stated they were largely symbolic gestures, especially given the number of exemptions permitted (Hoffmann and Fafard 2020a, 2020b; PHAC 2020f; Allin et al. 2022).

On 14 March 2020 the federal government issued a travel advisory to avoid all non-essential travel outside Canada and all cruise-ship travel. Canadians were urged to return home via commercial means while those means were still available. By 16 March, only Canadian citizens and permanent residents could enter Canada. The Canada-US border was closed to non-essential travel on 18 March. At this time, international commercial flights could land at only four airports (Toronto, Calgary, Vancouver, and Montreal). On 8 June foreign nationals who were immediate family members of Canadian citizens and permanent residents, and who did not have COVID-19 symptoms, were permitted entry to Canada to visit immediate family members (CBSA 2020).

Mandatory self-isolation for fourteen days for all travellers returning to Canada was implemented on 25 March 2020 and enforced under the Quarantine Act. By 14 April, travellers had to confirm they had a suitable place to isolate or quarantine. If they could not do so, the chief public health officer of Canada designated a place (PHAC 2020e). Temperature screenings were introduced at airports and railways in mid-June. As of 21 November 2020, travellers to Canada were required to register their information electronically through ArriveCAN (PHAC 2020c). Border control in Canada has been criticized for weak enforcement and many exemptions (Hill and Russell 2021; C. Tunney 2021b). For example, as of 26 January 2021, only 2.4 per cent of all international travellers required to quarantine were followed up on by an enforcement officer; 74.0 per cent of international travellers were deemed essential workers and exempted from the Quarantine Act (Hill and Russell 2021; C. Tunney 2021b; Allin et al. 2022).

Each province and territory implemented its own travel restrictions to limit the spread of COVID-19. Initially, self-isolation was voluntary until federally mandated; however, on 13 March 2020, the Government of New Brunswick mandated self-isolation for fourteen days for all international travellers returning to the province. By the end of March 2020, the Northwest Territories, Nunavut, Yukon, New Brunswick, Nova Scotia, and PEI had enacted regulations stating that anyone entering from outside the province or territory had to self-isolate unless exempt. As of 26 March, people wishing to return to Nunavut required approval from the office of the chief public health officer. As of 16 April, the Government of Manitoba prohibited travel to the northern part of the province and required self-isolation for all travellers entering the province.

On 3 July 2020 the Atlantic provinces launched the "Atlantic Bubble." This was a policy decision made among the four Atlantic provinces that allowed their residents to travel between them without the need to self-isolate for two weeks (*Globe and Mail* 2020a). Cases in the Atlantic provinces had been generally lower than in the rest of the country; the bubble allowed interprovincial travel without exposing the region to risk of increased cases from the rest of the country (Allin et al. 2022). The Atlantic Bubble continued until 24 November when cases started to rise, and the Government of Newfoundland and Labrador and the Government of PEI mandated self-isolation for individuals coming from the Atlantic provinces (Government of Canada 2022m; Newfoundland and Labrador Executive Council 2020; Prince Edward Island Health and Wellness 2020).

The ArriveCAN app was used during the pandemic to screen the public health information of travellers crossing the border, and it has continued to be used as a voluntary option for travellers to clear customs (Osman 2023). The Canadian government has been criticized about the business model to develop the ArriveCAN app, led by the Canada Border Services Agency (CBSA). GC Strategies, a two-person company, was issued contracts worth $44 million over two years to develop ArriveCAN and other projects across twenty departments. The House of Commons Committee on Government Operations found that once the work had been contracted to GC Strategies, the company then subcontracted it to other companies (e.g., KPMG, BDO Canada, Optiv, Macadamian Technologies, Level Access, and Distill Mobile) at rates of between $900 and $1,500 a day. GC Strategies kept a commission of 15 to 30 per cent (Osman 2023; C. Clarke 2023).

Originally, the projected cost of ArriveCAN was $80,000, but it turned into a $54 million project, including maintenance and ancillary costs (Clarke 2023). The prime minister himself criticized the contract for being "highly illogical and inefficient" (Osman 2023). On 20 October 2022, GC Strategies' managing partner told the House of Commons committee that the firm billed $4.5 million per year to staff the development, support, and maintenance of the app (Osman 2023).

ECONOMIC SUPPORT

Throughout the pandemic the Government of Canada spent $210.7 billion on COVID-19– recovery benefits, including CERB and the Employment Insurance Emergency Response Benefit / Canada Emergency Response Benefit ($74.8 billion), CEWS ($100.7 billion), Canada Recovery Sickness Benefit (CRSB) ($1.5 billion), Canada Recovery Caregiving Benefit ($4.4 billion), Canada Worker Lockdown Benefit ($0.9 billion), Canada Recovery Benefit ($28.4 billion), in addition to provincial and territorial programs (OAG 2022). Over two-thirds of Canadians over fifteen years old received income from at least one of the COVID-19 benefits. Of these, 27 per cent received emergency recovery benefits, and nearly 56 per cent received top-ups to existing federal programs (Statistics Canada 2022h).

Income inequality increased quickly at the start of the pandemic, with many workplaces closing their doors and laying off staff. No one was sure how long restrictions would be in place. In time, the COVID-19 benefit programs were successful in supporting Canadians. Poverty rates decreased in 2020, largely due to increased economic transfers, including enhancements to benefits (e.g., Canada Child Benefit) and pandemic relief programs such as CERB. Government financial programs decreased income inequality throughout 2020 and into 2021 with increases to household disposable income (Statistics Canada 2021b, 2021e, 2022i). Poverty rates decreased by half across all age groups in 2020 compared to 2015 (Statistics Canada 2022c). As government COVID-19–relief

funding changed, inflation and rent increases affected low-income earners, and debt-to-income ratios increased for low-income households
and income earners under thirty-five (Statistics Canada 2021b). There
were administrative errors, and many payments were made to people
deemed to be ineligible for the COVID-19 economic-support programs.
In the AG's evaluation of the programs, the lack of prepayment control
mechanisms in favour of post-payment assessments was a major factor
for overpayments. The next sections provide an overview of CERB and
EI benefits, protections for tenants, and the CEWS.

CERB and Employment Insurance

The federal government launched CERB to provide financial support to
Canadians who were unable to work due to COVID-19 (Government
of Canada 2021c). Over three million people lost their jobs in March
and April 2020 as non-essential businesses were ordered to close, and
an additional 2.5 million worked less than half their usual hours (CBC
News 2020d). The goal of CERB was to support workers to meet their
financial obligations, allow them to stay home to prevent further spread
of COVID-19, and reduce the impacts of COVID-19 on individuals and
the overall health-care system (OAG 2021a). Those eligible could receive
$2,000 a month. When the benefit launched, it retroactively started on
15 March 2020 and ran to 3 October 2020, spanning twenty-eight
weeks (OAG 2021a). The program was extended twice during this time.
To be eligible, the applicant had to be at least fifteen years old, reside
in Canada, be unable to work due to COVID-19–related shutdowns,
and have earned at least $5,000 in net income in 2019. Workers were
ineligible if they earned more than $1,000 in net income in a two-week
period within the monthly benefit-claim period, which discouraged people from seeking additional income while receiving CERB (Government
of Canada 2021c). Non-citizens, including permanent residents and
international students, were also eligible for CERB. On 22 April 2020
the federal government introduced the CESB to allow eligible students
who were unable to find work due to COVID-19 to receive $1,250 per
month for a maximum of sixteen weeks between 10 May and 29 August
2020 (Government of Canada 2020e). The Canadian government spent
approximately $74.8 billion on CERB and EI benefits (OAG 2022).

   The pandemic created an unprecedented need for an emergency
response benefit to launch quickly. This meant that rapid payment was
prioritized over prepayment control measures; instead, the decision was
made to focus on post-payment controls (OAG 2021a). Priorities were

to provide a flat-rate payment instead of one based on income, have minimal and clear eligibility requirements, enable applicants to provide attestations rather than supporting documentation, enable applicants to use their Social Insurance Number (SIN) to verify identity, and confirm eligibility post-payment. According to Employment and Social Development Canada (ESDC), it could have taken months to issue payments if standard prepayment control measures were in place. ESDC supported the use of attestations over formal documentation to simplify the process and ensure applicants could stay at home rather than going to different locations to secure documentation (OAG 2021a).

While it is unclear exactly how government determined how much to pay people through programs like CERB, impacts on recipient groups, economic sectors, labour supply, and gender-based analysis were considered in the development of the benefit program, as well as the EI sickness benefit for health-care workers affected by the SARS virus in 2003 (OAG 2021a). EI statistics were used to determine the average rate paid out in the previous year. Analysis was conducted on people excluded from existing EI programs and showed that those who did not contribute to EI, and people who needed to care for children while schools were closed, were ineligible for EI. The Department of Finance also reported that Canada's emergency benefit programs were comparable to COVID-19 emergency benefit programs implemented in other countries (OAG 2021a). CERB was more generous than social assistance programs, particularly when compared to disability support benefits. This called attention to inequities of government support for people with disabilities. For example, those eligible for the Ontario Disability Support Program could receive $1,169 per month (with one-time pandemic top-ups of $100 per month until the end of July 2020) (Graefe and Ferdosi 2021). Towards the end of October 2020 the federal government announced a one-time COVID-19 disability support payment of $600 (Government of Canada 2022m).

As of 4 October 2020, 8.9 million unique applicants had submitted a total of 27.6 million applications for CERB and EI benefits, meaning the same applicant applied for the benefits in multiple claim periods (Government of Canada 2021c). There was a high volume of applications from the outset of the pandemic, with over six million received in the first month – from over one in five Canadians over fifteen years old – demonstrating the demand for the program (CBC News 2020d). People aged twenty-five to thirty-four accounted for the majority of CERB applications, with slightly more male applicants than female (Government of Canada 2021c). Between 15 March and 3 October

2020, a total of $81.64 billion was administered through CERB and EI programs. Of this, approximately 91 per cent ($74.08 billon) was paid through CERB, and 9 per cent ($7.56 billion) through EI (Government of Canada 2021c, 2021h). Furthermore, as of October 2020, 708,440 unique applicants had submitted a total of 2,140,230 CESB applications. At this time $2.94 billion had been paid out to students through the CESB (Government of Canada 2020a).

Challenges to Supporting Citizens Quickly

The federal government was criticized for lack of fraud oversight during the early months of the pandemic. In June 2020 the Canada Revenue Agency (CRA) opened a phone line to accept reports of suspected fraudulent claims for the CERB and CEWS programs (Government of Canada 2020d). During the first seven months of the pandemic 1,610 people received CERB using a mailing address outside of Canada, accounting for $11.9 million of CERB payments (Bogart 2022). There are reasons a mailing address outside Canada could be used, for example someone may be considered a resident for tax purposes but reside abroad.

In March 2021 the AG reported that CERB payments of approximately $500 million were made to applicants who applied through both the CRA and ESDC, although this duplication accounted for less than 1 per cent of total payments (Turnbull 2021; OAG 2021a). Concerns were also raised about teenagers living at home accessing CERB. Over $636 million in CERB benefits was paid to approximately 300,000 teens aged fifteen to seventeen, also accounting for less than 1 per cent of total payments (Dawson 2021). The issue was addressed in updates to the program in April 2020, but the lack of prepayment-control measures was criticized. The Financial Transactions and Reports Analysis Centre of Canada found that criminal organizations also accessed CERB benefits (C. Tunney 2021a).

As of 30 November 2020, payments had been stopped for more than 30,000 potentially fraudulent applications, accounting for approximately $42 million (OAG 2021a). As of 4 October 2020, there had been over 830,000 voluntary repayments of CERB benefits from Canadians to the CRA (K. Harris 2020a). There were several reasons for the voluntary repayments; for example, recipients repaid payments made in error after the program's launch, such as double payments. Before the CRA sent out notices to repay CERB in May 2022, 341,000 Canadians had voluntarily repaid nearly $910 million; however, as of November 2022 nearly $1.2 billion was still outstanding (Major 2022b). There were calls to forgive CERB repayments, especially for low-income people.

Eligibility for CERB was adjusted slightly throughout the pandemic to address its shortcomings. On 15 April 2020 eligibility criteria for CERB and EI benefits were expanded to allow workers to earn up to $1,000 per month, and the EI Emergency Response Benefit was expanded to include seasonal workers and those who had exhausted their EI benefits (OAG 2021a). On 23 April the eligibility criteria were expanded to include self-employed fishers. As of 20 December 2020, of the approximately 141,000 individuals who had contacted the agency about rejected applications, only 11 per cent were actually eligible for CERB (OAG 2021a). In December 2022 the AG released additional reports evaluating the COVID-19–response benefits. The AG found that $4.6 billion in overpayments had been made to ineligible recipients of benefits for individuals, with half ($2.3 billion) having been repaid by recipients.

The former finance minister Bill Morneau supported CERB but also criticized the COVID-19 benefits program. In his book he stated that the prime minister and his advisors had overruled the recommendations of Finance Department officials and approved more generous payments than the department thought necessary; Morneau argued that the decisions were taken to support politically active groups and to meet the moment emotionally rather than by way of any rational economic analysis (Curry 2023a; Morneau 2023). With respect to CERB he noted that $500 a week exceeded the regular take-home pay of many part-time and low-income workers (Curry 2023a; Morneau 2023, 240), and he questioned whether seniors, many of whom had stable pensions, required additional assistance.

Protection for Tenants

The first form of support was targeted at homeowners and landlords through programs to pause mortgage payments, and then programs were introduced to target renters. Legislative changes were implemented at the provincial and territorial level to prevent renters from being evicted because of income loss due to COVID-19. In many provinces and territories, civil enforcement for evictions due to non-payment of rent had been suspended, landlords had been prohibited from increasing rent or charging fees due to missed payments, and evictions due to income loss had been prohibited by the end of March 2020 (Government of Alberta 2020c; Government of PEI 2020a; Government of

Northwest Territories 2020b). Some jurisdictions, such as Nova Scotia, also encouraged retail and commercial landlords to defer lease payments for three months for businesses that had to close due to COVID-19, and landlords were not permitted to seize property if the business had closed due to public health orders. Protections for tenants continued in many jurisdictions throughout the pandemic, especially while public health orders remained in place. For example, the Government of Yukon (2020b) announced that residential tenants who were under a health protection measure after 25 June 2020, or who needed to breach tenancy agreements because they were under a COVID-19 health protection order, would continue to be protected from eviction.

The Canada Emergency Wage Subsidy (CEWS)

The federal government first announced a wage-subsidy program in response to the pandemic on 18 March 2020. The Temporary Wage Subsidy for Employers paid employers 10 per cent of their employees' wages by reducing their remittances owed to the CRA. This program was expanded to the CEWS on 27 March as economic challenges increased due to COVID-19. The Canadian government spent approximately $100.7 billion on CEWS, as noted earlier.

The money was sent to employers with the goal of encouraging them to retain employees, to rehire people who had been laid off, and to ensure that workers had a steady income (OAG 2021b). The program subsidized up to 75 per cent of qualifying wages (up to $847 per week per employee) for all employers facing at least a 15 per cent decline in revenue in March 2020 or a minimum 30 per cent decline in April, May, or June 2020. The program was initially intended to run until 6 June 2020 but was extended three times into summer 2021 (OAG 2021b). On 15 May the criteria for CEWS were expanded to allow more types of employers to apply. By 17 July, program applicants no longer required a minimum percentage of revenue loss to qualify, and a top-up subsidy was added to support those most significantly affected by COVID-19. These changes were made to incentivize employers to rehire and to grow their companies; before that point, employers could deliberately slow growth to access the benefit. Like CERB, the program was administered by the CRA and overseen by the Department of Finance. The federal government approved 3,556,150 CEWS applications in total, with approximately 13 per cent (446,680) of these being unique applications, meaning the same applicant reapplied for multiple claim periods (Government of Canada 2022g). Most approved CEWS applications were for under $100,000; less than 0.16 per cent of total applications were approved for over $1 million. CEWS was estimated to cost approximately $97.6 billion by the end of the 2021–22 fiscal year and concluded by June 2021 (OAG 2021b).

There were criticisms. There were concerns raised about the interaction of CERB and CEWS, as employers found that many employees refused to work beyond fifteen hours in order to qualify for employment benefits. This particularly affected organizations that relied on seasonal workers, such as businesses in the tourism sector (CFIB 2020).

The CRA was criticized for not collecting employees' SIN information from employers and not having up-to-date tax and revenue information before issuing payments. This meant that recipients of other emergency response benefits could not be cross-referenced. The CRA was also not able to access data from the ESDC Work-Sharing Program and Temporary Wage Subsidy due to arrangements in their memorandum of understanding. This meant that the CRA had to rely on the accuracy of reports from employers and post-payment audits. The AG suggested that targeted audits could have been effective to strengthen the integrity of the program.

The CRA was also criticized by the AG for providing subsidy payments to organizations that seemed likely to fail before the pandemic or were at a high risk of bankruptcy, as well as to organizations that did not need assistance. Overall, approximately $37.7 billion in pandemic wage subsidies were awarded to businesses with tax debts, and $1 billion awarded to insolvent companies (Curry 2023b). The CRA identified 157,082 CEWS recipients with tax debts totalling $9.5 billion (Curry 2023a). According to the Bank of Canada, bankruptcy filings decreased by about 25 per cent between 2019 and 2020. Additional concerns have been raised that hundreds of publicly traded companies that received $3.6 billion in CEWS funds also experienced revenue increases throughout the pandemic and did not require government support (Cardoso and Brethour 2021). Data from the CRA show that $9.9 billion in CEWS funding was approved for publicly traded companies (Curry 2023b).

The AG recommended that at least $27.4 billion of payments to individuals and employers should be investigated further and cited the lack of prepayment control measures and complex post-payment processes as major factors for the overpayments.

The House of Commons Standing Committee on Public Accounts investigated the AG report's findings in January 2023. The commissioner of the CRA stated to the committee that preliminary reviews had suggested that it was not worth the effort to conduct a full review of the more than $15 billion in pandemic wage benefits made to the potentially ineligible recipients identified by the AG, and did not agree with some of her findings, including the $15 billion amount (Curry 2023b). The CRA supported its "risk-based" approach to enforcement, which reviews a sample of cases deemed to be most likely of concern with respect to fraud. The AG emphasized to the committee that a more aggressive and expansive review was warranted, given the very limited safeguards used to screen applications (Curry 2023b).

Economists have argued that the federal COVID-19 support programs pushed the Bank of Canada to increase interest rates in 2022, after large decreases in 2020 (Lundy and Rendell 2023). It is estimated that approximately 15 per cent of the inflation experienced in Canada, beyond the 2 per cent target, can be attributed to the federal COVID-19 support programs (Lundy and Rendell 2023).

Bank of Canada

The Bank of Canada, Canada's central bank, is a Crown corporation operating under the Bank of Canada Act. It formulates Canada's monetary policy, issues and distributes currency, and manages public debt programs and foreign exchange reserves with the aim "to promote the economic and financial welfare of Canada" (Government of Canada 2020b, 1).

Throughout the pandemic the Bank of Canada made credit more affordable and available to pay wages and purchase necessities while regular economic activities were disrupted due to COVID-19. The focus was to enable Canadians to be able to borrow money at low interest rates to support economic activity, such as paying employee wages (Bank of Canada, n.d.a; Poloz 2022b, 136). The interest rate was lowered to 0.25 per cent, which reduced loan payments on new and existing loans for consumers and businesses. There were concerns that unexpected increases in demand for cash could freeze business credit lines, which had occurred during the 2007–09 financial crisis (Poloz 2022b, 137). The Bank launched liquidity facilities and purchase programs to keep credit flowing and expanded its balance sheet by approximately 500 per cent between March 2020 and May 2021 (Dietsch and Best 2021). As economies reopened across the country in summer 2020 following the first wave of COVID-19, the Bank transitioned from purchasing long-term debt to supporting economic growth. The deep recession experienced in March 2020 was met with a quick economic recovery, according to the governor of the Bank of Canada (Macklem 2022).

Throughout COVID-19 the Bank of Canada coordinated with the country's major banks and financial institutions, the central banks of other Group of 7 (G7) countries, and international policy-makers and established foreign-exchange swap lines to ensure access to foreign currency. The Bank met with representatives from several countries, including China, Italy, and South Korea, to understand the impacts they faced and to learn what they could from their experiences (Poloz 2022b, 130).

The Bank of Canada also worked to ensure liquidity for other financial institutions that lent to individuals and businesses. It lengthened lending terms for banks, increased the range of acceptable collateral, and expanded eligibility for financial institutions to borrow money. The Bank also established a new standing term liquidity facility to support banks in managing liquidity risks while still providing credit to customers. The Superintendent of Financial Institutions lowered the amount of capital that banks were required to maintain as reserves, making $300 billion available for borrowing. The Bank committed to purchase at least $5 billion of Government of Canada bonds per week (Poloz 2022b, 138). The Canada Mortgage and Housing Corporation also committed to purchase up to $150 billion in insured mortgage pools (Talbot and Ordonez-Ponce 2020).

The Bank of Canada monitored several market indicators. The governor stated that the most significant domestic economic vulnerabilities stemmed from high household debt and inequities in the housing market. These issues are normal concerns for the Bank, but the pandemic made them more severe (Macklem 2021). Globally, the Bank looked to the international economic outlook to gauge trends in interest rates and investor appetite. It monitored the price of assets and the degree of credit spread, the yields of two different bonds or investments. A noted concern was that wider credit spreads could have an impact on Canadian businesses that depended on high-yield debt markets. The COVID-19 pandemic spurred digitization of the economy, both domestically and internationally. The Bank of Canada emphasized that this increased cybersecurity risks, as the interconnectedness of the global financial system and expanding digitization expose vulnerabilities to cyberattacks (Macklem 2021).

In a 2021 study, concerns were raised that the Bank of Canada seemed to prioritize the status quo at the expense of more progressive policies (Dietsch and Best 2021). The Swiss National Bank, for example, made progress on climate change by deciding to exclude coal-mining companies from asset purchases (Dietsch and Best 2021; Jordan 2020). There were also concerns raised about policies exacerbating inequality. Some of the liquidity injected to support the market ended up in the stock market and the housing market, further benefiting wealthy asset owners and pricing many Canadians out of the housing market (Dietsch and Best 2021). Low-income households with debt spent 31 per cent of income on debt repayment (Mulholland, Bucik, and Odu 2020, 6). Among indebted low- and moderate-income households, over 90 per cent have consumer debt but most do not have a mortgage, which is a much more stable and cheaper form of debt (Mulholland, Bucik, and Odu 2020, 8–9). The pandemic was expected to increase the risk of bankruptcy among households with high debt-repayment costs, particularly once COVID-19 relief programs had ended (Mulholland, Bucik, and Odu 2020, 7). In 2021 there was a 6.7 per cent decrease in rates of consumer insolvency and the lowest volume of insolvencies since 1995 (OSB 2022), but that trend changed during the pandemic. In 2022 there was an 11.9 per cent increase in insolvency filings compared to 2021, but this was lower than annual filings between 2001 and 2019 (OSB 2023). November 2022 saw the most significant increase in insolvency filings since March 2020 (CBC News 2023b). British Columbia and Ontario were the most significantly affected by consumer insolvency (OSB 2023).

Some criticized the Bank for keeping interest rates too low for too long, borrowing too much, and allowing its balance sheet to balloon (J. Cochrane and Hartley 2022; Rendell 2022). In 2022, for the first time in its history, the Bank of Canada was projected to report a financial loss and expected to take at least a few years to return to surplus (Rendell 2022). Governments' spending, together with lower interest rates and supply chain problems, contributed to a jump in inflation. The pre-pandemic inflation rate of the Consumer Price Index was 2.2 per cent, but by June 2022, it had reached 8.1 per cent, which reduced people's purchasing power. Significant contributing factors occurred prior to the pandemic, such as US inflation, changes in currency exchange rates, and high commodity prices.

Supply shortages were estimated to have caused up to 35 per cent of the inflation experienced beyond the 2 per cent target. As noted, government support programs were estimated to contribute a further 15 per cent. Thus, the Bank's intention shifted to curbing spending by limiting borrowing (Macklem 2022). The Bank's rate increased to 3.25 per cent in September 2022 (from 0.25 per cent in March 2020), which had significant impact on variable rate mortgages as well as various lines of credit. In December 2022 the interest rate increased further to 4.25 per cent.

Some people criticized major banks and financial institutions for their pandemic response. At the start of the pandemic many major banks did not believe tools such as deferred mortgage payments would be necessary (Poloz 2022b, 130). One study concluded that only three of the banks analyzed – RBC, Desjardins, and BMO – were noted for proactively supporting their clients and the broader community. The study indicated that most banks were not proactive in navigating the pandemic despite the severity of the economic situation and the financial easing measures taken by the Bank of Canada and the Superintendent of Financial Institutions (Talbot and Ordonez-Ponce 2020).

GOVERNANCE

COVID-19 had an impact on elections across Canada. For the federal election on 20 September 2021, voter turnout was 62.5 per cent, compared to 65.95 per cent in 2019. There was a 23.0 per cent increase in voters using advance polling stations in 2021 compared to 2019 (Elections Canada 2019, 2021).

New Brunswick, British Columbia, Saskatchewan, and Newfoundland and Labrador held provincial elections between March 2020 and March 2021. The elections in New Brunswick and British Columbia were called early by minority governments,[1] whereas Saskatchewan held a regularly scheduled election. Regulations in Newfoundland and Labrador meant that an election was required to be held by August 2021 because the elected premier had resigned (Garnett et al. 2021).[2] Election turnout was lower in these jurisdictions than prior to the pandemic. Turnout was 66.1 per cent in New Brunswick, 53.9 per cent in British Columbia, 52.9 per cent in Saskatchewan, and 48.2 per cent in Newfoundland and Labrador. The risk of exposure to COVID-19 was a factor in decisions to not vote, but not the predominate reason (Garnett et al. 2021).

The scrutiny provided by Parliament changed during the pandemic. It had only thirty-three sittings between January and June 2020, the fewest in a six-month period since the end of the Second World War. The House of Commons sat eighty-six times in 2020 and ninety-five times in 2021, less than the average 105 times between 2015 and 2019. Election years generally have fewer sittings; there were eighty-one in 2015 and seventy-five in 2019, for example. Between 2016 and 2018, the House of Commons met approximately 122 times each year (Parliament of Canada 2021).

The reduction in parliamentary scrutiny did not stop the federal government from acting; on the contrary, it committed to a $343 billion

Table 4.2 | Average number of legislative sittings in 2018–19 compared to 2020–21

Province/Territory legislature	Average legislature sittings, 2020–21	Average legislature sittings, 2018–19	Change (%)
Nova Scotia	17.5	46.5	–62.4
Saskatchewan	31.5	67.0	–53.0
Manitoba	34.5	68.0	–49.3
Yukon	35.0	60.0	–41.7
British Columbia	44.5	65.5	–32.1
New Brunswick	28.0	38.0	–26.3
Ontario	67.0	89.0	–24.7
Quebec	58.5	71.0	–17.6
Nunavut	35.5	42.5	–16.5
Northwest Territories	40.0	46.5	–14.0
Prince Edward Island	37.0	41.0	–9.8
Newfoundland and Labrador	48.0	53.0	–9.4
Alberta	86.0	91.0	–5.5

Provincial and territorial legislatures reduced sittings by 5.5 to 62 per cent (January 2020–December 2021).

Sources: Department of Health 2020; Government of Alberta 2020e; Government of British Columbia 2020b, 2020c, 2020d; Government of Manitoba 2020b, 2020c; Government of New Brunswick 2020a, 2020b; Government of Nova Scotia 2020b, 2020d; Government of Ontario 2020c; Government of PEI 2020b; Government of Yukon 2020a; House of Assembly Newfoundland and Labrador, n.d.; Legislative Assembly of Alberta, n.d.; Legislative Assembly of British Columbia, n.d.; Legislative Assembly of Manitoba, n.d.; Legislative Assembly of New Brunswick, n.d.a, n.d.b; Legislative Assembly of the Northwest Territories, n.d.; Legislative Assembly of Nunavut, n.d.; Legislative Assembly of Ontario, n.d.a., n.d.b; Legislative Assembly of Prince Edward Island, n.d.a, n.d.b; Legislative Assembly of Saskatchewan, n.d.; Locke et al. 2020; National Assembly of Quebec 2021; Nova Scotia Legislature, n.d.; Office of the Premier of New Brunswick 2020b; Office of the Premier of Ontario 2020; Ontario Solicitor General 2020; Prince Edward Island Health and Wellness 2020; Province of British Columbia 2020a, 2020b; Yukon Legislative Assembly 2021.

deficit and went more than two years without tabling a budget, a record length of time. After nearly two years of virtual and hybrid Parliament, the government put forward a proposal to continue the hybrid format. Many were concerned that this would allow elected officials to evade scrutiny and accountability, while others supported it, arguing it could be a positive process change and enable Members of Parliament (MPs) to attend Parliament from their offices or homes and address responsibilities in their ridings (Woolf 2021).

Provincial and territorial legislatures operated differently, including in their use of in-person, online, and hybrid meeting formats. Some continued to hold legislative house sittings, while others greatly reduced the sittings held throughout the pandemic. For example, the Nova Scotia legislature did not sit between 10 March and 18 December 2020 and had an over 82 per cent reduction in legislative sittings, whereas Alberta reduced average legislative sittings by 14 per cent in 2020–21 compared to 2018–19 (Nova Scotia Legislature, n.d.). Most provinces and territories decreased their average sittings by more than half in 2020–21 compared to 2018–19. Across all provinces and territories the average number of legislative sittings declined by approximately 28 per cent. Table 4.2 outlines the percentage change in average sittings between January 2020 and December 2021 and 2018–19.

Judicial proceedings across Canada were affected by the spread of COVID-19, and the justice system altered processes to accommodate virtual operations (Ministry of Justice, n.d.; Law Society of Saskatchewan 2020; Morawetz 2020; Alberta Court of Appeal 2020; Province of British Columbia 2020a). Courts suspended activities except for emergency proceedings. Regulations were altered, and decision makers had discretion to waive, suspend, or extend time periods related to their powers (Attorney General of British Columbia 2020a; Government of Alberta 2020d).

Governance boards for corporations and not-for-profit organizations also altered their operations. Changes were required to enable organizations to conduct official business remotely (Government of PEI 2020b; Government of British Columbia 2020c; Office of the Premier of Ontario 2020; Office of the Premier of New Brunswick 2020a; Government of Manitoba 2020c). Not every organization was able to transition easily to virtual operations. Concerns were raised that online meetings protected executives and directors from proper scrutiny, and investors called for new rules to be established for virtual annual general meetings (Trichur 2021).

CONCLUSION

After a slow start, governments' reactions to the pandemic in March 2020 were swift; major policy announcements were made daily. Many of these directives had immediate effect, on a scale that one could not have imagined days earlier. Governments' actions were also blunt: quarantine, lockdown, gathering limits, border closures, and income-support programs, such as CERB. When consequences are potentially catastrophic, conventional cost-benefit analyses do not hold – survival is the main concern. In the face of such uncertainty we should expect a degree of over-allocation of resources for particularly consequential failures; we should also tolerate mistakes if they are made with good intentions and with a capacity to learn and adjust – it is often better to be proactive. (For further discussion on the precautionary principle see chapters 9 and 11.)

There were mistakes in governments' economic programs. Income inequality initially increased and then decreased with the help of federal support programs; however, these impacts changed again in 2021 and 2022 as support programs were altered, inflation significantly increased, and mortgage and rental costs grew. Governments initially overlooked students, seasonal workers, and the needs of persons with disabilities; they subsidized non-viable businesses – in some cases, businesses that did not need the cash – and paid benefits to individuals who may not have needed them, including over 300,000 teens, many of whom lived at home with their parents. While some people repaid payments made in error, there was a level of fraud among claimants of government benefits. There were also inconvenient truths: while many lost their jobs and lived in precarious circumstances, some benefited financially during the pandemic through the housing and stock markets.

Most would agree that the crisis necessitated a significant economic response from government. Ultimately, the federal government borrowed approximately $700 billion. Perhaps the most significant criticism of the federal government's fiscal response to the crisis was that it borrowed and spent too much for too long (J. Cochrane and Hartley 2022). Together with the monetary policy of the Bank of Canada, this drove up inflation. While Canada experienced the second-lowest inflation rate among G7 countries (Hockaday 2022), it was still significant and by 2022 had caused economic uncertainty for most and hardship for many.

Governments did loosen standards for certain sectors as they started to understand better the challenges and trade-offs. Some rolled back certain health restrictions for some communities or types of business if case counts dropped to a certain level, for example. Governments such as those of Ontario and New Brunswick introduced colour-coded systems to categorize communities as high or low risk.

Normal democratic checks were reduced. It is often noted in emergency-response literature that non-democratic states address emergencies more effectively because they act decisively without reference to democratic accountability or individual freedoms (Paris and Welsh 2021). We certainly saw this in China's lockdown of Wuhan. While Canada's public institutions persevered, democratic accountability was curtailed. True, the prime minister met with the press frequently, but Parliament met much less frequently, and budgets were not tabled. The largest spending in Canada since the Second World War was not scrutinized by the House of Commons in the way it normally would be.

One aspect of control that was enforced aggressively by both democratic and non-democratic states was border control. After decades of growing global trade and political and economic agreements that saw a freer flow of goods, services, and people, governments found themselves unable to take responsibility for other jurisdictions and, as such, imposed rules strictly in their own jurisdictions and made it difficult for people to enter. Borders thickened across all Western countries and, in Canada, included restrictions on interprovincial travel. The aggressive stance was ironic because throughout the H1N1 episode, governments had underscored that closing borders had little impact on disease spread (B. Walsh 2009). There is a further paradox in that while most governments acted forcefully within their jurisdictions, they were never really free to act independently. Recall that Canada did not act with conviction until the CDC had acknowledged the gravity of its concerns at the end of February 2020. Within Canada, provincial and territorial cases, hospitalizations, and ICU occupancy were always being compared across provinces as well as to those of the US and Europe.

Governments' principal preoccupation was stability. Rules were enacted at least initially to contain the spread of COVID-19 and limit the pressure on ICUs in particular; the strong precautionary stance against disease spread created economic problems but also problems in parts of the health sector, notably LTC, mental health and addictions, and less urgent medical treatments.

Governments' standards were shaped by the conventions of containing disease transmission and constitutional responsibilities, all within a bureaucratic paradigm. Government bureaucracies have benefits and disadvantages (Hood 1998; Aucoin 1997). They can gather considerable resources and apply them to massive social and economic problems that markets on their own cannot adequately address. They can secure expertise and stability and clarify accountability in uncertain times. They can also standardize rules across massive geographic spaces in the name of fairness. There can be challenges. Bureaucracies can be slow and expensive; they are not very flexible. Massive operations often result in mistakes, and these mistakes can be swept under the rug in such a large organization. Standardization can lack nuance. The (at times) rigid top-down accountability structures can lead to part of the organization fixing a problem but, in so doing, creating problems elsewhere.

Once new rules and processes were in place, it was difficult for governments to roll them back. Different degrees of risk tolerance among the population, together with the tenuous nature of any improvement and a media culture ready to amplify mistakes and personal testimonies by anxious members of the public, made governments reticent to roll back precautionary policies, programs, and processes. There were rarely any clear processes or tools to guide governments in making these decisions other than perhaps watching case, ICU, and death counts and following the advice of public health officials and the lead of other high-profile jurisdictions.

This leads us to our final aspect of cybernetics, behaviour modification. However dramatic governments' declarations were, they had to compel behaviour change to be effective. Indeed, behaviours did change in light of governments' standards; as we will see, some changes were intended, some were not.

5

Behaviour Modification 1: The Public's Choices and the Cascading Impacts of Government Directives

Behaviour modification refers to the preferences, incentive structures, beliefs, and attitudes that shape systems; the capacity to modify behaviour of participants is the capacity to change systems. Behaviour modification is often the most difficult, intrusive, and controversial aspect of controlling a system. It can include subtle persuasion and nudging, to education and training, to enforcing restrictions, to incentives, penalties, and prison time. The most effective behaviour change occurs due to culture change when desired changes simply occur without much thought because it seems natural. Such behaviour-change methods are slow and expensive. While governments spend much of their time studying public problems and debating policies, they are often cautious when it comes to compelling behaviour change. It can be very unpopular and difficult to enforce.

There are three particularly striking aspects of behaviour change during the pandemic that we will focus on in this chapter. First, we will examine how quickly and willingly people accepted changes directed at containing the disease, like staying at home, socially distancing, and wearing masks. These demands were unprecedented in living memory. After two months of governments describing the virus as low risk, the change in narrative in March 2020 led to far-reaching public health directives that would effectively shut down much of society. There was considerable public anxiety, and people largely accepted the direction of public health officials and elected governments.

Secondly, the focus on containing the spread of COVID-19 led to effects across community health. Many health-care procedures were deferred; mental-health issues spiked, and physical activities decreased. Third and relatedly, there were significant changes in community living, in the number of marriages and births as well as in the products and services we bought and how we bought them. Most crime went down although some, like domestic violence, almost certainly increased. The not-for-profit-sector, often a critical support for the vulnerable, was highly constrained during the pandemic.

This chapter brings into focus how people responded to government directives and the cascading effects of those directives. Intended or not, governments' interventions included trade-offs in how people would live and the choices they would make to be better protected from COVID-19. For the most part, this chapter does not repeat the key outcomes data summarized in chapter 1, which focuses on the system and the case, hospitalization, ICU, and death counts, or people's willingness to be tested for COVID-19, which is captured in chapter 3. Chapter 9 has a more complete discussion of the economic impacts.

RESPONSES TO RESTRICTIONS:
PHYSICAL DISTANCING AND MASKS

Physical Distancing

When public health officials enacted physical-distancing measures – two metres, or six feet, between individuals – workplaces that were allowed to stay open needed to ensure that employees and customers were able to stay at a distance. Many installed plexiglass barriers between customer and employee, mandated mask-wearing, reduced the number of people in a space at one time, and marked the floor with directional arrows to ensure one-way foot traffic in narrow aisles. As businesses were permitted to reopen during the spring and summer of 2020, many of these changes stayed in place.

Such changes are easier to incorporate in some workplaces than others. Up to 40 per cent of the workforce worked from home and often met through online means. (For a more complete discussion about working from home see chapter 9.) It was much more difficult to separate workers at factories and warehouses, which became hotspots for COVID-19 outbreaks. In the US, Amazon reported 19,816 confirmed COVID-19 cases in a workforce of 1.37 million (1.5 per cent) between 1 March and 19 September (not including workers in contracted third-party delivery networks and not directly employed by Amazon; A. Palmer 2020). Amazon facilities in Canada were also affected, as COVID-19 outbreaks occurred at multiple facilities in Ontario (T. Grant 2021).

Many organizations cancelled events due to COVID-19 restrictions or made the transition to virtual events. According to Canada's destination-marketing organization Destination Canada (DC 2020b), 84 per cent of 2020 events were cancelled (e.g., conferences, concerts, festivals). COVID-19 restrictions changed how organizations conducted their meetings and events. Many industry leaders found benefits in virtual meetings, including reduced event costs and increased diversity in audience participation from wider geographical areas. At the same time, just over 50 per cent of event marketers were challenged by the logistics of virtual events, and 68 per cent believed it was more challenging to provide networking opportunities virtually (Bizzabo 2020).

Limits on the size of social gatherings were part of many COVID-19 regulations, including event sizes, sport spectators, and visitors to households. Both organizations and families made the transition to online events to remain in contact. Significant life events such as graduations, weddings, and funerals were celebrated with few or no attendees, or online.

The pandemic altered how people mourn. In the early stages there were high rates of COVID-19 transmission among funeral attendees. In early April 2020 more than half the known cases in Newfoundland and Labrador were connected to one funeral home (McKenzie-Sutter 2020). Many funeral homes upgraded technology to enable virtual services (MacLean 2021a). In some of the worst cases around the world many who died of COVID-19 needed to be buried with little or no ceremony (McCann 2020). For example, in India cremation pyres were created in parking lots, city parks, and other open spaces, in addition to crematoriums, to conduct a semblance of a funeral ceremony (Sethi 2021). There are many significant religious and cultural implications for death that were challenged due to the pandemic, as well as many social gathering traditions in the mourning period that have been disrupted and, at times, transformed (Mikles 2021).

Masks

Early in the pandemic, procuring PPE such as medical masks for health-care workers was a significant undertaking. Deputy Prime Minister Chrystia Freeland described the market dynamics as "the Wild West" (Reynolds 2020, para. 12). As jurisdictions sought PPE for health-care and other essential workers, guidance on public masking changed. The CDC and PHAC changed their advice on mask-wearing (Gollum 2020), for instance, following a change in early April 2020 by the WHO, which began recommending the use of non-medical masks in public spaces. Within a week of the CDC announcement, the number of Americans who reported wearing a mask in public increased from 38 to 62 per cent (Gollum 2020).

Mandatory mask-wearing regulations for non-health-care professionals began with the travel and transportation sector. Early on, most mask regulations focused on travellers, especially in airports. As of 3 June 2020, all people involved in federally regulated transportation in Canada needed to wear masks – including travellers and employees (Transport Canada 2020a). Mandatory masking regulations varied from province to province. Nova Scotia became the first to enact province-wide universal masking in all indoor public spaces on 31 July 2020 (Government of Nova Scotia 2020c). From this point on, mandatory mask regulations were implemented across the country.

Most people came to accept wearing masks. Between 3 and 19 April 2020 the number of masked people in public areas increased from one in five to one in three across Canada (Jedwab 2020a). By May, 65 per cent of people agreed that they should wear a face mask in public; 81 per cent agreed that masks should be worn for personal services, such as hair salons (Gollum 2020). By July, wearing a protective mask while grocery shopping increased from one in five to nearly two in three (Jedwab 2020b). In addition to more members of the public wearing masks voluntarily, many retailers and transportation organizations such as Uber required customers to wear masks (Gollum 2020).

Not everyone sees risk the same way; there were some nuances. Fear of the virus influenced whether someone wore a mask, with those least afraid of the virus being the least likely to wear one (Jedwab 2020a). Women and people born outside Canada were more likely to wear a mask, whereas men, people born in Canada, and francophones continued to be less likely to wear a mask than other groups (Jedwab 2020b). By July 2020, people living in urban or suburban areas, and those over fifty-five, were more likely to wear a mask than other groups; people living in rural areas were less so. In some respects this can be seen as rational; COVID-19 rates were often lower in rural communities and there is more space to distance from others. Polling also revealed conflicted feelings about wearing masks. By September, 87 per cent of respondents felt that wearing a mask was a civic duty; despite the high level of support, 21 per cent also said wearing a mask was an infringement of personal rights and freedoms, which represented a 6 per cent decrease from July 2020 (Berthiaume 2020a).

Although a subject of debate throughout the pandemic, mask-wearing lowers virus transmission according to many studies (Howard et al. 2021; Brooks and Butler 2021; Cheng et al. 2021; Leech et al. 2022).

In a 2020 study, Leffler et al. found that mandatory mask-wearing in Canada lowered the number of new weekly cases by 22 per cent. Leech et al. (2022) studied ninety-two regions (countries and US states) and found that mask-wearing lowered transmission by 19 per cent on average. The efficacy of mask-wearing, however, can also depend on people doing it consistently and in combination with other measures, such as social distancing.

Enforcement of Directives

For the most part, behaviour changes resulted from public health disseminating information to the public and establishing directives, and the public voluntarily following these directives. Still, at times, these directives had to be enforced. Specific directives and enforcement mechanisms varied by jurisdiction, as well as the degree to which directives were enforced by authorities. Between March 2020 and January 2021 there were nearly 38,000 reported violations of provincial or territorial COVID-19 regulations. By the end of June 2020, Canadians had accumulated approximately $13 million in COVID-related fines. According to the Canadian Civil Liberties Association (CCLA), nearly 77 per cent of all fines at this time were assessed in Quebec. Ontario had the second-highest number of fines at this point, followed by Nova Scotia and Alberta (Deshman 2020; A. Russell 2020). The number of fines in Quebec and Ontario is not surprising as they are Canada's most populous provinces, but Nova Scotia issued the most tickets per capita (CCLA and Policing the Pandemic Mapping Project 2021a).

A study by the CCLA indicated a large increase in such fines during the second wave towards the end of 2020 compared to the first wave (Snyder 2021). CCLA's study found that, overall, Manitoba and Quebec were the most punitive but, unlike in the first wave, Nova Scotia had become the least punitive of the jurisdictions studied (CCLA and Policing the Pandemic Mapping Project 2021b; Snyder 2021). During the second wave Ontario, British Columbia, and Nova Scotia issued between 0.21 and 0.28 tickets per 1,000 people between October 2020 and February 2021. During this time Quebec issued 0.51 and Manitoba 0.69 tickets per 1,000 residents (CCLA and Policing the Pandemic Mapping Project 2021b). Data on COVID-19 fines are inconsistent due to varied reporting requirements, but it is informative to see that the control mechanism in place was not applied consistently across the country. The CCLA argued that strict measures, such as the evening curfew in Quebec and the use of a private security firm to levy fines in Manitoba, were not the most effective measures for COVID-19 containment. The CCLA empha-sizes that before vaccines were distributed in Canada, Quebec had some of the highest rates of cases, and Manitoba struggled to contain cases, compared to provinces of similar size (Snyder 2021).

In 2021 the number of violations dropped compared to 2020, to approximately 24,224 violations and/or calls to the RCMP related to provincial and territorial COVID-19 regulations (Statistics Canada 2022o). The number of fines associated are unknown, and, in fact, by the end of 2021, more than $1.5 million worth of COVID-19 fines in Ontario were unpaid (Hristova 2022).

With respect to fines for violations of the federal Quarantine Act, the PHAC website noted 19,000 tickets had been issued across Canada between March 2020 and September 2022 (PHAC 2023; CBC News 2022a). The PHAC does not track whether fines have been paid. Fines varied from $825 to $5,000. In 2022 a traveller entering the country without a pre-arrival COVID-19 test was the most common federal COVID-19 offence (CBC News 2022a).

Although regulations were put in place to empower police, not all regulations were embraced by police forces. At times, police opted not to issue tickets at mass protests, choosing instead to keep order (Gatehouse 2020a; Villani 2020; Warick 2020; CBC News 2020c). In Alberta, for example, police officials felt they received mixed messages from the provincial government and were concerned that government saw the issuing of fines as heavy handed and did not want the courts overburdened (CBC News 2021a). A group of fifteen active and four retired police officers from several forces in Ontario challenged the constitutionality of COVID-19 restrictions (Loriggio 2021). The group claimed that enforcement of the restrictions was a breach of a police officer's oath to uphold the Constitution of Canada and that restrictions on interprovincial travel violated the Charter of Rights and Freedoms. They also claimed that the regulations were too broad and vague to enforce uniformly and fairly. The position of the Toronto Police Service was that the emergency legislation was lawful.

CASCADING EFFECTS ACROSS HEALTH CARE

Health-Care Disruptions and Undiagnosed Diseases

COVID-19 disrupted health care for many individuals and delayed thou-sands of diagnoses and treatments for severe diseases, such as cancer and heart disease – both leading causes of death globally. In 2020 cancer caused 26.4 per cent and heart disease caused 17.5 per cent of deaths in Canada, with higher mortality rates in lower-income neighbourhoods (Statistics Canada 2022b). Scientists estimated that lockdown measures used to contain COVID-19 could increase risk of obesity, heart disease, and chronic illnesses such as diabetes (Clemmensen, Petersen, and Sørensen 2020). Ischemic heart disease is a leading cause of death around the world, for example, and caused 16 per cent of global deaths in 2019. Heart disease also had the largest increases in mortality globally since 2000 (WHO 2020j).

COVID-19 caused disruptions to diagnoses of heart disease, especially in economically disadvantaged areas (Einstein et al. 2021). A survey of in-patient and outpatient centres performing cardiac procedures across more than one hundred countries found that procedures had decreased 42 per cent in March 2020 compared to March 2019, and 64 per cent in April 2020 compared to March 2019. The decrease in procedures was greater in countries with lower GDP where there was an additional 22 per cent reduction in cardiac procedures and less availability of PPE and telehealth (Einstein et al. 2021). Between 2021 and 2022 in Canada the leading causes of hospitalization were giving birth (2.1 days), COVID-19 (10.1 days), heart failure (9.2 days), heart attack (4.9 days), and substance use disorders (5.4 days) (CIHI 2023).

Globally, cancer accounted for ten million deaths in 2020 (WHO 2021b). Early detection can help prolong life, but disruptions to healthcare systems meant that many people did not seek or could not obtain timely screening or treatment (*Lancet* 2021). According to Statistics Canada, a six-month delay in primary screening for colorectal cancers could lead to 2,200 cases and 960 more cancer deaths. For breast cancers a six-month delay could lead to 670 more cases diagnosed at an advanced stage and 250 more deaths between 2020 and 2029 in Canada (Statistics Canada 2021h).

Signals from other Western countries revealed similar disturbing patterns at the start of the pandemic. A UK study found that 45 per cent of those with potential cancer symptoms did not contact their doctor during the UK's first wave of the pandemic (March–August 2020), and approximately 40,000 fewer people than normal started cancer treatment (*Lancet* 2021). In April 2021 the UK National Health Service reported that over 4.6 million people were on surgical wait-lists, the majority of which were cancer patients, and 300,000 were waiting for more than twelve months (100 times higher than the pre-pandemic wait-list; *Lancet* 2021). Delays in diagnosis due to COVID-19 could result in approximately 3,500 avoidable cancer deaths in the UK (Hogan and Glanz 2020). A study conducted in Australia's state of Victoria found there were approximately 2,500 missed cancer diagnoses in the first six months of the pandemic (*Lancet* 2021). One-third of European countries partially or completely interrupted cancer-care services early in the pandemic (WHO 2021d). Experts fear similar trends in Canada (Hogan and Glanz 2020).

In Canada thousands of surgeries deemed non-essential, non-urgent, or elective were cancelled and delayed. The governments of Ontario and British Columbia officially called for hospitals to cancel non-urgent surgeries, and indeed many hospitals and clinics decided to cancel surgeries and procedures to maintain surge capacity (Zussman 2020; Crawley 2021b). Between the start of the pandemic and December 2021 an average of 35,000 fewer surgeries were performed in Canada each month compared to previous years (CIHI 2021a). The biggest declines were in cataract surgeries and in hip and knee replacements. Other procedures with significant delays included sight restoration, less essential heart surgeries, and diagnostic imaging (Canadian Medical Association 2020). By spring 2021, models in Ontario indicated that the province had a surgical backlog of 250,000 procedures (CityNews Toronto 2021).

Physical Activity

The lockdowns enacted by governments generated negative consequences for healthy living. During the pandemic many people changed their behaviours regarding alcohol and cannabis consumption, physical activity, and healthy eating. Increases in alcohol and drug use, and deaths due to overdose, contribute to the significant cost of diseases and chronic conditions (*Lancet* 2020). In Canada younger adults who were born in the country were more likely to increase these negative health behaviours compared to older and immigrant Canadians. Adults who reported negative financial impacts due to COVID-19 were also more likely to increase all these negative health behaviours (Zajacova et al. 2020; MHCC 2021). Nearly one in four Canadians who consumed alcohol before the pandemic believed their consumption increased during the pandemic, while nearly one in five decreased their consumption (Statistics Canada 2021a). Approximately one in three who consumed cannabis before the pandemic increased their consumption during the pandemic, while 12 per cent reported a decrease in consumption. Young people (fifteen to twenty-nine years old) were most likely to decrease their consumption of alcohol (33 per cent of respondents) and increase their consumption of cannabis (43 per cent of respondents) (Statistics Canada 2021a).

As fitness and recreational facilities closed during lockdowns, many people needed to find alternative ways to exercise. Some turned to in-home gym equipment, and others engaged in recreational activities outdoors. Revenues from health and fitness equipment more than doubled between March and October 2020 (Shaban 2021); treadmill sales increased by 135 per cent, and stationary-bike sales tripled. Peloton, a major supplier of stationary bikes, reported a 232 per cent increase in revenue in 2020 compared to 2019, with high demand especially in spring and summer 2020. Many people used technology to engage in fitness activities, such as online classes and fitness apps. Sensor Tower, a mobile app marketing intelligence agency, reported 2.5 billion health and fitness app downloads globally from January to November 2020, a 47 per cent increase from the same period in 2019, while digital sales for Nike increased by 84 per cent compared to 2019 (Shaban 2021).

Cycling and hiking were also popular forms of exercise in 2020, especially once national and provincial parks reopened. In Canada national parks experienced an overall 2 per cent increase in visitors in 2020 compared to 2019 (Parks Canada 2021). National parks closest to urban centres experienced a considerable bump in numbers (Bain 2021).

There were concerns that changes in physical activity due to COVID-19 lockdown measures could lead to increased risk of chronic diseases such as cardiovascular disease, obesity, diabetes, and cancer. Before the pandemic one in five Canadians was estimated to meet a minimum 150 minutes of physical activity per week (Colley, Bushnik, and Langlois 2020). Studies noted that active people maintained or increased their physical activity during the pandemic, whereas inactive people became less active (Zajacova et al. 2020). This behaviour poses a risk of increased cardiovascular disease. A survey conducted in April 2021 found that only 8.8 per cent of respondents were able to manage mealtimes properly, and 42.3 per cent of Canadians had gained unintentional weight since March 2020 (Charlebois and Music 2021). If Canadians reduce their physical activity by 40 per cent, researchers estimate there will be nearly 4,850 additional people who will develop cardiovascular disease by 2023 (Manuel et al. 2021).[1]

Mental Health

The 2021 *World Happiness Report* reported that most developed countries saw a decline in mental health during the pandemic compared to 2017–19 data (Helliwell et al. 2021).[2] COVID-19 had especially worsened pre-existing mental-health inequalities across age, gender, and ethnic lines (Helliwell et al. 2021). In the UK, women reported the most significant declines in their mental health across all age groups. Both women and men aged sixteen to thirty-four reported larger than average changes in the quality of their mental health. Men aged thirty-five to sixty-four reported the least amount of change in quality of mental health between 2019 and 2020 (Helliwell et al. 2021). There are concerns that the increased burden on mental-health services in the future will heighten mental-health inequalities (Helliwell et al. 2021). The estimated cost of mental-health issues resulting from COVID-19 in 2020 was approximately $20,000 per person per year in the US (Cutler and Summers 2020).

Similar trends were observed in Canada. In 2021 all age groups (over twelve years) self-reported decreases in their mental health, especially women and young adults aged eighteen to twenty-four. Adults over sixty-five reported the least amount of change in their mental health throughout the pandemic (Statistics Canada 2023a).

In fact, Canadians have been reporting declining mental health since 2015. Between 2015 and 2021 the prevalence of anxiety and mood disorders increased by 2.6 per cent and 1.7 per cent respectively, especially among women, and has been highest in Ontario, Saskatchewan, and the Atlantic provinces (excluding Prince Edward Island). MHCC estimated the economic impacts of poor mental health to be $50 billion annually ($23.8 billion being non-dementia-related care), or approximately $1,400 per Canadian in 2016 (MHCC 2017).[3] Mental health and addictions have been growing public health concerns, especially over the past ten years and with increased attention on the opioid crisis. There are many barriers to accessing mental-health services, including cost, which in Canada generally falls to the individual or private insurance because coverage is not required under the Canada Health Act. Federal government investment in mental-health care has been increasing due to evolving social perceptions and attitudes about mental health and addictions. In 2015, Canada spent 7.2 per cent of the total health-care budget on mental-health services. This was lower than that of other G8 countries at the time; for example, England spent 13.0 per cent of its health-care budget on mental-health services (MHCC 2017). The pandemic brought even more attention to the issue.

During the pandemic the federal government created a web-based mental-health and addictions portal, "Wellness Together," to support Canadians dealing with mental-health issues due to COVID-19. The portal offers resources such as online courses, peer support groups, counselling resources, and information. Wellness Together had been accessed by 428,000 Canadians by 10 September 2020. Nearly half of the users were children and young people, and 42 per cent of texting users identified themselves as 2SLGBTQIA+ (Government of Canada 2022a, 156). Community organizations also take on the provision of many mental-health and addictions services (Eaton 2021).

In July 2020 the number of service requests to Canada's suicide-prevention service, Crisis Services Canada,[4] had doubled since March 2020 (PHAC 2020d). MHCC (2021) reported that 38 per cent of Canadians self-reporting their mental health said it had declined due to COVID-19, with 10 per cent reporting suicidal thoughts, and 4 per cent having tried to harm themselves. Despite the decrease in suicide rates overall, there were 3,675 more police-reported suicides and attempted suicides between 2019 and 2020, and an increase of 4,563 calls between 2019 and 2021 (Statistics Canada 20220).

Based on available data, suicide claimed the lives of 3,839 Canadians in 2020, a decline of 14.7 per cent from the nearly 4,500 reported in both 2019 and 2018. Based on reporting delays, however, this figure could be underestimated by 5 to 16 per cent. Deaths by suicide, accident, and homicide often require lengthy investigations, creating delays in reporting the data to Statistics Canada (2022c).

Kids Help Phone is a volunteer-led service that provides online and telephone-based counselling to youth across Canada. During 2020, Kids Help Phone received over four million requests for support – more than double the number of calls and texts received in 2019 (Yousif 2020; Kids Help Phone, n.d.). Towards the end of 2020, Kids Help Phone received more than 800 requests a day, with approximately ten of those being active suicide rescues. Most of these requests came from Ontario, Alberta, and British Columbia (Yousif 2020; Kids Help Phone, n.d.). Experts speculate that the increase in people reaching out for suicide rescue and mental-health support may have contributed to the decline in suicide rates (Shah 2021). Experts also note that the "pull-together effect" (Fletcher 2021b, para. 24), or the increased sense of community support during the pandemic, may have made people feel more connected to their community (Shah 2021).

Overdose-related deaths are also key to assessing suicide data. There are cases in which overdoses are incorrectly reported as suicides, and vice versa. Overdose deaths have increased in Canada in recent years and significantly so during the pandemic, especially in Indigenous communities (Fletcher 2021b; CDC 2020a; Bokat-Lindell 2021; CBC News 2021k). There was an increase in deaths due to accidents and substance-related harms in 2020. There were 4,604 deaths due to accidental poisonings, including overdoses, in 2020, which was nearly 20 per cent higher than in 2019 (3,705), comparable to the height of the pre-pandemic opioid crisis in 2017 (4,830) and 2018 (4,501). The largest increase in deaths occurred in people aged forty to forty-four. There were also increases in alcohol-induced deaths in 2020.[5] Among people under forty-five, such deaths increased by nearly 50 per cent (542) over the 2017–19 figures (360). There was also a 17.5 per cent increase in the number of alcohol-induced deaths in people aged forty-five to sixty-four in 2020 (1,946) compared to 2017–19 (1,656) (Statistics Canada 2022b).

CASCADING EFFECTS ACROSS CONSUMER BEHAVIOURS AND THE COMMUNITY

Family Life: Marriage, Babies, Divorces, and Pet Adoptions

There were many changes to family life due to COVID-19, such as decisions to get married and grow families. Despite the various restrictions on social gatherings, about 176,000 Canadians married between 2019 and 2020 (Statistics Canada 2021d), which represents a decrease from each of the previous five years. At the beginning of the pandemic there was speculation that lockdown measures would result in a baby boom as seen in past crises when people were confined together for short periods, such as power failures, storms, or terror attacks (M. Kearney and Levine 2020b). In fact, the historical perspective on these matters should be interpreted differently. The Great Recession of 2007–09 and the Spanish flu of 1918, which are likely better points of comparison with COVID-19 due to their duration and economic and social consequences, resulted in a reduction in births (Kearney and Levine 2020b). Like these events, the circumstances of COVID-19 did not generate a baby boom. In fact, Canada's fertility rate dropped to a record low of 1.4 in 2020, with the lowest number of births recorded since 2007 (Statistics Canada 2022e). The pandemic also altered Canadians' plans for children: 14 per cent delayed their plans to have children, while 11 per cent reduced the number of children they intended to have (Statistics Canada 2022e). According to data from the Brookings Institution, the primary reasons for delaying were financial hardship and uncertainty, the closure of schools and daycare centres, and stress (M. Kearney and Levine 2020a; Fostik and Galbraith 2021, 3). Data from the US, Italy, France, Germany, Spain, and the UK indicate that women in these countries made similar decisions (Broster 2021).

The number of divorces in Canada in 2020 decreased by 25 per cent from 2019, the largest year-over-year decrease since the Divorce Act was enacted in 1968 and the lowest rate recorded since 1973 (Statistics Canada 2022f, 1). While many law firms reported increased demand for divorce services and enquiries about proceedings, with firms in Ontario reporting a 40 per cent rise (Bowden 2020), temporary closures and disruptions to court services contributed to a lower divorce rate in Canada (Statistics Canada 2022f, 2). In the US there were increases in the use of online divorce contracts and web searches for ending a relationship or initiating divorce proceedings. The UK, China, and Sweden experienced similar patterns (Savage 2020). Globally speaking, divorce rates increased by approximately 30 per cent during the first year of the pandemic (E. Lloyd 2021).

Online dating increased during the pandemic because people were no longer able to meet others at school, work, or events. At the beginning of the pandemic online dating platforms such as Tinder experienced a 10 to 15 per cent increase in use between February and March 2020 (Karantzas 2020). Tinder also experienced its busiest year in terms of user engagement (Shaw 2021; Tinder Newsroom 2021).

With fewer weddings and children being born, people needed company, hence the surge in pet adoptions. Many shelters in Canada experienced high demand for pet adoptions as people worked from home and were under stay-at-home orders (CBC News 2020g). Online searches for "pet adoption," "dog adoption," and "cat adoption" peaked between April and May 2020 and were 250 per cent higher than the average for the previous five years (J. Ho, Hussain, and Sparagano 2021). It is estimated that approximately 3 per cent of Canadian adults, who did not have a pet before the start of the pandemic, had adopted one by June 2021 (Coletto 2021). Abandonment and acts of animal cruelty were also reported during the pandemic. The data suggest that the uptake in pet adoption offset the rate of abandonment in shelters at this time. Rumours circulated during the pandemic that animals such as dogs could be reservoirs for COVID-19, which influenced animal cruelty around the world (J. Ho, Hussain, and Sparagano 2021). There were pet kidnappings for ransom. Many pet owners may not have taken their pets for checkups and elective procedures, which could have an impact on the long-term health of these animals. There were also reported shortages of veterinary care products and pet food during the pandemic (J. Ho, Hussain, and Sparagano 2021). Following the easing of lockdown measures and the return to work, many shelters spoke out about the increases in pet abandonment they had experienced (CBC News 2022b; G. Jaeger 2022; H. Lee 2022).

Retail Consumer Behaviour

When stay-at-home orders were announced, many people raced to stores to stock up on supplies. In the week of 11 March 2020, grocery sales increased by 38 per cent, which is 16 per cent higher than the usual busiest shopping week of the year – the lead-up to Christmas and New Year's Day (Statistics Canada 2020b). New consumer behaviours emerged to prepare for the pandemic as early as the end of January when international headlines noted the virus spread. Sales of hand sanitizer were up by 477 per cent at the end of January, and by 639 per cent in the week of 14 March, over the previous year (Statistics Canada 2020b). Mask and glove sales increased by 122 per cent at the end of January, and by 377 per cent in the week of March 14, compared to the same weeks in 2019. Canadians also bought more dry goods and storable foods. Purchases of rice had increased by 239 per cent by the end of the week of 14 March, compared to 2019 (Statistics Canada 2020b). Purchases of baking supplies, such as flour and yeast, also increased as stay-at-home orders continued (Van Rosendaal 2020). News about toilet-paper stockpiling spread across the media and quickly became an Internet sensation. Despite the prevalence of the headlines, toilet-paper purchases in Canada had peaked by the end of the week of 14 March, with an increase of 241 per cent over 2019 (Statistics Canada 2020b).

Although common before COVID-19, online shopping surged during the pandemic as consumers sought alternatives to going personally to stores. Market observers expect online shopping to continue to grow after the pandemic, particularly among younger generations. A survey conducted in Toronto, Vancouver, and Montreal found that younger generations such as Gen Z bought more of all types of goods online. The survey also found that people who worked from home were more likely to buy goods online – even before the pandemic started (Gooding and Moro 2020). Many businesses pivoted to e-commerce for retail. There were increases in e-commerce transactions between 2018–19 and 2020 (January to May 2020) across every product category. The most significant increases were in electronics and appliances, furniture and home furnishings, sporting goods, hobbies, books and music, and food and beverages (Aston et al. 2020).

There was a 1.3 per cent decrease in total commodities and services purchased between 2019 and 2020, followed by an 11.8 per cent increase between 2020 and 2021 (Statistics Canada 2021n). Generally, products for domestic use had a bump in sales, whereas products for use outside the home saw a decrease. There were increases for specific products and services through retail stores between 2019 and 2020, such as soft drinks and alcoholic beverages, cannabis products, home furniture and furnishings, housewares, appliances and electronics, many sporting and leisure products, recreational vehicles, home health products, infant care products, personal and beauty products, hardware, tools, and garden products (Statistics Canada 2021n). Specific products and services that faced decreases in retail sales between 2019 and 2020 included clothing, footwear, jewellery, luggage, publications, audio and video recordings, game software, motor vehicles, and motor vehicle parts and accessories (Statistics Canada 2021n). Most of the categories that suffered drops in 2020 bounced back somewhat at retail stores in 2021. As people saved money by staying at home, there was also an increase in the purchase of some luxury items. Between 2020 and 2021 there were significant increases in sales of vehicles, clothing, footwear, jewellery, and luggage.

In any high-dread context with a risk of social disorder there is interest in people's propensity to buy guns for security (Quigley 2008). There were reports of surges in gun purchases in the US early in the pandemic, particularly in areas severely affected by COVID-19 (Perkel 2020). Data on background checks showed that 85 per cent more guns were sold in March 2020 than in March 2019, with many recent gun owners being first-time buyers and 76 per cent reporting protection as their primary motivation (N. Schwartz 2020). In Canada there has been a similar trend of increasing gun ownership, although not to the same degree. Gun-control regulations in Canada make licensing, purchasing, and protocols to obtain permission to carry a gun more time consuming and difficult than in most US states. Thus, a minority of gun buyers during the pandemic were first-time buyers. Handgun ownership in Canada is subject to additional regulations, and only 25 per cent of Canadian gun owners are licensed for handguns (N. Schwartz 2020).

In Canada some of the leading motivations for buying guns were concerns about the supply chain of guns and ammunition as well as concerns about acquiring permits with government offices being closed, meaning the people who would normally wait until the summer to make purchases were buying earlier. Canada experienced surges in sales of sporting guns and ammunition, whereas the US had an increase in handgun sales during the pandemic (N. Schwartz 2020).

Travel and Vacation

Travel was significantly restricted but did not stop altogether. Restrictions on travel, including border closures and policies on entering different jurisdictions, changed throughout the pandemic (see chapter 4). Just over 25.8 million international travellers entered Canada in 2020, of whom over half (56.4 per cent) were Canadian residents (Statistics Canada 2022l).[6] There was a nearly 85 per cent decrease in non-resident travellers entering Canada between 2019 and 2020. Canadians returning from abroad throughout the year decreased by 74 per cent in that period. Most of this travel was holiday related or specifically to visit friends and family. In 2021, international travel was down by about 27 per cent from 2020 (Statistics Canada 2022l). For the most part, people did not stray far. (For further discussion on changes in travel and tourism see chapter 8.)

Crimes: Data, Fines, and Enforcement

Aside from the fines for COVID-19 violations noted previously, most crime rates went down; Statistics Canada shows that reported crimes decreased by 9 per cent in 2020. There were decreases in assaults, thefts, vehicle-related crimes, property crime, and residential breaking and entering (Statistics Canada 2022o). Fraud incidents decreased by 9 per cent, but nearly 40 per cent of Canadians experienced a cybersecurity attack during the pandemic, such as phishing attacks, fraud, and hacking (CBC News 2021e; for further discussion on fraud incidents see chapter 9). The police-reported crime rate inched up in 2021 but was similar to 2020 across many categories.

Police reported increases in wellness checks for Mental Health Act regulations, suicide and attempted suicide, and overdoses (Statistics Canada 2022o). The total number of service calls rose by 8 per cent, especially for wellness checks and calls for domestic disturbances and mental health. Violent crimes, including assaults, dropped significantly; reported sexual assaults decreased by 20 per cent, and reported assaults declined by 9 per cent. The utterances of threats by a family member increased by 2 per cent at this time (CBC News 2021e). Crime rates began to increase between May and July 2020 as businesses reopened, but were lower than during the same period in 2019.

The number of reported domestic-violence cases did not change much during the pandemic, but it is important to note that these cases often go unreported. According to a report by the Canadian Femicide Observatory for Justice and Accountability (CFOJA 2020), 160 women and girls were killed violently in Canada during 2020, 146 in 2019, and 164 in 2018 (CBC News 2021l). Of the killings that involved a male accused, at least one in five of the victims were Indigenous, although race-based data were not available for many cases (CFOJA 2020).

Caremongering, Donations, Volunteerism, and the Not-for-Profit Sector

The first #Caremongering Facebook group started in eastern Canada, and within weeks similar groups had been created in every Canadian province and territory, with 96 per cent being created less than a week after the WHO had declared COVID-19 to be a pandemic. As of 4 May 2020, a study identified nearly 195,000 members across 130 #Caremongering Facebook groups in Canada. They described themselves as "grassroots networks to assist vulnerable people in the community by offering and seeking support, sharing reliable information, and spreading goodwill in the local community during the COVID-19 pandemic" (Seow et al. 2021, 4).

While people were generally more concerned about the welfare of their communities, on balance volunteerism dropped during the pandemic. Many not-for-profits struggled financially to meet high demands for services and worked to adapt their programming (Canada Helps 2021). According to a survey, 37 per cent of respondents decreased their donations to charities during the pandemic; only 9 per cent donated more than usual. Four in five survey respondents preferred donating to local charities than to larger, national organizations (Angus Reid Institute 2020a; Canada Helps 2021; World Vision 2021). The survey also found that the WE Charity scandal had affected trust in charitable organizations.[7] At least one in five charities, primarily small organizations, cancelled or reduced programs in the first few months of the pandemic.

A year after the start of the pandemic, revenues were down for 55 per cent of charities (Canada Helps 2021). In some respects, not-for-profit and charitable organizations had different experiences during the pandemic. In a survey in February 2021, 33 per cent of organizations reported laying off staff, whereas 23 per cent reported hiring new staff. By April 2021, 64 per cent of surveyed organizations had reported decreases in volunteers (Charity Village 2021). Social services organizations were the least likely to experience changes in staff; arts and culture, and children and family, organizations were the most likely to see reductions (Volunteer Canada 2020). Many not-for-profit organizations applied to CEWS; nearly 40 per cent of survey respondents reported that they had accessed the program or at least had planned to apply. Of organizations that used CEWS, 63 per cent would have had to lay off staff had they not received the subsidy (Charity Village 2021). (For further discussion on CEWS see chapter 4.)

CONCLUSION

On the surface, the response to public health directives during the pandemic in Canada is a remarkable story of public compliance. In light of the dread and uncertainty of a pandemic, people sought reassurance. Most people followed public health advice and directives. Generally, they respected the concept of physical distancing even if they did not adhere to the two-metre measure exactly; most also eventually wore masks. There were some fines for non-compliance with health directives, but they were few and were largely confined to young people who were understood to be low risk. There were many different motivations to comply with the orders, including civic duty and fear of contracting the disease. While heavy-handed enforcement had some impact at times, it is not clear that it was always necessary. In fact, trust in both governments and fellow citizens was an indicator of how the public behaved in response to restrictions (Klein 2022; COVID-19 National Preparedness Collaborators 2022).

There were positive spinoff effects. With so many people at home, so few businesses in operation, no cars on the road, and no drinking establishments open, most crime rates went down. People saved an inordinate amount of time when they no longer had to commute to work. Pollution decreased because people used their cars less frequently. People found new ways to spend their time. They exercised at home. There was an increased interest in nature as people tried to get out of the house. With so little travel available, most used holiday time to reconnect with local family and friends. They renovated their homes with the cash they saved from not going out, and they adopted pets from shelters to bring an extra spark of life into those homes. As we saw time and again, technology played an important role. Retail sales increased for products and services geared towards domestic use and available for purchase online. Online communities, like #Caremongering, sprang up to help the vulnerable.

There was, of course, a much more troubling side.

To start, every province and territory had a stretched health system. Focusing so many resources on containing the spread of one disease meant that there were significant trade-offs and cascading effects. Other, more common diseases with high mortality rates were neglected. Experts estimate the consequences will be felt for years. Efforts to have surge capacity in hospitals meant that surgeries and procedures were delayed. Some diseases will likely become more common because of a decrease in physical activity and an increase in substance abuse and generally unhealthy activities, particularly among the least healthy. While suicide rates decreased, mental-health issues skyrocketed. Social and economic hardship took a profound toll on many people: fear of disease transmission, loneliness, financial pressures, and strains on personal relationships became apparent; there was a spike in demand for divorces and separations; weddings and births were down. People were locked in, and social outlets were closed. Domestic abuse is difficult to track but likely increased.

People also experienced the pandemic differently. While older people were much more vulnerable to death when it came to COVID-19, many people, and young people in particular, faced challenges with their mental-health issues. Women's mental health was more negatively affected than men's; young women struggled more than most. Children and young adults could not go to school. There was a somewhat chaotic shift to online learning with modest success, but it created increased pressure on teachers and parents, and women in particular, and academic drift and isolation for many kids.

Places for social and spiritual relief and renewal – places of worship, community centres, schools, sports teams, arts and culture venues, local pubs and restaurants – were all closed to in-person gatherings. Some organizations were able to transition to online, which met with some success, but there is little doubt that many people felt lonely and isolated.

What started as a sprint became a marathon, making these social and economic issues worse. There was constant pressure from the business sector and community generally for governments to declare reopening plans, particularly between waves. Although people embraced opportunities when public health guidelines were relaxed, the relief was short lived as the second and third waves struck even harder, and many wanted strict health guidelines reinstated. People's lives were in perpetual suspension.

6

Behaviour Modification 2: The COVID-19 Vaccine

Vaccine approval was a significant turning point in the effort to contain the virus. From the early stages it was viewed as the way out of the COVID-19 pandemic. Developing and distributing the COVID-19 vaccine required considerable action from governments, industry, and the population, and therefore we treat it under behaviour modification. There are many unique dimensions to the development and distribution of the vaccine; for this reason we include it as its own chapter.

Despite the controversies about the way President Donald Trump's administration addressed COVID-19, few would dispute the incredible success of Operation Warp Speed (OWS), the public-private partnership established in the US to accelerate the development, manufacture, and distribution of COVID-19 vaccines, therapeutics, and diagnostics. The US government, as well as governments around the world, spent billions to develop and distribute the vaccines at record speed. Within eight months of vaccines being available, 80 per cent of the Canadian population over the age of twelve had received two doses (Government of Canada 2022k). Once double-vaccinated, people were thirty-six times less likely to be hospitalized and thirty-three times less likely to be in the ICU (Netherlands 2021; PHAC 2021l, slide 7).

Yet problems arose. Governments looked after their own first in a phenomenon termed "vaccine nationalism," which is perhaps not surprising, but there were far-reaching impacts of this approach. It was a two-track pandemic response in which poorer countries were left behind. Promises from wealthy countries to support low-income countries to vaccinate their populations were slow to be met.

In Canada there were access issues; it became clear that not everyone could easily access a local vaccine clinic or make a vaccine appointment for a myriad of reasons. The vaccine-hesitant, 28 per cent of the population at one time, had reservations about the vaccine despite the fact it had been available for months at that point. Over and above the 28 per cent, there was a further 10 per cent – anti-vaxxers – who adamantly and consistently refused to accept the vaccine. They were harder if not nearly impossible to sway. There is no one reason why people were opposed to vaccination. Generally, both the vaccine-hesitant and the anti-vaxxers had lower levels of income and trust in the system. Anti-vaxxers also tended to be politically right of centre and more individualistic in their orientation (B. Anderson 2021).

Some populations who were most at risk to get COVID-19 and experience severe symptoms (e.g., Black, Indigenous, and other visibly racialized people; see chapter 1) were also likely to be hesitant to get the vaccine, especially early on. The development of trust and relationships in these communities, as well as focused initiatives, was needed to increase vaccination participation among these groups.

While the vast majority of the population supported the vaccine, there were divisions over whether governments could compel someone to take a vaccine. As ICUs filled with those who chose not to be vaccinated, tolerance among the vaccinated towards the unvaccinated dropped; pressure mounted for the remaining people to either be vaccinated or accept significant restrictions in the way they lived and worked. This led to conflict, culminating in anti-vaccine mandate protests across the country in support of the self-named Freedom Convoy, notably blocking US border crossings and the streets around Parliament in Ottawa, which ultimately led to the federal government invoking the Emergencies Act.

This chapter reviews the development, distribution, and take-up of the COVID-19 vaccine. It examines which groups were most likely to get the vaccine and why, as well as various attitudes that prevailed among the vaccinated and unvaccinated.

THE GLOBAL RACE TO DEVELOP A VACCINE

Humans have been developing vaccines for over a thousand years. The earliest forms of vaccine development occurred in China around 1000 CE for smallpox inoculation. The 1930s saw advancements with antitoxins and vaccines against diphtheria, tetanus, anthrax, cholera, plague, typhoid, and more. Towards the middle of the twentieth century, polio vaccines were created; researchers worked to develop vaccines for other diseases affecting children, including measles, mumps, and rubella. In fact, the dramatic change in life expectancy in the twentieth century came about because of a significant decrease in infant mortality, largely due to improved access to clean water, increased sanitation practices, and vaccines. The Ebola vaccine is a more recent noteworthy development (History of Vaccines, n.d.).

Vaccines can often take ten to fifteen years to develop, from discovery to successful clinical trial and ultimately distribution (Altman 2020; Felter 2021; Kashte et al. 2021, 721; History of Vaccines, n.d.). Developers of the COVID-19 vaccine sought to condense this process to one to two years (Kashte et al. 2021, 722). Typically, 90 per cent of vaccines in clinical trials do not make it to market distribution (Altman 2020). Before the COVID-19 vaccines, the fastest development and approval was for the mumps vaccine in the 1960s, which took approximately four years (P. Ball 2020; Cagle 2021; Kashte et al. 2021, 722). COVID-19 vaccine development was the first time that the global scientific community mobilized on such a scale and was able to expand so quickly on existing coronavirus and vaccine research, including for SARS and MERS (Padron-Regalado 2020, 256–7; Cagle 2021; Felter 2021; Georgieva et al. 2021; Kashte et al. 2021, 722; National Institutes of Health, n.d.).

To expedite the process, the US government relied on the overlapping of development stages, including starting production on vaccines that were still in clinical trials, and committing to purchase vaccines before clinical trials had been finalized. COVID-19 spurred the development of RNA- and DNA-based vaccines, which can be mass produced quickly (Felter 2021; LaMattina 2021). While mRNA vaccines and technology have been studied for the flu, Zika virus, rabies, and cytomegalovirus and used in cancer research, for COVID-19 this was the first time that mRNA vaccines were available commercially to use in humans (CDC 2021; Felter 2021).

The first vaccine approved for emergency use to protect against COVID-19 was Pfizer and BioNTech's on 2 December 2020 in the UK (Ball 2020; Kashte et al. 2021, 722). Shortly thereafter, the Pfizer vaccine was approved by other regulatory agencies, including the WHO on 31 December 2020 (Kashte et al. 2021, 712). The first human trial in the US was started by Moderna in March 2020, which became the second vaccine approved for use in the US, on 18 December 2020 (Kashte et al. 2021, 722; National Institutes of Health, n.d.). Johnson & Johnson entered the market in February 2021 following a hold put on distribution. The AstraZeneca vaccine was approved in the UK on 30 December 2020; however, instances of blood clots changed recommendations to restrict use by age in some countries. In addition to these, there were an estimated 180 potential vaccines in development by pharmaceutical companies, academic institutions, and government agencies (Felter 2021).

The US Food and Drug Administration fully approved the Pfizer vaccine on 23 August 2021 (Gilmore 2021). On 16 September 2021, Health Canada granted Pfizer and Moderna vaccines full approval.

Cost of Vaccine Development

Partnerships between research institutions and public, private, and not-for-profit organizations supported vaccine development and distribution. The US and Germany were leaders in funding COVID-19 research and development (McCarthy 2021). The US allocated $18 billion through OWS to develop and distribute as many COVID-19 vaccine doses as possible (LaMattina 2021; Felter 2021). A virtual EU summit in mid-2020 resulted in $8 billion being pledged by world leaders, organizations, and banks to fund COVID-19 vaccine research.

COVID-19 vaccines were primarily developed by private companies with the support of public funds. Over $900 million of public funds were invested in Moderna and Johnson & Johnson. Pfizer and BioNTech received $800 million in research and development funding (McCarthy 2021). Some vaccine companies were state owned; in China, for example, two-fifths of the country's vaccine industry (Felter 2021) comprised state-owned firms such as Sinopharm. OWS enabled Moderna to develop and distribute its first product and helped fund the Johnson & Johnson and AstraZeneca vaccines. To speed up distribution, the US supported a waiver of patent for the COVID-19 vaccine, as did many member countries of the World Trade Organization, although this was not agreed to unanimously (Felter 2021; McCarthy 2021).

While vaccine doses were provided free of charge to the recipient, each dose costs between US$10.00 and US$19.50 in public funds under "pandemic pricing" in Canada and the US (Mitchell 2021; Refinitiv StreetEvents 2021, 19). Typically, vaccines such as these could have a market value of $150 to $175 per dose (Mitchell 2021; Refinitiv StreetEvents 2021, 19; Fang 2021).

The Government of Canada used public funds to cover the cost of vaccine procurement and distribution. The Canadian Armed Forces were deployed to support vaccine distribution efforts in remote areas, and the federal government provided logistical and supply chain support. On 25 March 2021 the government introduced a bill to provide a one-time payment of up to $1 billion to the provinces and territories on an equal per capita basis to support distribution through the COVID-19 Immunization Plan. As of April 2021, the federal government had spent $13.7 billion on vaccine efforts, including development, procurement, and distribution (Government of Canada 2021k).

Global Development and Distribution

Global manufacturing capabilities for vaccines were below what was needed, with only about a dozen countries able to produce COVID-19 vaccines early on, including the US, the UK, Germany, Belgium, the Netherlands, South Korea, Australia, Mexico, India, Argentina, China, and Russia (Felter 2021; *Globe and Mail* Editorial Board 2021). In addition to manufacturing challenges, vaccine doses needed to be transported and stored at ultra-low temperatures, which further complicated vaccine distribution (e.g., –90°C to –60°C) (Government of Canada 2023a). By 2021, the Government of Canada had made investments to redevelop domestic vaccine manufacturing capacity (Rabson 2021).

Countries such as Canada and the US established contracts for vaccine doses to inoculate their populations (Kashte et al. 2021, 712). Unsurprisingly, high-income countries started vaccinations first, at the beginning of December 2020. Some wealthy countries purchased enough doses to vaccinate their entire populations multiple times over by the end of 2021, and some Canadian provinces and territories were able to offer third doses of vaccines in summer 2021 (CBC News 2021h). During the first two years of COVID-19, Canada purchased the most doses of vaccine per capita in the world (Habibi and Lexchin 2021; Berthiaume 2020b).

In January 2021 the WHO raised concerns about the high risk that many low-income countries would not have access to vaccines until 2024 (Zahar and Sondarjee 2021; *Economist* 2021c). In February 2021 the WHO director general, Dr Tedros Adhanom Ghebreyesus, emphasized that leaving large areas of the global population unvaccinated would be "ethically, epidemiologically and economically unacceptable" (York 2021b, para. 5; Felter 2021).

Indeed, poorer countries, home to 60 per cent of the global population, were unable to acquire adequate vaccine supplies (Ghebreyesus 2021). Low-income countries started vaccinations in mid-February 2021. Approximately 90 per cent of the population of sixty-seven countries, however, were unable to receive a COVID-19 vaccine in 2021 (Office of the High Commissioner of Human Rights 2020, 2). By the beginning of May 2021, Canada had approximately 33 per cent of its population vaccinated, compared to 120 countries that had only 0.06 per cent of their populations vaccinated (M. Walsh and York 2021). Some called this a "two-track pandemic" in which rich countries had access to necessary resources and poorer countries were left behind (Pearce 2020).

Despite their improved public image during the pandemic, vaccine producers demanded considerable flexibility from countries when they were seeking vaccines; the agreements were largely confidential. After a legal battle in South Africa compelled disclosure of agreements, court documents showed that the government was liable for at least US$734 million in payments under four vaccine deals in 2021, including advance payments of nearly US$95 million (York 2023). South Africa was forced to adhere to considerable indemnification and confidentiality obligations, waive sovereign immunity, had no guarantee of delivery, and required a vaccine compensation program before any doses were supplied. The agreements constrained the capacity for local manufacturing and to share doses with other countries. The contracts showed that Pfizer charged South Africa 32 per cent more (US$10.00) than the "cost price" charged to the African Union (US$6.75). The Serum Institute of India charged South Africa double the price per dose of COVISHIELD (US$5.35) paid by the European Union and required payment in advance (York 2023). In addition to charging more than the price paid by the EU and non-profits, Johnson & Johnson prohibited South Africa from imposing any export restrictions on its vaccines, including doses that were filled and finished in South Africa. This meant that Johnson & Johnson could export some of the South African doses to Europe without penalty at the height of the pandemic (York 2023).

The WHO established a universal vaccination plan through COVAX, supported by 180 countries, to offer vaccine doses free of charge to low-income countries. Although by this point wealthy nations had pledged to donate more than one billion vaccine doses, the supply was slow in coming. By September 2021, less than 15 per cent of those doses had been delivered to the recipient countries, including only 5 per cent of Canada's pledged forty million doses. By the end of 2021, COVAX had distributed only seventy-seven million doses of its goal to distribute two billion (CBC News 2021d).

By the end of February 2022, 64 per cent of the global population had received at least one vaccine dose, but there were still large gaps between upper-middle-income countries and lower-income countries. In high- and upper-middle-income countries, 79 per cent of the population had had at least one dose, compared to only 13 per cent in low-income countries. At this time, Africa faced the lowest vaccination rate of any continent with 17.4 per cent of the population having had at least one dose (Holder 2022). Global Affairs Canada emphasized that donations of vaccines were managed by COVAX and that delays in distributing the vaccines once they left Canada were out of the federal government's control (York 2021a).

Many vaccines were wasted from expiration, improper storage, damaged vials, misalignment of supply and vaccine eligibility policies, and logistical challenges. An informal Canadian Press survey of health ministries across the country found that Canada wasted over one million vaccine doses, representing approximately 2.6 per cent of the total supply delivered to the provinces and territories (Djuric and Osman 2021). There are gaps in the data and varied reporting processes for each province and territory, but it is estimated that 0.45 per cent of these wasted vaccine doses had expired.

DISTRIBUTION AND PRIORITIZATION IN CANADA

The first COVID-19 vaccination in Canada was administered on 14 December 2020 to an eighty-nine-year-old living in an LTC facility in Quebec City; later the same day the vaccine was administered for the first time in Ontario to a personal support worker (Aiello and Forani 2020).

Advice about who should get vaccinated and when changed throughout the pandemic and varied by jurisdiction. For example, as of mid-July 2021 the Government of the UK did not recommend that children and teenagers under eighteen get vaccinated, unless they or someone they lived with was immunocompromised. People under eighteen often did not suffer severe cases of COVID-19, and therefore the risks of vaccination were seen to outweigh the benefits (Department of Health and Social Care 2021; Kirka 2021; Roxby and Triggle 2021; Walker and Davis 2021). In mid-September the UK government's position changed to advise vaccinations for people between the ages of twelve and fifteen, which was called for by regional chief medical officers of health (Walker and Davis 2021).

The debate about who should be vaccinated first persisted throughout the pandemic. Should the people most likely to spread the virus get it first, or those who were the most vulnerable to death and serious illness? Across Canada, prioritization of the COVID-19 vaccine was primarily based on age and type of employment, such as health care and other essential workers. The decision to prioritize the COVID-19 vaccine by age, starting with the elderly and making the vaccine available

Table 6.1 | Provincial and territorial vaccination rates, as of 3 April 2022

Rank	Proportion with at least one vaccine dose (%)	Proportion with two vaccine doses (%)	Proportion with at least one vaccine booster dose (%)
Newfoundland and Labrador	94.8	90.9	55.3
Nova Scotia	88.2	83.4	50.4
Prince Edward Island	87.8	84.1	47.0
New Brunswick	86.0	81.2	47.7
Quebec	84.8	82.1	49.5
British Columbia	84.7	81.2	48.3
Canada	83.3	80.0	46.4
Yukon	83. 1	79.8	45.3
Ontario	82.9	79.8	47.5
Manitoba	81.9	78.5	42.0
Nunavut	81.5	70.6	35.3
Northwest Territories	80.4	76.8	41.0
Saskatchewan	79.8	75.6	40.7
Alberta	78.2	74.2	35.6

Atlantic Canada had some of the highest vaccination rates. Children under the age of twelve were the last group to be eligible for COVID-19 vaccines.
Source: Government of Canada 2022i.

to younger populations successively, meant that the vaccine generally became available in phases from oldest to youngest. Consideration was also given to how the virus was spreading and where.

The federal government was criticized for its slow start with the vaccine rollout. The lack of domestic manufacturing capacity meant that Canada had to wait to receive doses, while countries like the UK and the US produced vaccines and distributed them quickly. Vaccine-storage requirements, such as ultra-low temperatures, and the limited number of vaccination clinics or locations contributed to the delays in Canada (Dangerfield 2021). At that time, provinces such as Quebec, British Columbia, and Ontario facilitated vaccine distribution directly

Table 6.2 | Vaccinated Canadians by age, as of 3 April 2022

Age group (years)	At least one dose (%)	Two vaccine doses (%)	At least one booster dose (%)
0–4	<0.1	0	0
5–11	56.2	39.7	<0.1
12–17	85.9	82.2	14.6
18–29	87.4	83.7	33.7
30–39	86.9	84.0	41.0
40–49	89.3	87.2	50.5
50–59	92.2	90.5	62.1
60–69	93.1	91.6	73.6
70–79	94.1	92.9	80.6
≥80	96.8	95.3	83.5

People over fifty had some of the highest vaccination rates, including at least one booster dose. Children under the age of twelve were the last group to be eligible for COVID-19 vaccines. *Source:* Government of Canada 2022i.

in LTC facilities (A. Miller 2021b). As of 3 April 2022, Canada was the eleventh-ranked country in the world for COVID-19 vaccination rate, behind Cuba, Chile, Singapore, Qatar, Uruguay, South Korea, Italy, Denmark, Cambodia, Belgium, and Australia (Ritchie et al. 2022b). By 3 April 2022, 80 per cent of Canadians had had at least two doses of vaccine (table 6.1).

Each province and territory developed its own vaccination plans, including prioritization and timelines to expand vaccine eligibility to additional population groups. Generally speaking, vaccines in Canada became available to people eighty years and older in mid-December 2020. By mid-April 2021, many jurisdictions had opened vaccinations to people over the age of eighteen, and by the beginning of June 2021, access had been expanded to people over the age of twelve. Vaccines for children between five and eleven years old were approved in October 2021 (Public Services and Procurement Canada 2021). As of 3 April 2022, people aged eighteen to twenty-nine had the lowest vaccination rate of those over the age of twelve (Government of Canada 2022k). Uptake in vaccine boosters waned after April 2022, with only 17 per cent of Canadians receiving a vaccine booster dose between April and October 2022 (Weeks 2022). Table 6.2 shows the percentage of vaccinated Canadians by age group as of 3 April 2022.

Some provinces adjusted their vaccination plans according to the supply and the trends in infection rates. For example, the intense third wave of COVID-19 motivated the Government of Ontario to target vaccinations in areas where COVID-19 cases were rising rapidly. This meant vaccines were made available based on postal code in addition to age (Office of the Premier of Ontario 2021).

Similar to the significance of international borders on global vaccine procurement, provincial and territorial borders within Canada were an important consideration for allocating domestic vaccine supply. For example, in February 2021 vaccine doses intended for New Brunswick, Nova Scotia, and PEI were diverted to the Territories, which were vulnerable if cases surged (Willick 2021).

Most people received their shots willingly and did not need to be encouraged. In time, however, different jurisdictions, organizations, and businesses encouraged people to get vaccinated by offering incentives such as cash, lotteries, scholarships, free alcohol, and free cannabis (Jiménez 2021; Deschamps 2021; MacLean 2021b; J. Keller 2021; Government of Alberta, n.d.b). In the private sector, insurers, food businesses, and tech companies offered deals to those who had been vaccinated. Manitoba offered a grant of up to $20,000 to community organizations that encouraged vaccinations where vaccination rates were low (Malone 2021).

To Mandate or Not to Mandate

Most people were willing to be vaccinated. Vaccine mandates were tools to encourage individuals to be vaccinated and to ensure jurisdictions could enforce them. Mandatory vaccination is not new in Canada. In Ontario, for example, children and staff in schools must be vaccinated for diphtheria, tetanus, polio, measles, mumps, rubella, meningitis, and whooping cough unless there is a valid reason for exemption. Children in Ontario born from 2010 onwards must also be vaccinated for chickenpox (Kupfer 2021). New Brunswick and Ontario are the only provinces with vaccination mandates for schools; this legislation has been in place since 1982 (Born, Yiu, and Sullivan 2014). In the US the earliest vaccination mandate for schools was implemented in the 1850s to address the spread of smallpox (Phillips and Rendall 2021).

The Government of Canada mandated COVID-19 vaccines for all employees of federally regulated agencies, including Crown corporations. This meant that all airline, marine travel, and train employees were required to be vaccinated (Stone and Leung 2021). Those who travelled on federally regulated services would also have to be vaccinated. In mid-October 2021 anyone entering the House of Commons was required to be vaccinated, including all MPs, staff, press, and public visitors (Aiello 2021).

Vaccinations for employees were also mandated by many private businesses, such as major financial institutions, including TD, CIBC, RBC, and Scotiabank. Employees who refused to get vaccinated by the deadline would have to be tested regularly and to complete training on the benefits of COVID-19 vaccination (Baystreet Staff 2021). At the end of August 2021 nine corporate law firms announced that they would mandate vaccinations (Kerr 2021).

Some jurisdictions in Canada mandated vaccines for health-care workers. In British Columbia, Alberta, Ontario, Saskatchewan, Manitoba, and Nova Scotia, health-care workers had to either be vaccinated or tested regularly for COVID-19 (McKenzie-Sutter 2021; CBC News 2021h, 2021i; MacLean 2021c; C. Dickson 2021; Long 2021; CTV News Edmonton Staff 2021; Saskatchewan Health Authority 2021). Many facilities such as hospitals and LTC facilities mandated that their employees be vaccinated.

In some jurisdictions this also applied to education workers. The Northwest Territories, Yukon, New Brunswick, Nova Scotia, and Newfoundland and Labrador mandated their public service employees to be vaccinated in October 2021 (J. Wilson 2021; Government of Nova Scotia 2021b; CBC News 2021b, 2021i; B. MacKinnon 2021a; Treasury Board Secretariat, n.d.). Concerns were raised in some jurisdictions about staffing shortages due to vaccination policies, particularly in health care (Weichel 2021). As a result, in early November some jurisdictions, including Ontario and Quebec, backtracked on these decisions and decided not to mandate vaccination for health-care workers (CBC News 2021g; Ross and Lofaro 2021).

Vaccine Passports

Proof of vaccination requirements, also called vaccine passports, was implemented to permit vaccinated people to travel, access services, and attend events. This was met with mixed reactions. Some said vaccine passports were a good way to ensure that vaccinated people – those least likely to develop severe COVID-19 symptoms – could return to a sense of normalcy. Others believed that limiting services to those with vaccine passports coerced people into getting the vaccine and infringed on the rights of people who chose not to be vaccinated, whether it was for a medical or other reason (Stone and Cyr 2021). Equity, privacy, and surveillance concerns were raised about immunization records, such as vaccine passports and data storage (Murdoch 2020). There was also concern that vaccine passports could contribute to a "split society" in which some would be able to access services and others would not (Murdoch 2020, para. 4).

The definition of *vaccine passport* and what it entailed also varied (A.M. Jones 2021). The federal government developed a system to allow Canadians to prove that they had been vaccinated in order to travel internationally (Freeman 2021; A.M. Jones 2021). Provinces and territories decided how the system would be implemented in their jurisdictions. The governments of British Columbia, Alberta, Saskatchewan, and Ontario raised objections to a COVID-19 vaccine passport within Canada, whereas other provinces accepted it or implemented similar programs early on (Stone and Cyr 2021; Freeman 2021; A.M. Jones 2021).

International travellers to Canada were also required to be vaccinated before entering the country. Although many people followed these regulations, attempts were made to cross the border with falsified COVID-19 documentation, such as test results and vaccination records. By the end of October 2021, Canadian border officials had identified 374 suspected falsified COVID-19 test results at ports of entry – 187 at land borders and 160 at airports – and intercepted 92 suspected fake proof-of-vaccination credentials (Wong 2021).

Most people supported vaccination passports to access non-essential services, especially for international travellers. In May 2021, 79 per cent approved of a vaccine passport for international travel, but only 55 per cent approved of a vaccine passport to access non-essential services and events (A.M. Jones 2021). In September 2021 the Ontario Human Rights Commission stated that proof-of-vaccination policies, such as vaccine passports, were "generally permissible" as long as people with legitimate exemptions could be "reasonably accommodated" (Rocca 2021, para. 1). Despite these concerns, and with some variation in the motivation and reach, all provinces and territories implemented a vaccine passport system in the fall of 2021. By the end of March 2022, many provinces had announced that their vaccine-passport programs would be ending.

BEHAVIOURS AND ATTITUDES TOWARDS
THE COVID-19 VACCINE

When it comes to the unvaccinated, people are put into different categories. Vaccine hesitancy is a delay in accepting or rejecting vaccination "regardless of the accessibility of vaccination services" (Kashte et al. 2021, 729). Someone would be considered vaccine hesitant if, for example, they had concerns about side effects and wanted to wait for more information to be available. Anti-vax is a stronger position. Anti-vaxxers are opposed to vaccinations and are not typically open to persuasion. Although a small minority, the anti-vaxxer population can threaten the mission to achieve herd immunity, particularly by spreading misinformation and by mounting protests, as governments would learn (Stecula, Pickup, and van der Linden 2020; Kashte et al. 2021, 730; Ullah et al. 2021, 94). At times, people with legitimate concerns about the vaccines who were hesitant to be vaccinated were labelled as anti-vaxxers. These attitudes are not limited to the COVID-19 vaccine. For example, in 2019 the worst measles outbreaks in recent history were connected to people's refusal to be vaccinated. Some people do not get vaccinated for fairly benign reasons. When mandatory flu vaccination was implemented in Denmark, many people indicated that they did not get the vaccine because they did not feel they became sick often, they did not see the vaccine as essential, or they blamed forgetfulness or lack of time (Kashte et al. 2021, 730).

There are many reasons why someone may hesitate to get a vaccine. Often these factors relate to confidence or trust, complacency, convenience, calculation of risk, and the degree to which someone accepts ·collective responsibility. Confidence can relate to the levels of trust in the effectiveness and safety of vaccines, the institutions distributing the vaccines, and the motivations of decision makers in vaccine policy development. Complacency means that the perceived risk of the disease is low enough that vaccination is not considered necessary. Convenience refers to the levels of availability, affordability, and accessibility of the vaccine, as well as information about the vaccine. Calculation refers to an individual's risk assessment of the disease and the vaccine. Collective responsibility is the degree to which an individual is willing to get the vaccine to protect others (Government of Canada 2021a). Vaccine hesitancy also occurs among health-care practitioners, as 15 per cent of those surveyed expressed hesitancy towards the COVID-19 vaccine at one point (Government of Canada 2021a). Between November 2020 and mid-April 2021, vaccine hesitancy decreased by nearly half, and support for vaccines doubled; 8 per cent said they would never take the COVID-19 vaccine, compared to 11 per cent in November 2020 (B. Anderson 2021). Vaccine hesitancy continued to decrease throughout the spring and summer, but vaccine refusal remained consistent. As of June 2021, 18 per cent of the population was still vaccine hesitant, and 10 per cent continued to refuse the vaccine (Parkin et al. 2021).

There were hiccups. Dr Caroline Quach-Thanh, former co-chair of the National Advisory Committee on Immunization (NACI), in May 2021 reflected on how guilty she would feel if her sister died of a blood clot after Quach-Thanh advised her to take the AstraZeneca vaccine. The comment caused a stir in the public health community; the comment was seen to be careless if not irresponsible, knowing that many people are motivated by emotion rather than rationality when it comes to decisions about vaccines (Kirkey 2021). NACI is a fourteen-member panel that provides recommendations about the vaccines (e.g., dosing schedules and priority populations) but does not set vaccine mandates, and the vaccines themselves are approved by Health Canada. NACI recommendations are not binding. NACI did not typically have a public-facing role but started holding technical briefings during the pandemic. Following Dr Quach-Thanh's statement, however, the committee's public-facing role was even further reduced. NACI's expertise is impressive, it was often seen to make the right call on many difficult decisions, but the members are not experts in risk communication (Kirkey 2021). The episode revealed how disciplined the risk message had to be and that the popular press was not a good place to speculate or raise doubt about key messages.

A study of over fifty countries found that vaccine refusal was connected to strong feelings of invincibility and higher focus on individualism rather than obligation to community, especially in countries such as Canada, the US, and the UK that tend to focus on individual rights and freedoms (Ibbitson 2021).

Vaccine hesitancy also varied by vaccine type. Confidence in the Pfizer and Moderna vaccines started to increase at the beginning of March 2021, whereas confidence in AstraZeneca and Johnson & Johnson vaccines declined. Of respondents who were vaccine hesitant, 26 per cent indicated concern about receiving the AstraZeneca product and wanted to wait until another option was available (B. Anderson 2021).

Vaccination mandates and proof-of-vaccination policies became an election issue in many jurisdictions. Dr Anthony Fauci speculated that a key issue in the US was the degree to which the vaccine was politicized.

The way a person or jurisdiction voted in the 2020 presidential election was a key indicator of vaccination rates, and vaccination rates in turn became a key factor in predicting state elections (Masket 2021; Honderich 2021; Leonhardt 2021b). In the 2021 Canadian federal election, vaccinations became a political issue, and although every party supported vaccinations, each had a different approach to mandatory vaccines, incentives, and proof-of-vaccination policies (Boynton 2021). There were many socio-economic, ethnic, gender, and race factors that correlated with attitudes towards vaccines and willingness to get vaccinated. For a more complete discussion and more data on public attitudes please see chapter 10, "Opinion-Responsive Hypothesis."

Truck Convoy and US-Canada Border Protests

In early 2022 the self-named Freedom Convoy protested measures requiring truck drivers to be fully vaccinated as of 15 January to enter Canada, or to test and quarantine on arrival (PHAC 2021c, para. 4). A week later the US mandated that all Canadian truck drivers were required to be vaccinated to enter the US. The group's vague demands were understood to be an end to vaccine mandates and all pandemic restrictions or the resignation of government leaders, especially Prime Minister Trudeau. Their demands were at times incoherent and lacked an understanding of Canadian law (Jackman 2022).

On 22 January, convoys formed in BC, Alberta, Ontario, and Newfoundland and drove to Ottawa. On 29 January, 8,000 to 15,000 people converged on Parliament Hill (J. Dickson, Walsh, and Hunter 2022). About 3,000 gathered the next day, and just 250 by 3 February (CBC News 2022e). Some stayed for three weeks; participant numbers increased during the weekends. Although some claimed that as many as 50,000 trucks were headed to Ottawa (Warmington 2022), only about 250 reached the city; they honked incessantly until a court-granted injunction on 7 February ordered the silence of truck horns downtown (C. Tunney 2022a). The group displayed hate symbols, desecrated the National War Memorial and a statue of Terry Fox, harassed residents, and went maskless into businesses, causing some to close temporarily (Anderssen 2022). The atmosphere on Parliament Hill was "largely party-like" (Globe Staff and Wire Services 2022, para. 7).

Organizers raised $10 million through GoFundMe, $1 million of which was released before the page was shut down on 4 February for violating GoFundMe's rules against violence and harassment (Boisvert 2022b; GoFundMe 2022). Through GiveSendGo $12 million was raised, with 43 per cent of donations and over half the donors being from the US (Cardoso 2022). Access to this money was frozen on 10 February (E. Thompson, Rocha, and Leung 2022).

Related protests blocked the Canada-US border. In Coutts, Alberta, where $44 million in goods passes daily, a two-week highway blockade disrupted tens of millions of dollars of trade (CBC News 2022c). When it was broken up, police seized weapons and arrested thirteen people; four were charged with conspiracy to murder (M. Grant 2022). A six-day blockade of the Ambassador Bridge between Windsor and Detroit cost $3 billion to $6 billion in trade, primarily of automotive parts and machinery and electrical equipment (La Grassa 2022). These economic threats were shut down somewhat quickly compared to the Ottawa protest. Smaller border protests happened in Manitoba, Saskatchewan, and BC (CBC News 2022d).

In Ottawa organizers allegedly told police chief Peter Sloly that the protest would last through the weekend of 29 January (Tasker 2020c). It was unclear who the official organizers were. Sloly said that the initial police response was successful because violence was avoided (Gollum 2022), which made sense given comparisons with the 6 January 2021 rioting at Washington's Capitol Building (Moscrop 2022; Austen and Isai 2022). While not violent, Ottawa protesters became "increasingly more difficult to manage" (Ottawa Police Service 2022, para. 7). They set up tents, a stage, and hot tubs. Sloly said that 1,800 more officers were needed (Gilmore and Lord 2022). While the location gave the impression it was a federal issue, responsibility fell to Ottawa police, who seemed slow to act. It became embarrassing for the prime minister, particularly given international media coverage (Panetta 2022; Gillies and Crary 2022). It was arguably a fringe movement that "got lucky" from policing failures and media attention but was unlikely to sustain momentum (Kitroeff and Austen 2022, para. 19). According to our media analysis (see chapter 10), over 500 articles were written about the Freedom Convoy by the *Toronto Star*, *National Post*, and CBC News in January and February 2022. By 14 February, 64 per cent of Canadians had opposed the demand to end all pandemic restrictions, and 70 per cent had opposed the protesters' approach and behaviour (Angus Reid Institute 2022). A proposed class-action lawsuit was filed against protesters for a claim of over $3 million (Crawford 2022). Although governments denounced protesters, Saskatchewan and Alberta started to drop COVID-19 restrictions soon after protests started (Quon 2022); rules requiring a PCR test before entering Canada were also eased (S. Harris 2022; PHAC 2022a). Governments said that decisions were science driven, but it was clear people were becoming frustrated by restrictions generally and governments needed to think about lifting them, especially as other Western countries were lifting theirs. One poll showed that 46 per cent of Canadians believed the protesters' frustration was legitimate and worthy of some sympathy (*Economist* 2022).

The political winner was unclear. Several Conservative MPs took photographs with protesters (Shield 2022); others disagreed with the group's lawlessness (Silver 2022). The Liberal Party of Canada also experienced division. Liberal MP Joël Lightbound argued that the government had been using the vaccine mandate issue to gain political support, rather than to protect public health, since the 2021 election (Tasker 2022b). Prime Minister Trudeau invoked the Emergencies Act, a controversial first, on 14 February 2022 (C. Tunney 2022b). Peter Sloly resigned on the next day (Lapierre 2022). The New Democratic Party (NDP) supported the Act's use, but the party was divided; it was described as betraying "the legacy" of opposing the War Measures Act in 1970 (Rabson and Woolf 2022, para. 30). Invoking the Emergencies Act was opposed by the Bloc Québécois and the Conservatives (Major 2022a). The prime minister said that the military would not be deployed and that the Act would be used to freeze bank accounts funding the protests, to ensure towing services removed trucks, and to give police more authority (C. Tunney 2022b). Starting on 16 February, police warned protesters to leave or face arrest, charges, and seizure of vehicles. Access to the area was restricted (Globe Staff 2022). On 18 February, Ottawa police, Ontario Provincial Police, Toronto police, Vancouver police, RCMP, and Sûreté du Québec swept downtown Ottawa (Cecco 2022; Mehrabi 2022; Raymond 2022), arresting almost two hundred protesters, including several organizers (CBC News 2022e).

The Act was lifted on 23 February. The federal government faced legal challenges from civil liberties organizations and the government of Alberta, which argued that it was an overreach; international news sources, like the *New York Times* and the *Economist*, agreed. An inquiry and report were required within 360 days of its revocation (Government of Canada 2022e). While Justice Rouleau concluded that the federal government was justified in invoking the Emergencies Act, he also noted several failures in policing, intelligence, and indeed federalism in a crisis (Rouleau 2023).

COVID-19 CASES AMONG THE
VACCINATED AND UNVACCINATED

The Freedom Convoy was the culmination of a tension that had been brewing for several months between the majority, who were vaccinated, and those who were not. The fourth wave of COVID-19 was described as a wave of the unvaccinated (Woo 2021b). After one dose, COVID-19 vaccines were 60 per cent effective at preventing infection and 80 per cent effective at reducing hospitalization. After two doses, they were 92 per cent effective at preventing infection and 96 per cent effective at reducing hospitalization (PHAC 2021k, 20). According to PHAC (2021m), unvaccinated people were ten times more likely to get COVID-19 and thirty-six times more likely to be hospitalized.

"Breakthrough" cases of COVID-19 are those that occur in fully vaccinated individuals. According to PHAC, breakthrough infections of COVID-19 accounted for 0.5 per cent of all reported cases from the start of the vaccine rollout to the end of June 2021 (Lao 2021b). Of a total of 2,700 breakthrough COVID-19 cases, 0.0018 per cent of fully vaccinated people died of COVID-19.

The Omicron variant had three times the genetic mutations of prior variants. This enabled it to spread more easily than the original COVID-19 virus and earlier variants, even among vaccinated people. It was estimated that one person with Omicron could infect four other people, a rate far higher than that of previous variants. Although the Omicron variant generally caused less severe disease and a lower risk of death than the Delta variant did, public health officials were concerned by the higher transmissibility (Semeniuk 2021; CDC 2022b; Woo 2022).

Tolerance of the Unvaccinated

Most people supported regulations to encourage vaccination. Approximately 75 per cent of survey respondents indicated they support regulations, such as vaccine passports and mandatory vaccinations, to enter public spaces (Angus Reid Institute 2021c; Lao 2021c).

Support for regulations and incentives for vaccinations varied by political affiliation, region, and age. For example, 93 per cent of respondents identifying with the Liberal Party supported regulations and incentives for vaccinations, compared to 67 per cent of respondents identifying with the Conservative Party (Angus Reid Institute 2021c; Lao 2021c). Among respondents who thought governments should have done nothing to encourage vaccination, 7 per cent identified with the Liberal Party, 12 per cent with the NDP, and 33 per cent with the Conservative Party (Angus Reid Institute 2021c).

Among respondents in Saskatchewan, 37 per cent believed that governments should do nothing to encourage vaccinations. In Manitoba it was 30 per cent. In British Columbia, Ontario, and Atlantic Canada there was majority support for regulatory measures to encourage vaccination. Support for regulations or incentives was high among all age groups but was lowest among young people (Angus Reid Institute 2021c).

Tolerance towards unvaccinated people wore thin. Among vaccinated respondents, 83 per cent indicated they had no sympathy for unvaccinated people who contracted COVID-19 (Angus Reid Institute 2021c). There were concerns that limited tolerance towards the unvaccinated, and polarization of vaccinated and unvaccinated, would further alienate those who were vaccine hesitant or against vaccines altogether (Lao 2021c).

During the fourth wave a disproportionate part of the burden on hospitals and ICUs was from unvaccinated COVID-19 patients, and many medical procedures and treatments were affected. At the start of September 2021 there were 465 people in ICU due to COVID-19 across Canada (Ritchie et al. 2022a; PHAC 2021e). By the end of the month an additional 315 people were in the ICU with COVID-19, and the weekly average had increased to 769 ICU admissions (Ritchie et al. 2022a; PHAC 2021c, 1). ICU admissions due to COVID-19 were rising in Alberta, Saskatchewan, and New Brunswick. In Alberta, hospitals and ICUs were overwhelmed with COVID-19 patients in what the premier described as a "crisis of the unvaccinated" (CTV News Calgary Staff 2021, para. 2). At this time ICUs would have operated at 155 per cent capacity without the additional surge capacity (Herring 2021). All elective surgeries in Alberta were cancelled in early September 2021 due to lack of resources caused by COVID-19 (C. Tait 2021). In British Columbia one-third of ICU beds were occupied with COVID-19 patients at the end of September 2021 (Carrigg 2021). At the same time, New Brunswick hospitals were also under pressure, with 70 per cent of all ICU beds occupied (B. MacKinnon 2021b). In Quebec in August and September 2021, people aged forty to forty-nine made up the majority of hospitalizations, followed by those aged fifty to fifty-nine; people aged twenty to twenty-nine also reached their highest hospitalization rate at this time at 8.9 per cent (Jonas 2021b). By the end of September and into October 2021, Saskatchewan had cancelled organ-donation and organ-transplant procedures and nearly two hundred surgeries a day (Quon 2021; *Globe and Mail* 2021). COVID-19 patients at this time occupied 70 per cent of ICU beds (Giles 2021).

A survey of health-care professionals and patients highlighted concerns about delayed medical treatment and diagnosis, particularly for heart and stroke patients. Two-thirds of respondents living with a heart condition, effects of a stroke, or vascular cognitive impairment had at least one medical appointment delayed or cancelled (Woo 2021a).

COVID-19 was identified as a preventable condition that strained Canada's health-care system and ICU capacity. As a 2016 CIHI report highlights, however, many conditions that result in ICU admission are preventable, and if these conditions are treated earlier, they can be managed in less intensive settings, including treatment for diabetes and chronic obstructive pulmonary disease. In this sense, the media's vilification of the unvaccinated in ICUs was an oversimplification of a more complicated situation, but the strain on hospitals and ICUs due to the infectious nature of COVID-19 and the availability of vaccines left little patience for people choosing to not be vaccinated.

CONCLUSION

Governments had an indispensable role to play in vaccine development and distribution. Public investment stimulated markets to develop the vaccine at record speed; government regulations ensured that the necessary standards were met without unnecessary slowdowns. Canada was vulnerable because it could not develop its own vaccine supply; it signed contracts early on with several international pharmaceutical companies to ensure that it could secure an adequate supply for the country.

Governments also had an important role to play in encouraging people to get the vaccine, and it did so with success. After a slow start, Canada is among the most COVID-19–vaccinated nations in the world, which required considerable investment to address complex logistics, underpinned by important ethical considerations about who should receive the vaccine first. Governments' decision to prioritize front-line workers, those who lived in LTC facilities, other vulnerable groups, and then generally by age seemed reasonable to most people; there were few objections. Focusing on vulnerable communities sooner, however, could have improved outcomes; 90 per cent of Ontario cases, for example, resided in 10 per cent of the province's postal codes, with highly concentrated populations and large proportions of newcomers, a fact that was overlooked for too long (CBC News 2020i; H. Chung et al. 2020, 14; Gatehouse 2020b; Habib 2021).

In some cases, however, the challenge of distributing the vaccine went beyond logistical challenges. Persuading people to take the vaccine in some cases was necessary. It is virtually impossible to know definitively why so many people were either slow to get vaccinated or did not get vaccinated at all. Risk psychologists have studied vaccine hesitancy for decades; more research will be compiled in the post-pandemic era.

Trust in the vaccine, governments, and public health seemed to be important variables in understanding participation rates. To establish trustworthiness, people and organizations need to convey openness, knowledge, and concern (R. Kramer 1999, 572, 586–7). To many people in Canada, governments and public health could not have been more transparent, and doctors typically are among the most trusted people in society. Nevertheless, the vaccine stage is a powerful reminder that openness, knowledge, and concern are not necessarily objective, verifiable matters; perspective, social context, and experience are also factors.

Some have been marginalized before and therefore doubt those in power. Many vaccine-hesitant people had lower levels of income and education; many were also Indigenous or Black. It is a powerful irony that people who were most vulnerable to contracting COVID-19 and at times paid the highest price during the pandemic, in health and wealth, were often the least likely to get the vaccine. That they would act against their personal interests by failing to get vaccinated reinforces the notion that the system does not connect well with them or their lived experience. Programs that targeted Indigenous populations and low-income neighbourhoods showed success, but they were slow to start.

For some, not getting vaccinated seemed like a rational decision; the risk was low, particularly for young people. As the vaccine rollout continued, many of the vaccine-resistant were White men earning moderate to high incomes (Ibbitson 2021). This type of argument – that the pandemic carried low risk for some – was given little attention in the mainstream media as coverage amplified the most tragic stories.

A small but determined group was hostile, raising doubts about the vaccine and the role of governments. These types of doubts are not new when it comes to large, uncertain risks (van Prooijen and Douglas 2018, 901; Roulet 2020; Dacombe 2021; Kashte et al. 2021, 730). Conspiracy theories flourish, particularly in social media echo chambers. The episode produced some powerful ironies. Anti-vaxxers' use of the pro-choice slogan "my body, my choice" enraged many in the pro-choice movement and sparked heated exchanges across many media outlets (Harrison Warren 2021; Schultheis and Grieshaber 2021).

Despite the media attention the Freedom Convoy was a small and disorganized group with incoherent demands and mixed-to-little knowledge of how the parliamentary system worked. While the conflict over vaccine mandates arguably represented a conflict in world views, the government did not have an adequate process in place to address the conflict. The episode did, however, expose poor security practices on and around Parliament Hill.

Despite the media's focus on people's choice not to get vaccinated and thereby unnecessarily requiring an ICU bed, many people in ICUs have preventable diseases – COVID-19 is not unique. The singular focus on COVID-19, however, placed the blame for overcrowded ICUs squarely on the unvaccinated. As time went on, tolerance for diversity of views about the vaccine dropped. Orders of governments converged to pressure people to become vaccinated through various standards, penalties, and incentives.

While there was general enthusiasm for vaccines, Canada and other Western countries made only modest gestures towards poor countries. When Canada reclaimed part of its donation to COVAX to increase domestic supply, most of the world had not yet had a single shot and would not for years. Canada was able to offer third doses to Canadians while many countries worked to administer first doses.

As is often the case in public policy, the pandemic was a reminder that there are scarcely any absolute rights and wrongs, or at least they continue to elude us. Public policy is often understood as what seems reasonable at the time; it is highly susceptible to current circumstances, context, and framing and is constantly shifting. Future efforts to contain COVID-19 variants will certainly be more modest than what we experienced in 2020 and 2021; so, too, might any effort to contain future pandemics. Having lived through COVID-19, we will think about and experience pandemics differently. After our two case studies, we will review these shifting contextual pressures that drove the governments' response to COVID-19.

PART THREE

Case Studies:
Long-Term Care and Tourism

In this section we examine two case studies during the COVID-19 pandemic using the Hood, Rothstein, and Baldwin (2001) framework. Chapter 7 examines one of the most noted failures in terms of health care during the pandemic: long-term care. In the chapter we set the case up by detailing how governments regulate LTC facilities and the broader social and economic context in which that governance occurs. With that context in place, we detail the chronology of COVID-19 in LTC facilities, primarily in the first two waves of the disease. This includes a review of audits and studies that detail the failings of facilities across the country. We connect these shortfalls with the broader context outlined in the chapter.

Turning from health care to the economy, chapter 8 examines one of the sectors most affected during the pandemic: tourism. As in the LTC case, we use in this chapter the Hood, Rothstein, and Baldwin framework to examine the context and governance of the sector and how that relates to the various vulnerabilities that were exposed in the sector during COVID-19.

7

Caring for the Vulnerable: Long-Term Care, Short-Term Thinking

Canada's COVID-19 pandemic was dominated by the tragic narrative of LTC homes. In the first wave alone there were over 840 outbreaks in facilities across the country, accounting for over 80 per cent of COVID-19–related deaths in Canada by the end of May 2020 (CIHI 2020c, 1). Conditions in certain LTC homes and the pressures faced by staff elicited outrage and passionate calls for government action. The disproportionate effect of the pandemic on Canadian LTC homes brought unprecedented attention to the management of LTC and what we owe to vulnerable members of society. In the aftermath of the outbreaks, questions about the structural weaknesses of the LTC system have come to the fore.

This chapter explores the social and economic context shaping the governance of LTC in Canada. We describe the policy landscape and the attitudes and behaviours of the major players with reference to the three components of the cybernetics control system: standard setting, information gathering, and behaviour modification. We then explore how well Hood, Rothstein, and Baldwin's (2001) three hypotheses of regulatory change explain this governance structure. The second half of the chapter reviews the LTC sector's experience during the first and second waves of the COVID-19 pandemic. We conclude our review with observations about pandemic response, LTC audits, and the market and demographic pressures that continue to shape the system.

DEFINING LONG-TERM CARE

LTC is a complex and fragmented system in Canada. It is regulated on a provincial and territorial basis, with significant variation across and within provinces and territories in the definition of care needs

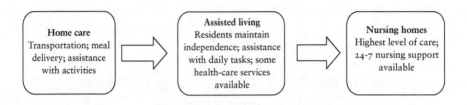

Figure 7.1 | The spectrum of long-term care: home care, assisted living, and nursing homes. *Source:* Adapted from Banerjee 2007, 6–7.

and governance structures. It is generally understood as representing "a range of services that addresses the health, social and personal care needs of individuals who ... have never developed or have lost some capacity for self-care. Services may be continuous or intermittent, but it is generally presumed that they will be delivered for the 'long-term' that is, indefinitely to individuals who have demonstrated need, usually by some index of functional incapacity" (F/P/T subcommittee 1988, as quoted in A. Banerjee 2007, 6).

LTC is generally divided into three categories defined by the level of support or the venue in which care is delivered. *Home care* refers to services delivered at the individual's residence, or in some cases as a scheduled appointment in a separate location. Individuals who receive home care typically have an adequate level of independence and benefit from informal caretaking services from family or friends. Home care is a range of services including personal care, mobility and transportation assistance, and emotional support and companionship. It may also include medical and nursing services. Specific services and how they are funded differ between provinces.

Secondly, *assisted-living facilities*, *supportive-living facilities*, or *retirement homes* are appropriate for individuals who require assistance with certain daily tasks but do not require intensive medical care. In assisted-living facilities, residents can maintain their autonomy and access personal care, homemaking, health care, and wellness services such as recreational programming intended to support social well-being. In some cases, they offer a spectrum of care to support residents as their needs become more complex.

Nursing homes, also called residential care, care homes, or LTC homes, represent the highest level of care for residents whose health-care or personal-care needs are too intensive or complex for them to maintain the independence necessary in assisted living or home care. Nursing homes have 24-7 professional nursing support. This chapter will refer to this category of care as *nursing homes*, while LTC is used as an overarching term to refer to all categories of the spectrum of care. (See figure 7.1.)

People in LTC are more likely to be female and tend to be sixty-five years of age or older. The correlation of age with the use of LTC services is not absolute (Statistics Canada 2020f, 1).

REGULATORY CONTENT

Standard Setting

The federal government is involved directly with LTC support only through its subsidy program for veterans and the First Nations and Inuit Home and Community Care program (Canadian Health Coalition 2018, 6). LTC is not subject to the overriding principles of the Canada Health Act.

LTC is a provincial and territorial responsibility (Government of Canada 2021f, sec. 92) delegated to the ministry or department of health. In New Brunswick the Department of Social Development and the Department of Health share responsibility (Keefe, MacEachern, and Fancey 2017, 3). In each province, governance is devolved to regional authorities, which range in number and size; provinces also change their structures from time to time.

LTC has accounted for a small proportion of the public spending on health-care services, about 15 per cent in the 2016–17 fiscal year (OECD 2019a, 161). This was 1.3 per cent of Canada's gross domestic product, less than the OECD average of 1.7 per cent (OECD 2019a, 239). LTC spending in Canada has grown at a slower rate than the OECD average (OECD 2017, 215). Compared to the OECD average, a larger proportion of funding is directed towards publicly subsidized assisted-living and nursing homes (OECD 2019a, 239). Ontario is the only province with more growth in home- and community-care budgets than in in-patient care (National Institute on Ageing 2019, 45–6).

Nursing homes are subject to statutes, regulations, and directives that affect their operations. In Ontario the strict regulation of many non-medical tasks adds an administrative burden that workers described as "more counting than caring" (Daly et al. 2016, 57). Other provincial and territorial legislation allows more room for interpretation, detailing general care tasks but not dictating as strictly who must undertake them or when.

The labour force is a notable exception to the high degree of regulation. As of 2015, personal support workers (PSWs) made up 58 per cent of the nursing-home workforce and provided 75–80 per cent of direct care (Estabrooks et al. 2015, 48). PSW is not a registered profession and has no regulatory or professional authority governing it. PSWs in Canada are 90 per cent female, and 67 per cent are older than forty-one years of age (Chamberlain et al. 2019, 40). In 2015 more than half were not born in Canada and spoke English as a second language (Estabrooks et al. 2015, 47).

Most jurisdictions require formal college-level training for PSWs, but the lack of national standards prior to the pandemic led to a patchwork of training curricula. Nova Scotia and British Columbia required the highest minimum classroom and clinical hours, at over 745, compared to Alberta's 485 (Association of Canadian Community Colleges 2012, 23). Despite variation, overall education levels improved, with a much higher proportion of PSWs holding a post-secondary certificate in 2015 compared to 1990 (Pyper 2004; Chamberlain et al. 2019). In some cases, immigrants with professional training, such as nurses, work as PSWs due to difficulty having their credentials recognized (Harun and Walton-Roberts 2022, 11).

Nursing homes are subject to detailed building standards, with a trend towards single-occupancy rooms in recognition of the benefits to the psychosocial and clinical health of residents (Calkins and Cassella 2007, 175). British Columbia permits shared rooms for only 5 per cent of a nursing home's maximum occupancy (Government of British Columbia 2022b, sec. 25). There is a high degree of compliance (Office of the Seniors Advocate British Columbia 2018, 20). Facilities built decades ago, such as Nova Scotia's Northwood facility constructed in 1962, often have shared rooms. Ontario has standards for single or double rooms, but a high proportion of older buildings are exempt from current standards (Stall et al. 2020, e949).

Information Gathering

Information gathering in the LTC sector is fragmented and shared among many different actors within and outside the system. The formal aspect of information gathering is inspection audits of nursing homes that are undertaken, typically annually, by the province or regional health authority. Manitoba and Newfoundland and Labrador do not post inspection results publicly (Frampton 2013). The detail of reports varies considerably; Ontario's resident quality inspections are the most comprehensive (Ontario Ministry of Long-Term Care 2019).

A significant portion of information gathering is undertaken by semi-independent and non-governmental organizations, including advocacy groups. Lobbying organizations also play an important policy intermediary role in interpreting and communicating academic studies (Kemper 2003, 437–8). National studies comparing data across jurisdictions are limited because of reporting differences (Berta et al. 2006, 193).

Wait times for nursing home spaces vary considerably within and across provinces. In 2018 over 32,000 Ontarians were waiting for nursing-home space (Ontario Long-Term Care Association 2019, 2), with a median wait time from the community of 161 days (Health Quality Ontario, n.d.). British Columbia has fewer people on wait-lists (Office of the Seniors Advocate British Columbia 2018, 23), and median wait times vary from 14 to 2,627 days (Office of the Seniors Advocate British Columbia 2018, ii). From 2005 to 2015 the number of nursing-home beds fell by 12.2 per cent, even as demand increased (*Globe and Mail* Editorial Board 2022a). Demand is estimated to more than double, to 454,000 beds, by 2035 (Gibbard 2017, 9).

Behaviour Modification

The two major mechanisms for behaviour modification in LTC are training standards to modify staff behaviour, and enforcement through inspections to modify administrative behaviour. Inconsistent application of each mechanism results in a compliance regime that is not as robust as it may appear.

PSW curricula do not represent true working conditions, with reports of a disconnect between classroom learning and the pace of work in LTC. During staff shortages experienced staff disregard safety protocol in the name of expediency (Kelly 2017, 1434–5). Education programs for mid-career PSWs cause workers to miss wages while paying program fees and incurring transportation costs (Luz and Hanson 2015, 152). Training programs do not prepare students for a shortage of stable, full-time positions (Kelly 2017, 1434). Less than half of the PSWs in Ontario and less than a third in Quebec have full-time jobs (Ontario Ministry of Long-Term Care 2020, 8; Montpetit 2020). Some staff work multiple jobs because part-time work offers low salaries and minimal benefits (Ontario Ministry of Long-Term Care 2020, 11; Chamberlain et al. 2019, 40). High turnover is exacerbated by emotional exhaustion and burnout (McGilton et al. 2014, 918, 922; Ontario Ministry of Long-Term Care 2020, 9). Some studies suggest that the burnout rate is consistent with health-care professions in other settings (Leiter and Maslach 2009, 331). Others find that the unique circumstances in LTC result in higher risks of burnout (Estabrooks et al. 2015, 52; Chamberlain et al. 2017, 61; McGilton et al. 2014, 923).

Implementation of standards can be affected by the scarcity of available resources. Infection prevention and control is one area in which LTC facilities have repeatedly failed to meet recommended standards, some of which are mandatory for accreditation. Despite the recommendation to have one full-time infection-control professional for every 250 beds (Morrison 2004, 5), nursing homes report a mean of 0.6 and a median of 0.3, and few of these professionals are certified by Canada's Certification Board of Infection Control and Epidemiology (Zoutman, Ford, and Gauthier 2009, 359). Low IPC budgets and limited access to both physicians and clerical support have been identified as obstacles to fulfilling recommendations (Gamage et al. 2012, 153).

Inspections are limited by their inconsistent application and minimal enforcement capacity. Historically, Ontario conducted mandatory annual resident quality inspections (RQIs) but amended this system in 2018 to instead conduct inspections in response to specific complaints or incidents (Crea-Arsenio, Baumann, and Smith 2022, 130); in 2019 only nine of 2,800 inspections were RQIs (Pederson, Mancini, and Common 2020).

When non-compliance is found, facilities are often given an opportunity to take voluntary corrective action. Stronger penalties are rarely enforced due in part to the high need for LTC and the lack of alternative providers.

REGULATORY CONTEXT: MARKET FAILURE HYPOTHESIS

Canada's LTC sector is a mix of public and private providers. Of the 2,039 nursing homes in Canada, 46 per cent are publicly owned, 28 per cent are for-profit facilities, and 23 per cent are not-for-profit (CIHI 2020b; see figure 7.2). These numbers are approximate because a breakdown of private facilities in Quebec is not available. For-profit facilities constitute a growing trend. In British Columbia over half of nursing homes built since 1999 are for-profit facilities (Office of the Seniors Advocate British Columbia 2020, 10). Quebec has shown growth in private facilities since 1999 (Gouvernement du Québec 1999, 14). Ontario is the most commercialized province (Daly 2015, 36, 38).

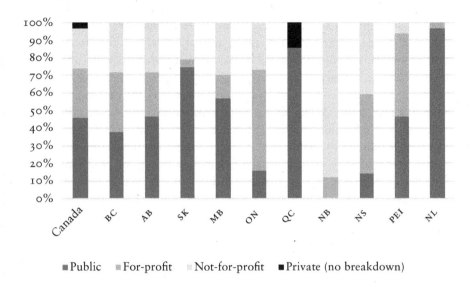

Figure 7.2 | Nursing home ownership by province, 25 May 2020.
Forty-six per cent of nursing homes are publicly owned. *Source:* CIHI 2020b.

The need for formalized LTC is partially a function of labour-market changes. Unpaid caregiving is undervalued despite its economic contribution, estimated to be upwards of $4 billion annually (Jacobs et al. 2013, 108). Caregiving roles were traditionally filled by otherwise unemployed women; as female labour-force participation grew, the pool of people providing full-time informal care shrank. Thirty-five per cent of employed Canadians provide informal care to a friend or family member (Government of Canada 2015, 6). Young and middle-aged women are more likely to remain in the workforce while providing care (Y. Lee and Tang 2013, 468). At higher levels of care intensity, this is not as feasible, and retirement is more likely (Jacobs et al. 2014, 77). The loss of an informal caregiver is one of the primary predictors of transition to nursing-home care (Garner et al. 2018, 20).

Information Costs

Information costs refer to the costs of assessing the probability and severity of risks. A scenario in which individuals need further support but cannot or do not know where to obtain information about available options would be a high-cost situation. Generally, information costs are high for those seeking to make informed choices about what care they need or are entitled to as they age, due largely to the number of sources, different standards across jurisdictions, and, at times, lack of transparency in reporting. This makes it difficult to learn about the system in a comprehensive manner.

The number of people who live at home but need further support is difficult to estimate. Eligibility requirements vary by jurisdiction, and there are no comprehensive databases tracking wait-lists (Gibbard 2017, 6). Additionally, defining a "need" for nursing-home care is subjective. Unfamiliarity with options, difficulty navigating the health-care system, or contextual factors, such as the death of a spouse or living in a rural area, can influence individuals who do not require full-time care to move to nursing homes by default (National Institute on Ageing 2019, 67; CIHI 2020a).

Opt-Out Costs

Opt-out costs are the costs of avoiding or reducing one's exposure to risk, which in the context of LTC generally refers to vulnerable populations securing appropriate care as they age or their needs change, to minimize the risks of long-term conditions or, simply, aging. One component of opt-out costs is the legal framework that gives people recourse if negative outcomes occur due to negligence. If a recipient of LTC experiences harm from care staff or management, there is legal recourse in the form of a tort claim. Facilities owe residents a "duty of care" – a legal responsibility to make efforts to avoid acts that could reasonably be expected to cause harm – and must uphold a reasonable "standard of care" (Pinkesz 2020, para. 2, 4). If either is violated, the claimant may be entitled to compensation, and the LTC home may be liable. Usually they are covered by liability insurance in case of claims of medical malpractice or negligence (Meckbach 2020b). Limits on the amounts of damages that may be awarded and a high threshold for establishing negligence reduce the financial burden on LTC homes (Law Library of Congress 2009, 1).

Opting out of risk exposure also depends on one's ability to pay to avoid risk. In terms of who pays for LTC, it was largely an afterthought in the context of health care. The evolution of universal public health insurance, like most policy, is a product of incrementalism and compromise, not necessarily reflecting evidence-based decisions on how to best direct funds. The Canada Health Act (1984) insures only the health-care portion of LTC expenditures, leaving the rest to provincial and territorial administration or the private market. The definition of "medically necessary" services is based on old legislation and is ambiguous, affecting the delineation of federally insured health services (Flood and Thomas 2016, 399, 411). Provinces and territories can choose to insure extended health services, including nursing-home intermediate care, adult residential care, home care, and ambulatory health-care services.

A range of services further complicates opt-out costs. Rates for a room can be $1,800–$3,400 per month (Fernandes and Spencer 2010, 310; Picard 2021, 52). Private home care can cost $25–$100 an hour. Some expenses are paid by individuals, but much is publicly funded. In Ontario 91 per cent of clients pay nothing for home-care nursing services, while 79 per cent pay nothing for other home-care services (Closing the Gap Healthcare Group Inc. 2019, sec. 4ii).

There is considerable variation in ability to pay. The mean disposable income of Canadians over sixty-five was $48,817 as of 2018 (OECD 2020b). As of 2016, 12.2 per cent of Canadians sixty-five and older lived in poverty, less than the OECD average (OECD 2019b, 187). Among Canadians aged fifty-five to sixty-four, 75 per cent have $100,000 or less in savings, while 44 per cent have less than $5,000 (Janes 2023). In contrast, over half of Canadians aged fifty-five to sixty-four have accrued employer pension benefits (Shillington 2016, 3), and some live in expensive real estate. The transfer of wealth as the baby-boomer generation dies is expected to be the largest in history (M. Hall 2019, para. 2).

Demand for some services outpaces supply, and more than one-third of people with self-reported home-care needs were unable to access sufficient services in 2015–16 (Gilmour 2018a; 2018b, 3). In other areas, resources are allocated inefficiently; only 30 per cent of those eighty-five and older in nursing homes require such robust supports (Garner et al. 2018, 16; Picard 2021, 55).

REGULATORY CONTEXT:
OPINION-RESPONSIVE HYPOTHESIS

Canadians' average age has increased every year since 1971 (Statistics Canada 2020a, 1, 4). In 2011 the first members of the baby-boomer generation turned sixty-five. As they age, Canada will experience significant demographic and economic change. Seniors over sixty-five years of age make up 17.2 per cent of the total population (see figure 7.3) but are predicted to reach 21.4–23.4 per cent by 2030 (Statistics Canada 2019b, 14). Consequently, LTC is expected to become a growing concern.

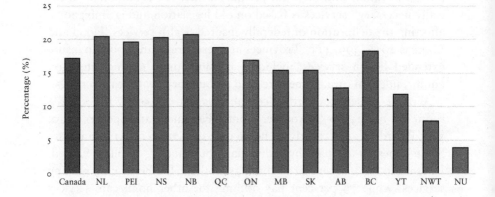

Figure 7.3 | An aging population: proportion of seniors sixty-five years of age and older, by province, 2018. *Source:* Statistics Canada 2019b.

As a result of economic pressures and immigration, certain regions, like Atlantic Canada, will be more affected by aging than the Prairies and territories (Saillant 2017, 15:08, 19:44; Statistics Canada 2019b, 38, 50). Longer lifespans come with rising acuity levels, meaning that more nursing resources are required to provide care, and there is a higher prevalence of chronic conditions that can limit an individual's independence (Chappell 2011, 6).

Traditionally, a cultural taboo around death has inhibited meaningful conversation about how individuals would like to be supported in their final years (Llewellyn et al. 2016, 308). Recent discourse around medical assistance in dying suggests that Canadians are becoming more engaged in discussing end-of-life care (Angus Reid Institute 2020b; R. Jones 2021b). Canadians largely agree that a "good death" means appropriate support and not dying alone (Heyland et al. 2006, 630).

Public opinion is largely in favour of policies that expand access to health care. Most people are worried about growing health-care costs due to an aging population; over half believe that many people will delay retirement to pay for health care in their old age (Ipsos and Canadian Medical Association 2019, 4, 7). Three in five Canadians report being unprepared to care for family members who require LTC (Ipsos 2015, 1), and informal caregivers who receive financial assistance report the need for more (Statistics Canada 2020e, 2). Sixty per cent of Canadians believe that nursing homes should be a health

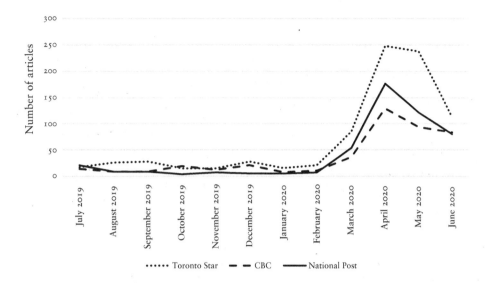

Figure 7.4 | Media coverage of senior residences, long-term care, assisted living, seniors' homes, or retirement homes, July 2019–June 2020. LTC coverage was minimal before the 2019 federal election.
Sources: Toronto Star; CBC News; *National Post*.

priority; support is especially strong among those over fifty-five years of age (Ipsos 2017, 7). In the 2019 federal election two-thirds of older Canadians were prepared to vote for the party with the most convincing policies to improve the health system, which included increased funding to help provinces cover health care for seniors, and a new family care benefit so that seniors could afford care options (Ipsos and Canadian Medical Association 2019, 3). Non-medical LTC services receive less overall support, but the priorities of older Canadians are of particular significance; until 2018, the baby-boom generation represented the largest portion of the electorate.

Apart from occasional investigative pieces (L. Lloyd et al. 2014; Welsh 2020), media coverage of LTC does not reflect the importance ascribed to it by polling data. As figure 7.4 shows, there was no spike in mentions of LTC terms in major Canadian newspapers in the lead-up to the 2019 federal election.

REGULATORY CONTEXT:
INTEREST GROUP HYPOTHESIS

The interest group hypothesis (IGH) analyzes the distribution of costs and benefits of regulation to determine the level of intervention that can be explained by organized interests lobbying to maximize their own benefit (Hood, Rothstein, and Baldwin 2001).

The for-profit LTC market is concentrated but still relatively modest compared to oligopolies in other sectors, like finance or telecommunications. The five largest chains in Canada, owning and operating 18.9 per cent of nursing homes and 23.8 per cent of beds, are Extendicare, Revera Inc., Sienna Senior Living Inc., Chartwell Retirement Residences, and Schlegel Villages. Financial data show stable profit margins of 9–13 per cent annually (Harrington et al. 2017, 5). In 2020, a challenging year for the sector, many operators met their corporate targets, even paying bonuses to top executives (Milstead 2021).

Private companies are playing an increasingly larger role. Accreditation of nursing homes is voluntary. Forty-two per cent of LTC homes are not accredited by Accreditation Canada (Health Standards Organization 2021). Accredited facilities are likely to be in an urban area, part of a chain, and owned by a for-profit corporation (McDonald, Wagner, and Gruneir 2015, 55). For-profit providers make up an increasing proportion of the market. Fifty-six per cent of Ontario nursing homes are owned by for-profit providers, 82 per cent of which are large chains (Daly 2015, 50; Harrington et al. 2017, 5). Elimination of preferential funding for not-for-profit providers and onerous regulatory and reporting tools have forced smaller, independent homes to contract out their management to large for-profit companies (Daly 2015, 51).

Staffing is the largest expenditure for private owners, though for-profit facilities spend less on direct care and consistently provide fewer hours per patient than public or not-for-profit facilities do (Office of the Seniors Advocate British Columbia 2020, 6; McGrail et al. 2007, 57; Berta et al. 2006, 189). Wages for PSWs are lower in the private sector than in public nursing homes (Office of the Seniors Advocate British Columbia 2020, 28; Montpetit 2020, 17).

The benefits of intervention are diffused across recipients of LTC services, their families, and staff. Nursing-home residents have minimal ability to mobilize, and families have limited regulatory influence (Annable 2020, 4). Advocacy groups, like CanAge, represent the interests of seniors. With partners in academia and in the delivery of senior support services, CanAge is an important part of the government's information-gathering strategy, appearing at committee meetings in the Senate and the House of Commons. Another advocacy group, the Canadian Association of Retired Persons (CARP), is advocating for home care that focuses on person-centred care, updated standards, and a worker-recruitment drive.

Staff can mobilize through union membership. By international standards Canada has high rates of unionization in the LTC workforce (Lowndes and Struthers 2016, 377). Membership is fragmented across several different unions, most of which are not devoted to PSWs or LTC staff.

In sum, standards in LTC vary as each jurisdiction has its own model with a range of structures (public, private, for profit, and not-for-profit). Operations of nursing homes tend to be strictly regulated, though the workforce is largely unregulated. Information gathering is fragmented among many actors, with differences in types of data collected and disclosed. That said, a multitude of inquiries and reports offer evidence of a system in need of change (Picard 2021, 2). Behaviour modification is modest, with inconsistent application of training standards and weak enforcement through inspections.

A market failure hypothesis is one possible explanation for this control mechanism. Information costs are somewhat high; it is difficult to learn about the system in a complete manner, and people generally do not concern themselves with LTC until they or someone they know urgently requires care. Opt-out costs vary due to a range of funding and ability to pay. It is unlikely that a market failure is the most effective predictor of regulatory change for LTC, given there are policies that could lower information costs by centralizing information, or that could lower opt-out costs by implementing stricter standards and audits to protect a vulnerable population. In terms of public opinion, media coverage of LTC is low, but polling data indicate that people support the expansion of services. If the opinion-responsive hypothesis explained the control mechanism, a population with high electoral influence would pressure the sector to improve, which may be seen as the population ages. At this point, there has been limited regulatory change. The IGH has moderate explanatory value, but it could be increasing. There are some interests, like LTC providers, on which the costs of regulation are concentrated. A growing private sector benefits from low regulation that permits limited transparency and low wages for staff. The benefits of LTC regulation generally rest with residents, their families, and staff, but these groups have limited advocacy and representation. Should service provision become more concentrated in a handful of organizations with strong lobbying capacity, these problems will become more pronounced. High regulation can also make it easier for large companies, with the capacity to meet regulations, to establish oligopolies.

LTC in Canada is a fragmented system with long-standing problems, weak mechanisms to modify standards and behaviour, and a vulnerable population with limited influence. From these contextual pressures it is evident that the system was akin to a tinderbox that the COVID-19 pandemic ignited.

CHRONOLOGY OF THE FIRST WAVE

Close living quarters and shared caregivers are conducive to the spread of respiratory diseases (Lansbury, Brown, and Nguyen-Van-Tam 2017, 356–7). Influenza and pneumonia are consistently in the top ten causes of death in Canada, and older populations are significantly more vulnerable. In 2019, influenza deaths in people sixty-five years and older accounted for nearly 90 per cent of all influenza-caused deaths (Statistics Canada 2020l), though the proportion that occurred in LTC facilities was not reported. Influenza hospitalization and death rates are higher in LTC compared to those of seniors living in the community, which can be partly attributed to the poorer baseline health of LTC residents (Menec, MacWilliam, and Aoki 2002, 629). Influenza outbreaks are common and can be widespread (Mahmud et al. 2013, 1056; Government of Canada 2006), so it is not unprecedented that respiratory illnesses cause death in nursing homes. The mortality rate of COVID-19 in nursing homes, however, was high, reaching 3–4 per cent in June 2020, compared to a 0.1 per cent mortality rate from a typical influenza (Estabrooks et al. 2020, 11).

On 5 March 2020 a nursing home in North Vancouver reported that one of its staff members had tested positive for COVID-19 (Hager and Woo 2020). On 6 March another health-care worker and two residents tested positive. Canada's first LTC outbreak was declared, followed two days later by its first official COVID-19–related death.

In anticipation of hospital overload as seen in Wuhan or Italy, early provincial government strategy in Alberta, Ontario, and Quebec focused on increasing surge capacity by transferring patients who no longer required the intensity of hospital resources to LTC homes or temporary wards. Both Ontario and Alberta amended policies to be able to transfer patients more easily to the first available LTC bed. In two months Ontario hospitals transferred approximately 1,600 patients to nursing homes and 600 to assisted living (K. Grant and Ha 2020). Quebec relocated patients to temporary wards in hotels, decommissioned hospital buildings, or private LTC facilities. By early April it was evident that the initial hospital surge would not occur to the same extent as it had in Wuhan or Italy, but that LTC homes would be a battleground. Quebec and Ontario suspended hospital transfers in mid-April (Ha 2020; M. Anderson et al. 2020).

There were some success stories. LTC homes with few cases had strong leadership and set new standards early without formal direction from government (Lavoie-Tremblay et al. 2022; Baumann et al. 2022). In January 2020 a nursing home in Montreal required staff travelling from abroad to stay home until they were determined to be COVID-free (Bains 2020). A non-profit group operating four nursing homes in Toronto cancelled social gatherings within the homes and put staff returning from visiting Asia over the holidays on a paid fourteen-day quarantine (S. Ho 2020). Within two days of the WHO declaring a pandemic, these nursing homes prohibited non-essential visitors and began restricting resident movement (S. Ho 2020). LTC homes that demonstrated successful infection management also took early steps to modify staff behaviour: offering full-time hours to part-timers to prevent staff working in multiple homes (Bains 2020); conducting recruitment drives among nursing and PSW students, retirees, and non-union hires; and training housekeeping staff to cover non-medical tasks, freeing certified staff for other duties (S. Ho 2020). Placing an early focus on PPE, these facilities reached out to suppliers in China to avoid the looming domestic shortage (S. Ho 2020); provided staff with training related to PPE use, sanitation protocol, and infection control; and had dedicated IPC teams available to answer questions (Bains 2020).

The inability of other LTC homes to prevent or slow outbreaks was exacerbated by staffing problems. British Columbia issued a health order restricting workers to one facility (K. Grant and Stone 2020). Ontario issued similar guidance, then orders, to restrict circulation (Stone, Howlett, and Ha 2020). In contrast, Quebec issued a decree on 25 April permitting its health ministry to redeploy LTC workers to fill gaps at other homes, which likely caused several outbreaks (McKenna 2020).

The pandemic exerted pressure on an already stretched workforce as staff self-isolated, tested positive, or stayed home out of fear. In extreme cases like Quebec's CHSLD Résidence Herron, only three staff remained to oversee 133 residents on the morning of 29 March (Derfel 2020a). Provinces attempted to boost their workforce with medical students, retired nurses, and volunteers from shuttered services, with limited success (Grant and Stone 2020). Wage increases and bonuses were used to attract and retain PSWs. In British Columbia standardization of pay regardless of facility ownership resulted in wage increases in private facilities. All provinces accessed the $3 billion federal fund for essential worker wage top-ups, though each had a different payment plan and definition of "essential worker." British Columbia, Ontario, and Quebec retroactively paid a $4 per hour top-up for a sixteen-week period; Alberta settled on one-time payments of $1,200 (French 2021). With average wages of $18–$21 per hour, hiring companies that offered $30–$35 an hour for positions at a different facility or in home care attracted PSWs away from their current positions (Stone and Keller 2020; Hendry 2020).

Both Ontario and Quebec asked for extra support from the Canadian Armed Forces (CAF), an expense of $53 million paid by the federal government (Brewster 2020). Starting on 16 April, a total of 1,350 soldiers were deployed to twenty-five nursing homes in Quebec, mainly around Montreal (*Globe and Mail* 2020c). On 22 April Ontario asked for assistance in five nursing homes: Eatonville Care Centre, Hawthorne Place Care Centre, Altamont Care Community, Orchard Villa, and Holland Christian–Grace Manor – private, for-profit facilities, three of which were accredited. Forces were later deployed to Downsview LTC Centre and Woodbridge Vista Care Community, too. Both missions released reports detailing conditions witnessed by CAF personnel. The Ontario report is graphic in detailing poor hygiene standards, poor compliance with IPC guidelines, and insufficient PPE (CAF 2020b). It identifies inadequate staffing and incidents of elder abuse and neglect like "forceful feeding," ignored calls for help, and skipped meals (CAF 2020b, B-1/3). The Quebec report details problems of insufficient staffing with high rates of absenteeism, poor IPC compliance and training, and inadequate supplies (CAF 2020a).

Several provinces took over the administration of poorly performing private LTC homes. Alberta Health Services temporarily took over the day-to-day operations of one facility and transferred management and operations of a second to another organization after outbreaks among staff rendered them unable to care for residents (J. Russell 2020). Quebec placed Résidence Herron under trusteeship; the facility had the appearance of a "concentration camp" with dehydrated, soiled, and unfed residents (Derfel 2020b, para. 1, 15). SEIU Healthcare, an Ontario union, called for the provincial government to take over the operations of Eatonville Care Centre and Anson Place Care Centre, where more than fifty-four residents died (Stone and Howlett 2020).

The government initially declined. Five days later those two facilities received military assistance. Following the release of the CAF report in May, Ontario announced that it would assume control of four of the five homes listed in the report as well as one in Mississauga (CBC News 2020e), eventually transferring the management of nine facilities temporarily to local hospitals. Deaths in these facilities represented one in four of all LTC deaths in Ontario during the first wave (K. Howlett 2020).

Unions used legal means to influence the pandemic response of nursing homes. SEIU Healthcare turned to the Ontario Labour Relations Board for emergency measures to protect front-line workers. The board ordered three nursing homes to take more steps to provide appropriate protections for staff, and mandated weekly in-person inspections by the Ministry of Labour (Grant and Howlett 2020). The Ontario Nurses' Association alleged that four private facilities were restricting PPE and not following proper infection protocols; the Ontario Superior Court of Justice issued a court order for them to comply with public health directives and rectify health and safety issues (Ontario Nurses' Association 2020).

As the pandemic took its toll, families of victims began to seek redress for their losses. By 30 June 2020, ten proposed class-action lawsuits had been launched on behalf of residents and their families in four provinces, alleging negligence in the form of non-compliance with infection protocol and substandard care (Top Class Actions 2021). The defendants were private owners or operators of LTC homes, occasionally in conjunction with a government body (Zanoni 2020). The first lawsuit to be filed was against Résidence Herron and alleged a "wanton disregard for the life, safety and dignity of its residents" (Kugler Kandestin 2020, para. 2); lawyers reached a $5.5 million settlement with the facility's owners in April 2021 (S. Banerjee 2021). The number of class-actions lawsuits grew as more information emerged (Top Class Actions 2021).

CHRONOLOGY OF THE SECOND WAVE

After a respite in the summer, the virus's second wave disproportionately affected LTC. From 1 September 2020 to 15 February 2021, more LTC facilities experienced outbreaks, and 62 per cent more residents were infected compared to the first wave (CIHI 2021a, 7). As seen in table 7.1, however, Quebec and Nova Scotia showed a decrease in resident deaths.

Quebec premier François Legault announced in June 2020 a campaign to recruit and train 10,000 new orderlies by mid-September in

Table 7.1 | Long-term-care homes affected by the first two waves of COVID-19

Province	Resident deaths, first wave (1 March 2020–31 August 2020)	Resident deaths, second wave (1 September 2020– 15 February 2021)	Change (%)
QC	4,613	3,103	–32.7
ON	2,072	2,225	+7.4
AB	153	1,013	+562.1
BC	120	567	+372.5
NS	57	0	–100.0
SK	2	84	+4,100.0
MB	3	465	+15,400.0
NF	0	0	0.0
NB	2	13	+550.0
PEI	0	0	0.0
CAN	7,022	7,470	+6.4

In Canadian LTC facilities the second wave caused 6.4 per cent more deaths than the first wave. *Source:* National Institute on Ageing, as quoted in Howlett and Ha (2021).

preparation for subsequent waves (Mignacca 2020). This was complemented by implementing IPC teams in LTC homes (Howlett and Ha 2021), which prevented fatalities in facilities but potentially neglected other forms of elder care (Hendry and Shingler 2020; Span 2021). While people over sixty years of age made up the majority of COVID-19–related deaths in Quebec from September onwards, they died at home or in private seniors' residences. Nova Scotia planned measures for the second wave, but the peak of active cases was low and primarily affected people aged eighteen to thirty-five years (Luck 2020), with fewer than thirty cases in nursing homes (CIHI 2021a, 9).

Provinces with increased LTC cases and deaths delayed preparation or failed to implement changes from the first wave. More than half of Ontario's COVID-related nursing-home deaths, including its deadliest LTC outbreak, occurred in the fall and winter (Crawley 2021a; A. Russell 2021). Many workers left the sector between waves, citing financial constraints (Amin and Bond 2020). In July 2020 Ontario was aware that it needed "1000s" of PSWs (A. Russell et al. 2021b, para. 10), but programs to recruit workers and accelerate training were not launched until the fall (Government of Ontario 2020b, 2020d). In homes that experienced large outbreaks from mid-November to December 2020, 64.6 per cent of workers said there was not enough staff to provide daily hands-on care (Ontario Health Coalition 2020, 1). In addition, over one-third of Ontario nursing homes adhered to design standards from 1972 that permitted up to four beds per room (Stall et al. 2020, e949). Though the presence of COVID-19 in the surrounding community was the greatest indicator that an LTC home would experience an outbreak, crowded facilities experienced significantly larger outbreaks (Stall et al. 2021, 14). Ontario specified in October 2020 that new residents must be placed in single or "semi-private" rooms (Stall et al. 2021, 19), but the province lacked clear protocols for isolating infected residents. Some facilities planned to use spaces such as convention halls (Russell et al. 2021b); these efforts varied. Crowding was an issue in about one-fifth of subsequent outbreaks (Ontario Health Coalition 2020, 2).

Other jurisdictions that fared relatively well in the first wave were not able to sustain that success. In Manitoba there were only three LTC resident deaths in spring 2020, then 465 during the second wave. A private facility in Winnipeg with 54 deaths was not prepared for a major loss of staff, public health officials were not informed in a timely manner, and directives from the health ministry were confusing and unwieldy (Stevenson 2021, 21). A class-action lawsuit alleged that residents were left "dehydrated, malnourished and vulnerable" (Levasseur 2021, para. 3).

British Columbia was praised for its handling of the first wave, but it too managed poorly from September onwards, seeing a nearly five-fold increase in LTC deaths. An East Vancouver nursing home was understaffed, even with 87 additional workers, during a two-month outbreak. Forty-one of 114 residents died (Kane 2021). Staff, with few clear directives, struggled to keep residents isolated and care for those who were sick. Another criticism was that widespread testing was not prioritized in LTC facilities until January 2021 (J. Hunter 2021), though modelling found that its earlier implementation could have caught asymptomatic cases and prevented 25–55 per cent of outbreaks (Tupper and Colijn 2021, 7).

Attempts to reduce transmission led to residents experiencing prolonged social isolation. A September 2020 directive in Ontario clarified that "essential visitors" included designated caregivers. Rules did not expand until May 2021, when two people could visit a resident outside – meaning immobile residents still could not have any visitors (Jonas 2021a, para. 7). In British Columbia a policy allowing one designated visitor per resident meant that families had to make difficult decisions (CBC News 2020b). The well-documented effects of prolonged isolation on residents include worsening loneliness, depression, and dementia (King and Gollum 2021).

On 9 December 2020 Health Canada approved the use of the *Pfizer-BioNTech* COVID-19 vaccine, and then on 23 December the use of the Moderna COVID-19 vaccine (Tasker 2020b; R. Jones 2020). The first person in the country to receive a COVID-19 vaccine was Gisèle Lévesque, an eighty-nine-year-old nursing-home resident in Quebec City, on 14 December (Perreaux, Walsh, and Gray 2020). Later that day, Anita Quidangen, a Toronto PSW, was the first person in Ontario to get the vaccine (Powers 2020).

Before Canada received any shipments of vaccines, the NACI recommended that priority be given to certain populations: residents, staff, and family caregivers in LTC, retirement homes, and other congregate settings for older persons; adults over seventy years of age; healthcare workers; and adults in Indigenous communities (Sinha, Fell, and Iciaszczyk 2021). Each province and territory released vaccination rollout strategies, all with a target date for the first dose to be offered to LTC residents by March 2021 at the latest. Five provinces and one territory included family caregivers of residents as part of the prioritized group. In some cases priority seemed to be given to staff over residents. For example, by 5 January 2021, Ontario had given an initial dose of vaccine to around 4,000 (5.5 per cent) of 72,000 residents and 26,000 (26.0 per cent) of more than 100,000 staff (Sinha, Feil, and Iciaszczyk 2021). Ontario also faced criticism for shipping vaccines to hospitals, whereas Quebec placed half of its vaccine distribution centres directly inside LTC homes, ensuring residents would be inoculated quickly (A. Russell et al. 2021a).

Most LTC residents were vaccinated by March 2021, and the impact was felt quickly. Eight weeks after vaccinations began in Ontario, the estimated reduction in COVID-19 infection was 89 per cent in LTC residents and 79 per cent in workers. Mortality due to COVID-19 in residents was reduced by 96 per cent (K. Brown et al. 2021, 2). Attention then shifted to the quality-of-life issues resulting from social isolation (Ireland 2021).

AUDITS AND REPORTS

Several reports and audits have been published following the pandemic's impact on LTC. Insufficient staffing and training and poor IPC compliance are common problems detailed in facilities that experienced devastating outbreaks. Conditions witnessed by CAF personnel in Ontario in April 2020 include low staffing levels "such that it is impossible to provide care at a pace that is appropriate to each resident" (CAF 2020b, annex A 6e), and "little or no orientation for new staff resulting in low adherence to protocol" (CAF 2020b, annex B 6b). The CAF report on Quebec has similar observations and partly attributes poor adherence to standards to the high proportion of volunteers and new employees with limited training (CAF 2020a). Insufficient access to PPE did not help. At the Extendicare Parkside special-care home in Saskatchewan, where 194 of 198 residents tested positive in the second wave, Extendicare issued one mask per worker per day instead of the four required by the province (Ombudsman Saskatchewan 2021).

Infrastructure was a problem in several provinces. More than half the residents at Extendicare Parkside, built in the 1960s, lived in shared spaces of up to four people per room. Eliminating shared rooms would have led to 30 per cent less revenue for Extendicare (Ombudsman Saskatchewan 2021). In Nova Scotia's Northwood facility an outbreak that killed fifty-three residents was exacerbated by shared rooms and bathrooms; a review recommends, without specific targets, that occupancy be reduced permanently (Lata and Stevenson 2020, 2, 5). A report on the future of LTC in Alberta recommends revising design guidelines and phasing out shared rooms by 2027 (MNP LLP 2021). Some provinces will likely keep a small number of double or adjoining rooms for couples (Saskatchewan Ministry of Health 2009, 2).

Regulating staffing is a consistent theme. In June 2020 a policy briefing from the Royal Society of Canada stated that the workforce crisis was the "pivotal challenge" facing LTC (Estabrooks et al. 2020, 6). It recommends providing better pay and benefits for PSWs, setting minimum education standards, and emphasizing continuing education (Estabrooks et al. 2020). A report in Alberta recommends increasing direct hours of care in nursing homes, which would require 6,500 more jobs; the report emphasizes creating full-time positions over part-time (MNP LLP 2021, 47, 192). Another report recommends that the Ministry of Long-Term Care in Ontario develop a staffing strategy to address the root causes of shortages that occurred throughout the pandemic and consider ways to professionalize and regulate the role of PSWs (Lysyk 2021, 42). It also notes that Ontario's emergency plan was outdated, and recommendations made by the Auditor General three years ago to update and revise it regularly had not been implemented.

One policy briefing says that although an effective LTC sector includes home care, assisted living, and retirement homes, the need for nursing homes will not disappear. This suggests that increasing funding to improve home care is not the only solution to the problems facing LTC (Estabrooks et al. 2020). Few reports suggest the services to cut. The review in Alberta recommends changing the distribution of services by 2030 to decrease the portion of the population receiving care in facilities from 39 to 30 per cent and to increase home or community care from 61 to 70 per cent (MNP LLP 2021, 114).

CONCLUSION

Although the media coverage of LTC facilities during the first wave was profoundly disturbing for most, in non-pandemic times death and suffering occur regularly in LTC facilities, an experience not always on display in popular culture. In Ontario the average nursing-home resident dies within eighteen months of being admitted (Arya 2020). Public health was, in part, unlucky in its initial handling of COVID-19. The risk was uncertain, and early strategy focused on transferring hospital patients to LTC homes, based on experiences elsewhere. By April, however, it was clear that LTC homes would be an important battleground.

Though some nursing homes implemented risk-reduction measures nearly two months before the first case of the virus in Canada's LTC system, this forward thinking was unfortunately too rare. After the first wave of COVID-19 had subsided, the rate at which jurisdictions learned contributed to their success in containing the second wave, raising important questions about how the system establishes standards and enforces behaviours.

Midway through 2021, after vaccine distribution, the majority of Canadians with family and friends in LTC believed that their facility handled its COVID-19 response as well as "could be expected" (39 per cent) or "well enough overall" (42 per cent; Angus Reid Institute 2021a, para. 4). Almost one in five, however, said that their loved one's LTC facility failed in its duties. Liability for LTC failures is not consistent across jurisdictions. In Ontario, legislation protecting organizations from COVID-19 liability covers LTC facilities that take "honest measures" to follow public health guidelines (CBC News 2020f, para. 3).

Lawsuit immunity for essential-service providers in British Columbia excludes LTC homes (J. Hunter 2020).

The way forward is fraught with difficult decisions captured by the tensions inherent in the system. In cultural theory terms (see chapter 2), LTC sits between competing governance forces. Based on a history in the welfare system, it still has elements of a community service that cares for the vulnerable. It is expensive and difficult to organize on a large scale. It is also bureaucratic; various standards aim to emphasize fairness, but by its nature, bureaucracy can be highly depersonalized. Increasingly, the private sector has responded to the market's needs by treating people like customers who make demands for care and who pay for service. Market, not-for-profit, and bureaucratic influences all try to keep costs down, but each makes different assumptions about where to cut and what constitutes good governance.

Among older Canadians there is a pronounced resolve to avoid LTC facilities; 85 per cent of Canadians and 96 per cent over the age of sixty-five plan to live at home as long as possible (National Institute on Ageing 2021, 7). CARP (2021) is advocating strongly for improved home care. This still leaves vulnerabilities. During the first two waves of the pandemic in particular, the elderly living at home were largely overlooked, partly due to the focus on nursing homes (Picard 2020; Eligh 2020).

Addressing the needs of the elderly requires a broad scope. Government policies increasingly encourage people to stay at home longer with various tax incentives and home-care services (Greenard 2020; Government of British Columbia, n.d.; City of Toronto, n.d.). While advocates argue that home care is better and can be more cost-effective (Chappell 2011, 17), having people stay longer in homes creates other challenges, like a lack of housing stock for people entering the housing market. There is also dispute over which home-care costs should be publicly funded. Even if resources are diverted to home-care services, the need for facility-based care will not disappear. Patients with complex care needs require the full-time supports of facility-based care, and many home-care clients will eventually need such care.

In some respects, it would be an ironic conclusion to the pandemic if more money were spent on the last years of life; public health advocates have long argued for funding to promote health and prevent disease throughout a person's life (National Expert Commission 2012, 13, 18). Mental-health issues among younger people throughout the pandemic underscore the need for resources at different times in one's life, but there is not a lot of extra cash. Health is already the largest expense among provincial, territorial, and local governments, accounting for 37.2 per cent of spending (Statistics Canada 2020o, 2).

There is also financial disparity among the elderly. Irrespective of income, LTC serves a vulnerable population with limited self-advocacy. About 4.1 per cent of LTC residents in Alberta, for example, are incapacitated and with no surrogate decision maker (Chamberlain et al. 2019). This population is expected to grow given the increasing proportion of older adults, the higher rates of one-person households and childlessness, and the rising prevalence of dementias. Advocacy of workers is limited, too: few unions are focused exclusively on PSWs or LTC staff, whereas doctors and nurses tend to have stronger representation.

If a "good" death is important, reforms are needed, as reports have noted for decades. There are calls for a public system to be incorporated into the Canada Health Act or for building on existing regulatory provisions in the Act, using the approach of the 2017 Health Accord (Tholl, Hirdes, and Hébert 2020). Changing the Act would be a slow and expensive process. The private sector will likely continue to play an important role in an era when people are pushing for better-quality home care and more choice in services.

An increased role for the private sector must be accompanied by stronger standards (Roman 2023), including the accreditation of organizations, consistent audits with publicly available results, and the enforcement of legal and financial penalties if standards are not met. The sector needs to continue to professionalize with better pay, training, and stability for employees (Bulmer and Penny 2022; Colleges & Institutes Canada 2023). Although we think of LTC failures as a health issue, low wages and a lack of stable employment are economic issues and market failures. If society wants stronger LTC, the front-line workers require stronger representation.

The similarities in recommendations across audits following the pandemic are striking, with many calling for stronger pandemic protocols to be identified, shared, put in place, and enforced. Given the frequency with which people die of viral infection in homes, these risks need to be treated as complex. While a precautionary stance against viral infection is necessary, operators of LTC facilities require a stronger understanding and management of the variables that cause disease spread. Families and caregivers need to be aware of these plans and included in solutions. Crucially, we must put dignity at the centre of care. As COVID-19 demonstrated repeatedly, and dramatically in LTC, there is a need for greater concern for vulnerable populations. In the case of LTC, this will only grow as the population ages.

Tourism: The Higher It Rises, the Harder It Falls

The COVID-19 pandemic devastated tourism. With borders and businesses closed, flights cancelled, and large gatherings forbidden, the sector was effectively shut down overnight by the nature of the disease and various government interventions.

After decades of growth in global travel and tourism, arguably a feature of modernity (Butcher 2020), it all seemed to stop. While the pandemic was a global phenomenon, everyone's world seemed to shrink; everything suddenly became local. The decision to restrict travel to contain the virus saved lives but contributed to a worsening of people's subjective well-being[1] as social, health, and economic problems piled up and much-needed relief and renewal through holiday rituals were significantly curtailed.

Beyond this broad social impact, the pandemic exposed more clearly the economic importance of the sector. Tourism is one of the fastest-growing sectors in the world. It is a significant employer made up of several industries, including accommodations, food and beverage, recreation and entertainment, transportation, and travel services (Tourism HR Canada, n.d.e). Like the health sector, the tourism sector employs just over 10 per cent of Canada's workforce, although the average salary in the tourism sector is significantly lower (Statistics Canada 2020n, 2022l). It is also a highly fragile sector; crises are not new to it. Although COVID-19 is the most significant in the sector's modern history, there are several recent examples of events that have demonstrated the sector's vulnerability.

There are actually two realities in tourism: 1 per cent of tourism businesses are large companies like hotel chains and airlines that have significant staff, money, and lobbying capacity, and the other 99 per cent are small and medium-sized enterprises (SMEs), 98 per cent of which employ 100 or fewer employees (DC 2021a, 8; Tam, Sood, and Johnston 2021b, 4); they work in a highly competitive context, with low cash reserves, little influence, and precarious employment (DC 2021a). Food and beverage services account for more than 55 per cent of all tourism jobs (Tourism HR Canada, n.d.e). Many in the sector work part time for low wages and few benefits and are vulnerable to market changes (ILO 2022, 9). Job losses in this sector were larger than in any other; in May 2020 unemployment hit 30 per cent.

In contrast to the previous chapter on LTC, which was framed largely as a health issue throughout the pandemic with important economic dimensions, this chapter focuses on a sector that was devasted economically as a result of COVID-19 with important health-related dimensions. It reviews how governments regulate the tourism sector generally and the market, media, popular, and interest-group context in which it existed pre-pandemic. The chapter then summarizes how COVID-19 and government response had an impact on the sector.

The sector is considered non-essential. In fact, the episode reveals how important it is. Governments need to move beyond seeing the sector strictly as a short-term job creator to regarding it as a strategic sector that plays an important role in supporting people's well-being, employs many vulnerable people in urban and rural areas, and has significant sustainability challenges. Stronger partnerships between government bodies and industry can help address some of these challenges. Like the previous chapter on the vulnerable and LTC, we start by reviewing the standards, then focus on how the federal, provincial, and territorial governments gather information about the sector and change behaviour. We then look at how the vulnerabilities in the sector manifested throughout the pandemic and conclude with some lessons that the sector and governments should draw from the experience.

REGULATORY CONTENT

Standard Setting

In Canada, like most health policies, tourism largely falls under provincial and territorial jurisdiction, which makes it fragmented across the country. Health and safety laws, labour laws, building standards, and environmental and heritage policies are most relevant to the sector's operations. The regulation is relatively light touch; it focuses on private, mostly small businesses and entrepreneurs. The federal government is responsible for national border controls, including land, air, and sea, regulating the operations of national airlines, and determining travel tariffs and ticket taxes; national parks (Parks Canada); national security concerns; and aspects of environmental policy (Theckedath 2014, 6). The federal government also provides the tourism sector with funding for infrastructure investments and event sponsorships as well as for research and marketing.

Recently governments have been concerned about the sustainability of tourism. Targets 8.9 and 14.7 of the UN's Sustainable Development Goals (SDGs) address the international tourism sector's negative impact on destinations and cultures (UNWTO 2016, 14). The UN World Tourism Organization (UNWTO) also emphasizes that long-term sustainability requires a balance among the environmental, social, and economic dimensions. The environmental dimension is about respecting and managing the natural environment by using resources sustainably, including natural capital, and supporting ecological processes.[2] The social dimension relates to the preservation of destinations, including their values, heritage sites, and Indigenous communities, and to the sector's contribution to destinations through community development and safe work opportunities. The economic dimension is about sustaining tourism's economic impact, including employment opportunities, through professionalization of the sector, fair distribution of economic benefits, and measurement of tourism consumption and production, including visitor experiences (UNWTO 2016, 3; 2018, 19–20).

In 2019 the Government of Canada released *Creating Middle Class Jobs: A Federal Tourism Growth Strategy*. The strategy proposes targets for the tourism sector to achieve by 2025, which includes creating 54,000 new jobs, increasing revenues by 25 per cent, growing the number of international tourists during the off-season by one million, and directing tourism spending to regions outside Toronto, Montreal, and Vancouver (Government of Canada 2019a, 24). Like the health sector, which grew by 4.6 per cent in 2019, the tourism sector was growing pre-pandemic with expenditures up by 2.8 per cent in 2019 (DC 2019). Combined with a steady increase in tourism jobs (see table 8.1), the growth made these targets seem reasonable.

Information Gathering

Destination Canada (DC), a Crown corporation, performs global tourism market research and analysis to identify trends and set targets for the sector, most of which focus on the economic impact. It also markets Canada as a tourism destination at the national and international level, targeting Australia, China, France, Germany, Japan, Mexico, the UK, and the US (DC, n.d.b).

Overall, information gathering for the Canadian tourism sector focuses largely on its growth and contribution to regional economies. Section 1.4 of the United Nations' *International Recommendation for Tourism Statistics 2008*, a standard framework for collecting, compiling, and disseminating tourism statistics, emphasizes "a need for a holistic approach to tourism development, management and monitoring" (United Nations 2010, 1). From the beginning of the COVID-19 pandemic until March 2022 the federal government did not release any strategy progress reports.

Behaviour Modification

The federal government can influence behaviour in tourism through infrastructure investments and sponsorships. While each order of government plays a role in attracting and hosting events, such as conventions and festivals, the federal government contributes significant sponsorship funds to large events and invests in the infrastructure required to host them. These sponsorships can act as an anchor for small businesses. In *Budget 2019* the federal government allocated $60 million over two years to expand supports for artists and cultural events (Government of Canada 2019b, 208).

The federal government can also use infrastructure announcements to promote and enforce policy objectives. Indigenous representation and issues, national heritage, environmental standards, and rural economic development have all been a focus of the Canadian government's tourism strategy. Infrastructure developments, however, can take years to negotiate and build and can be expensive to maintain. As a result, the federal government has been criticized for contributing to the construction of projects but failing to contribute to their ongoing operating costs.

In collaboration with regional destination-marketing organizations (DMOs), DC is responsible for destination marketing and development, which in recent years has included a focus on sustainability. Some have noted that these do not address the underlying sustainability challenges associated with tourism, including economic leakage, the exploitation of cultures for the purpose of differentiation, and continued use of environmentally harmful modes of transportation, with emissions from tourism-related transport accounting for 22 per cent of global transport emissions in 2016 (de Lange and Dodds 2017, 1978; UNWTO 2019).

REGULATORY CONTEXT

Legal

There are several laws that shape the tourism sector. Liability, which falls under tort and contract law, is a primary concern for tourism businesses. While tort law focuses on wrongdoings that cause emotional and/or physical harm to an individual, or property damage, including cases of negligence, contract law is concerned with the terms of legal agreements, such as waivers and vehicle-rental contracts (Legal Information Institute, n.d.; Webster 2020).

The Canada Border Services Agency (CBSA) is the primary organization responsible for regulating the movement of people and goods in and out of Canada (Government of Canada 2021b, 2). In reaction to 9/11 and changes in US security legislation, the Government of Canada introduced counterterrorism legislation, which made border operations and international travel stricter and more complex (Carvin and Tishler 2020, 54; Bianchi and Stephenson 2018, 131–2). Following the implementation of the Western Hemisphere Travel Initiative (WHTI) in 2009, which mandated the use of passports for travel between the US and Canada, the number of American visitors declined by 6.7 per cent from the previous year (Statistics Canada 2018a). Furthermore, as demonstrated by human rights legislation, including articles 9 and 30 of the UN's Convention on the Rights of Persons with Disabilities, the accessibility of transportation, services, and cultural, recreational, and tourism activities is another legal consideration of the sector (United Nations Human Rights Office of the High Commissioner 2006, 9, 22–3). Providing inclusive tourism opportunities for people with disabilities and other vulnerable populations also aligns with the UN's SDGs and can contribute to the competitiveness of destinations (Darcy, McKercher, and Schweinsberg 2020).

Tourism's reputation as a largely low-paying, labour-intensive, and revenue-driven sector, with workers earning 47 per cent less than those in other Canadian industries (R. Robinson et al. 2019, 1015–16), makes employment law and employee rights potentially relevant aspects of the legal context. Employee rights, including "the right to be treated fairly in workplaces" (Government of Canada 2021m), are protected under the Canada Labour Code (1985) and equivalent provincial and territorial legislation. Historically, tourism workers have lacked representation and the capacity to pursue labour complaints, including against unfair and inadequate wages (ILO 2017, 23, 13).

Market and Market Failures

Mass tourism was born in the mid-1800s and grew exponentially during the twentieth century. Prior to the era of the industrial entrepreneur Thomas Cook, most people rarely ventured far from their village or the city in which they lived unless they were in search of work (Polat and Arslan 2019). The growth in mass industrial transportation technologies and middle-class wealth as a result of the Industrial Revolution led to increases in middle-class holidays. Following the Second World War, with a rise in households' disposable income and the introduction of paid vacation time for more working- and middle-class workers, tourism and travel became popular across Europe and North America. In the 1960s there was an increase in tourism infrastructure, such as hotels. To keep prices low and demand high, these developments followed the Fordism model, which emphasizes efficiency, standardization, mass production, and economies of scale (Butcher 2020, 908). The fragmented and unorganized nature of the sector, however, can undermine standardization.

Globally, tourism provided 330 million jobs and accounted for 10.6 per cent of total employment in 2019, including one in four new jobs created (WTTC, n.d.a). This employment translated to 10.4 per cent of global GDP (WTTC, n.d.a). The sector also grew by 3.5 per cent in 2019; the global health sector in comparison grew by 1.3 per cent (WTTC 2020, 1; World Bank 2022).

Prior to the pandemic the tourism sector was also growing in Canada. In 2016 the number of tourism workers in Canada outpaced various economic industries, including manufacturing, professional or scientific, construction, and public administration (Tourism HR Canada 2019). In 2019 the tourism unemployment rate ranged from 4.7 to 6.2 per cent, which was close to the national unemployment rate (Tourism HR Canada, n.d.d; Statistics Canada 2020k). Amid population declines in rural communities (World Bank, n.d.b), close to 58,000 Canadians in rural regions worked in accommodation and food services in 2019, an 11.8 per cent increase from 2018 (Statistics Canada 2021m).

Tourism generated $104 billion in revenue and was Canada's largest service export in 2019 (Government of Canada 2022f). Domestic and non-resident spending increased by 13.0 and 13.6 per cent, respectively, over the previous three-year period (table 8.1). Domestic tourism makes up the largest segment of Canada's tourism market. In 2019, domestic tourism accounted for more than 80 per cent of the total 116.5 million overnight visitors (DC 2019). Visiting friends and family accounted

Table 8.1 | Tourism spending and jobs in Canada, 2016 versus 2019

	Domestic spending on tourism ($ billions)	Non-resident spending on tourism ($ billions)	Direct jobs
2016	16.2	4.4	721,000
2019	18.3	5.0	748,000

Tourism spending and jobs were on the rise. The numbers reflect the average amount of spending and jobs recorded during the four quarters of each year. *Sources:* Statistics Canada 2017, 2020j.

for about 40 per cent of Canadians' domestic trips (Statistics Canada 2020d, 1).

International tourism in Canada also experienced its sixth year of growth in 2019 with 22.1 million overnight visitors. About 7.5 million tourists came from overseas, while 15 million came from the US – nearly two-thirds of all international visitors (Statistics Canada 2020q). The Indigenous tourism sector in Canada was also growing, with its market segment expected to increase from $1.7 billion in 2017 to $2.2 billion by 2024 (Fiser and Hermus 2019, 2).

While workers over the age of forty-five have some of the highest participation rates in tourism, the sector has also been a significant employer for youth (Statistics Canada 2020p, 2). For many Canadians, including students and individuals in transition, tourism provides flexibility, income, and, most significantly, entry to the workforce (Tourism HR Canada 2019). In 2019, youth aged fifteen to twenty-four accounted for 32.4 per cent (or 560,000) of the Canadian tourism workforce, more than double its 13 per cent share in the general labour force (Tourism HR Canada, n.d.e; WTTC 2019).

Due to its seasonal nature, tourism work is often temporary or casual. In 2019 there were 812,403 part-time jobs in tourism, accounting for 42.8 per cent of total direct and indirect jobs (Statistics Canada 2020m). Tourism employment can be considered exploitative due to the sector's poor working conditions and low wages; the growth of gig industries and services has also contributed to its precarity (T. Baum 2019, 46–8; R. Robinson et al. 2019, 1012). Gig industries' focus on performance and service delivery can lead to worker burnout (*Guardian* 2019). Despite representing 9.8 per cent of jobs in 2019, the tourism sector's workforce accounted for only 5.8 per cent of total employment income in Canada (Statistics Canada 2020n). Although the tourism sector has low entry barriers, it offers minimal protections for workers, many of whom come from vulnerable populations with limited options (R. Robinson et al. 2019, 1009). Like the health sector, tourism employs more immigrants and racialized persons than other sectors in Canada do, with these populations accounting for 26.0 and 27.5 per cent, respectively, of all tourism workers in 2016 (Tourism HR Canada, n.d.b). R.N.S. Robinson et al. (2019, 1010) suggest that the tourism sector "operates within two parallel and largely independent worlds," with formally regulated industries in one world and unregulated industries in the other.

In recent years the Canadian tourism sector has struggled to attract the workers it needs. Staff turnover is also high (Tourism HR Canada 2023). Pre-COVID-19 projections indicated that more than 10 per cent of tourism jobs would become vacant between 2010 and 2035 (Murray 2017, 2). The sector depends significantly on the Temporary Foreign Worker (TFW) Program: 7.2 per cent of TFWs work in accommodation and food services, and 4.5 per cent work in amusement, arts, information, and recreation (Y. Lu 2020, 4). Over the years, unstable working conditions have become a defining characteristic of the tourism sector that contributes to low worker-retention rates.

There are several market failures in tourism. Market failures relate to externalities, which can lead to negative economic, social, and environmental impacts (Costa 2011, 21). (For more discussion on market failures see chapter 9.) While the sector is highly responsive to fluctuations in the market, the overall size of the sector and the precarity and low wages of the work contribute to its unstable labour supply and significant consequences for those who work in tourism and for overall social stability. Tourism industries are also free riders, particularly when it comes to marketing and promotion (Costa 2011, 19). For instance, tourism activities often involve the use of public goods, which are subsidized by taxpayers; neither tourism operators nor tourists pay the full cost of what they consume or of the environmental impact they have.

PUBLIC OPINION

Affordability continues to dominate peoples' decision making. For example, a recent survey found that 61.8 per cent of people consider costs the most influential factor when booking travel, followed by time and convenience (E. Jones 2021).

Despite concerns over climate change, public opinion has become only marginally more concerned with the environmental impacts of global tourism (Ipsos 2019; Newman 2019). There has been increased demand for novel types of tourism, driven by changes in taste and functional need. Public interest in nature tourism, for example, which can relate to Indigenous tourism in Canada, has grown in recent years (Lee Kong 2023; ITAC 2022). Aging of the population has created greater demand for more accessible tourism and travel experiences. In 2019, seniors (65 years and older) accounted for 17.5 per cent of Canada's population, anticipated to grow to 20.0 per cent by 2025 (Statistics Canada 2020a). Since aging and disability are correlated, improving travel for people with disabilities can increase tourism. According to an Australian study, 44 per cent of people with disabilities travel regularly for leisure purposes (Convery 2021).

Media

Media coverage of the Canadian tourism sector is largely positive. Tourism marketing has benefited from the media, particularly in the age of social media (Zeng and Gerritsen 2014, 33). Much of the sector's marketing and image, however, derives from a somewhat superficial depiction of destinations and can often exploit cultural stereotypes (Caton and Santos 2008, 9). Media depiction of a place being dangerous, for example, can lead to long-lasting impacts on a destination's image and tourism sector (Avraham 2020, 712).

Both the tourism sector and the governments that promote destinations are sensitive to negative media coverage. The tourism sector is no stranger to the impacts of crises and related supply-and-demand shocks, which negative media coverage can intensify. The media's depiction of crises and impactful events "can be somewhat imbalanced … highly sensationalised … [and use] negatively phrased emotive headlines" (Walters, Mair, and Lim 2016, 8). Natural disasters, such as earthquakes and hurricanes, and crimes and political instability are the primary drivers of negative tourism stories (Rosselló, Becken, and Santana-Gallego 2020, 1, 4). For example, the 2010 earthquake in Haiti that resulted in more than 200,000 deaths (Trevelyan 2013), terrorist attacks that killed more than sixty people (mostly tourists) at a museum and beach in Tunisia in March and October 2015, respectively (BBC 2015), and the 2015 bombing of a Russian charter plane over the Sinai Peninsula in Egypt (Knell 2015), were all tragic and had significant impacts on tourism in these regions. As we will discuss, media coverage of the 2003 SARS outbreak in Toronto exaggerated the impact and spread of the disease, which affected tourism industries across Canada (Wall 2006, 150).

Interests

The tourism market is complex. The fragmented and interdependent nature of the sector contributes to this complexity (R. Robinson et al. 2019, 1010). While the sector includes several major companies, including airlines and hotel chains, 99 per cent of tourism businesses are SMEs, many of which operate near large infrastructure and holiday destinations. Further, many businesses that benefit from tourism do not identify as part of the sector, such as local boutiques, suburban restaurants, and dry cleaners that service hotels, because tourism represents only a portion of their overall revenue. Together, these characteristics of the sector constrain its ability to organize and lobby effectively. Many businesses focus on day-to-day operations, not strategic lobbying.

In Canada, tourism lobbying occurs at all orders of government; here we focus on the federal government. The Tourism Industry Association of Canada (TIAC), with more than 600 members, including regional DMOs, is the primary advocacy group for the Canadian tourism sector (TIAC, n.d.). Over the years, TIAC has advocated on a range of topics mostly focused on increasing low-cost labour supply. These include changes to the national visitor-visa process and the TFW Program, and more human resources to support employment across tourism industries in 2018–19 (OCL, n.d.d). In 2019 the Registry of Lobbyists reported more than thirty monthly communication reports with TIAC;[3] however, the organization did not receive any funding during the 2019 financial year (OCL, n.d.c).[4]

Past Crises and the Weak Relationship between Industry and Government

Past crises have shown the vulnerability of the sector. The year 2009 was particularly bad. H1N1, the financial crisis (2007–09), and the thickening of borders because of the WHTI had a significant impact: 9.2 and 12.8 per cent decrease in international tourist arrivals and spending, respectively – the lowest rate in fifteen years. In 2009 Canadian tourism revenues fell by 3.7 per cent, and domestic spending declined by 1.8 per

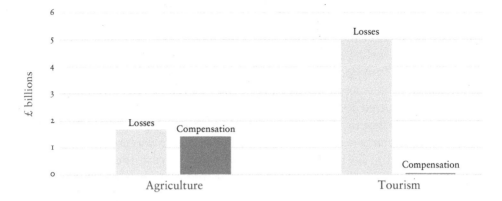

Figure 8.1 | Estimated losses and compensation for the tourism and agricultural sectors during the 2001 foot-and-mouth-disease outbreak in the UK. Compensation for the tourism sector was minuscule compared to financial losses. *Source:* National Audit Office 2002.

cent (Statistics Canada 2011). The number of international tourists also declined during the SARS outbreak in 2003–4, with a 12.6 per cent difference in arrivals between 2002 and 2003 (Statistics Canada 2018a).

Past crises have also demonstrated how fragmented the tourism industry can be and the consequences of this fragmentation. The 2001 foot-and-mouth-disease outbreak in the UK provides a salient example. The outbreak, which lasted seven months and led to the slaughter of more than six million animals, caused much of the British countryside to close to visitors and resulted in tourism losses estimated at between £4.5 billion and £5.4 billion (National Audit Office 2002, 25). Before the outbreak, tourism generated £64 billion in revenue annually, employed 7 per cent of the labour force, and accounted for 4 per cent of the UK's GDP, while the agriculture sector generated a much lower £15.3 billion, employed 1.5 per cent, and made up 1 per cent of GDP (Sharpley and Craven 2001, 535). The government's response to the crisis, however, was heavily weighted towards the farming industry, which received £1.4 billion in compensation, compared to only £50 million for non-farming businesses (figure 8.1). This imbalance may be attributed to various factors, including the relatively weak lobbying representation for the tourism sector compared to the agricultural sector's influential National Farmers Union

(Sharpley and Craven 2001, 536). Overall, the measures aimed at assisting businesses in the wider rural economy were considered relatively small-scale, piecemeal, and complex.

SARS provides a second example. The consequences of the SARS outbreak in Toronto were rapid and far reaching, with the cancellation of major conferences and events beginning in April 2003. These cancellations occurred despite confirmation from Ontario's chief medical officer of health that the risk of SARS transmission to the general population was extremely low (Wall 2006, 146), with its two waves being largely contained in hospitals. The outbreak, however, cost Toronto an estimated $500 million in tourism revenue and thousands of jobs (Wall 2006, 150; Black and the To3 Management Team 2004, 1). The Toronto hotel-occupancy rate fell to 46.6 per cent in April 2003 from 68.0 per cent the previous year. As Toronto is a major point of entry to other areas of Canada, the SARS outbreak caused setbacks for the national tourism sector, including a 14.0 per cent decline in international visitors, 13.0 per cent decrease in spending by international visitors, and a 2.4 per cent drop in employment (Wall 2006, 147).

At times, the way in which the threat of SARS was described was more damaging than the disease itself. The WHO travel advisory of 23 April 2003, which warned against all non-essential travel to Toronto, shaped perceptions of the city. Initially, politicians in the three orders of government were criticized by tourism industries for lack of leadership and failing to encourage travel to Toronto (Wall 2006, 146; G. Galloway and Lewington 2003). Ultimately, collaboration among all orders of government, public health, and the tourism sector was necessary to manage the recovery, which is cited as a tourism success story (Shier 2020).

In sum, the tourism sector generates significant revenue for local, regional, and national economies and accounts for about 10 per cent of jobs in Canada and globally. Tourism employment, however, is often precarious, seasonal, and provides low wages and benefits for its workers, many of whom belong to vulnerable populations, such as immigrants and the young. The sector's structure contributes to this instability, as most of its businesses are SMEs that lack organization and the capacity to lobby governments effectively. Together with governments' light-touch regulation of the sector, these characteristics challenge its strategic planning and risk mitigation, which make it particularly vulnerable during crises, including COVID-19, which we discuss next.

COVID-19 AND TOURISM

Impacts of COVID-19

The COVID-19 pandemic had a greater impact on the tourism sector than 9/11, the SARS outbreak in 2003, and the financial crisis (2007–09) had collectively (DC 2021a, 13). In some respects, COVID-19 gained international prominence because of the outbreak aboard the cruise ship *Diamond Princess*, which departed from Yokohama for a fourteen-day cruise to China, Vietnam, and Taiwan and returned to Japan on 20 January 2020 (CDC 2020b). (For further discussion on COVID-19 outbreaks see chapter 1.) The controlled environment of the cruise ship gave epidemiologists around the world the first glimpse of how easily transmissible and potentially fatal COVID-19 could be.

The federal government's advisory on 9 March 2020 against all cruise-ship travel, which had accounted for more than three million visitors to Canada in 2019 (Business Research & Economic Advisors 2021, 7), was the first of many travel-related regulations that would have an impact on the sector. On 13 March the Government of Canada formally postponed the upcoming cruise-ship season and on 14 March issued an advisory against all non-essential travel outside Canada. The federal government closed Canada's international border to non-Canadian and non-American travellers on 18 March and closed it to non-essential travel three days later (Statistics Canada 2020r; CIHI 2022a). Together, these regulations would change the nature of travel to and from Canada for the next two years and thereafter.

As a result of related public health orders and travel restrictions, travel to, from, and within Canada largely stopped in 2020, leading to significant uncertainty about the future of leisure travel. The number of international travellers to and from Canada dropped from about 96.8 million in 2019 to 25.9 million in 2020, a decrease of 73.3 per cent (table 8.2). Canada experienced the largest decline in international travel in April 2020 when the number of travellers declined by 92.0 per cent from March 2020 (Statistics Canada 2021o, 1). Air Canada's suspension of thirty regional routes in June 2020 compounded the drop in travel throughout the summer of 2020 (Air Canada 2020). Collectively, these changes in travel resulted in a 48.8 per cent drop in tourism spending in 2020 overall and a fall in the sector's share of GDP (Statistics Canada 2021g; Tam, Sood, and Johnston 2021b, 3). At the end of 2021 the total number of travellers to Canada was down by 80.6 per cent from 2019 and by 27.3 per cent from 2020 (Statistics Canada 2022l).

Table 8.2 | International travel to Canada, 2019–21

Type of traveller	2019 Total	2020 Total	Change, 2019–20 (%)	2021 Total	Change, 2020–21 (%)
Total non-resident travellers	32,429,771	5,068,350	–84.3	4,282,116	–15.5
Total Canadian resident travellers	56,157,406	14,605,347	–74.0	7,905,501	–45.9
Total other travellers	8,222,851	6,184,606	–24.8	6,598,645	6.7
Total international travellers	96,810,028	25,858,303	–73.3	18,786,262	–27.3

International travel was down by 73.3 per cent in 2020.
Source: Statistics Canada 2022l.

Following the largest month-over-month decrease in international arrivals since 1972, in late March and early April 2020 the hotel-occupancy rate fell below 20 per cent (Tam, Sood, and Johnston 2021b, 3), which caused the share values of hotel chains to drop (figure 8.2). While average occupancy rates grew throughout the summer, they were still half of 2019 levels (DC 2021a, 9). The industry experienced its worst performance in history during the first quarter of 2021, with an average occupancy rate of 27 per cent (Lanthier 2021). As a result, hotel revenues fell immensely; downtown Montreal, Toronto, and Vancouver collectively experienced a $2.3 billion decline (DC, n.d.a). Government policies regarding quarantine and housing the homeless provided some business to hotels (Gray 2020; Osman 2020), but overall the hotel-occupancy rate in Canada was 41.8 per cent in 2021, about a third lower than in 2019 (STR 2022a). By March 2022 there had been some modest improvements (STR 2022b).

While many businesses began offering their goods and services online, only about 40 per cent of tourism businesses were able to do so. In 2020 an estimated 83.4 per cent of tourism businesses experienced revenue losses; 44.9 per cent lost 40 per cent or more of their revenues, which is about double the rate of all Canadian businesses (Tam, Sood, and

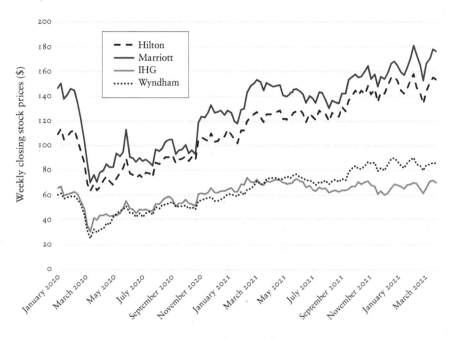

Figure 8.2 | Change in share values of major hotel chains, January 2020–March 2022. After the collapse, hotel shares mostly rose above pre-pandemic levels. *Source:* Yahoo Finance 2022a–d.

Johnston 2021b, 4). Although most tourism businesses were eligible for or received funding through government support programs (Tam, Sood, and Johnston 2021b, 8), many had to close their doors for good. Between March and December 2020, 50,559 tourism businesses closed, 60.6 per cent more than in the same period in 2019. As figure 8.3 indicates, by March 2021 the sector had started to show some signs of recovery (Tourism HR Canada, n.d.c).[5]

In 2019 the tourism unemployment rate in Canada ranged from 4.7 to 5.7 per cent, close to the total labour-force-unemployment rate (Tourism HR Canada, n.d.g). By March 2020, however, the tourism unemployment rate had reached 16.0 per cent, followed by 29.0 per cent in April before peaking in May 2020 at 29.7 per cent (table 8.3), significantly higher than the total labour-force rate, which was 8.5 per cent, 13.5 per cent, and 13.8 per cent during those months, respectively (Tourism HR Canada, n.d.g).

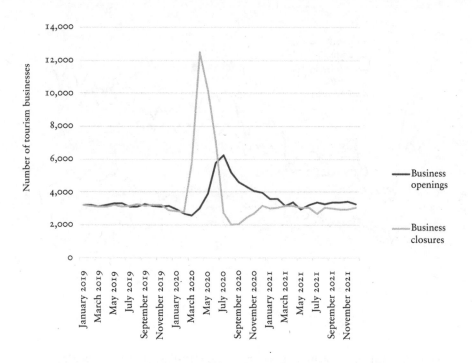

Figure 8.3 | Tourism business openings and closures, 2019–21. The number of tourism business closures peaked in spring 2020. *Source:* Tourism HR Canada, n.d.c.

Workers between the ages of fifteen and twenty-four, and twenty-five to thirty-four, were among those most affected by COVID-19 job losses in the tourism sector. The most substantial change in employment occurred in April 2020 when employment for these population groups was down by 60.7 per cent and by 39.7 per cent, respectively, compared to February 2020 (Tourism HR Canada, n.d.a). Immigrant workers, a particularly vulnerable population that accounted for about a quarter of tourism's total workforce before COVID-19, were also significantly affected (DC 2021a, 28; Tourism HR Canada, n.d.b). Following several years of growth, the Indigenous tourism industry lost an estimated 80 per cent of its jobs in 2020 because of the COVID-19 pandemic and various government health regulations (ITAC 2020, 9). Although tourism jobs improved in 2021, they were still down by about 20 per cent from 2019 (Statistics Canada 2021g; Tourism HR Canada, n.d.f).

Table 8.3 | Tourism unemployment rate, 2019–21

Month	2019 unemployment rate (%)	2020 unemployment rate (%)	2021 unemployment rate (%)
January	5.1	5.9	18.6
April	5.7	29.0	11.3
July	5.0	18.6	4.8
October	4.7	13.5	5.2

The tourism unemployment rate was larger than the national unemployment rate in 2020–21. *Source:* Tourism HR Canada, n.d.g.

By summer 2021, tourism was making a comeback. By July, the tourism unemployment rate was 4.8 per cent, on par with pre-pandemic levels (Tourism HR Canada, n.d.g). As of March 2022, the tourism unemployment rate was 5 per cent, 1 per cent lower than the total labour force rate (Tourism HR Canada, n.d.g).

COVID-19 had an impact on people's perceptions about travel. Generally, Canadians were willing to welcome visitors from nearby communities; they were less willing to welcome people from other parts of the country and even more cautious when it came to allowing people from other countries to visit their communities (table 8.4). Canadians' perceptions of travel varied largely by region and between urban and rural communities. Time also shaped people's perceptions of visitors, particularly international travellers. On average, Atlantic Canadians were less welcoming towards visitors from other provinces and countries, and Canadians from rural communities were less welcoming to visitors than were Canadians living in urban regions. As of March 2022, close to 50 per cent of Canadians were still uncomfortable welcoming international visitors to their communities (DC 2022b, 23).

In 2020, experts predicted that it would take several years for Canada to overcome the economic impacts brought about by the pandemic (Pittis 2020). An economic rebound coupled with global distribution of COVID-19 vaccines, particularly among wealthier countries with citizens more likely to travel, provided some cautious optimism that the sector would rebound more quickly than earlier forecast (*Toronto Star*

Table 8.4 | Canadians' level of welcome towards visitors,
May 2020–January 2022

Date	Canadians who welcomed visitors from nearby communities (%)	Canadians who welcomed visitors from other communities in the province (%)	Canadians who welcomed visitors from other provinces (%)	Canadians who welcomed visitors from the US (%)	Canadians who welcomed visitors from other countries (%)
11 May 2020	41.2	35.5	21.3	10.5	10.2
1 Sept. 2020	61.5	58.2	35.2	8.2	10.0
5 Jan. 2021	49.5	40.8	22.5	10.5	10.8
4 May 2021	57.7	48.7	28.2	18.0	14.7
7 Sept. 2021	72.8	68.2	52.5	25.3	21.8
11 Jan. 2022	66.3	62.5	47.2	27.8	23.7

Canadians were fearful of international visitors during the first two years of COVID-19. Destination Canada asked respondents: "To what extent do you agree or disagree with each of the following statements? I would welcome visitors travelling to my community ..." (DC 2020a, 7). The table represents the percentage of Canadians from British Columbia, Alberta, Saskatchewan/Manitoba, Ontario, Quebec, and Atlantic Canada who agreed or strongly agreed with the statements.
Sources: DC 2020a–b, 2021b–d, 2022a–b.

2021). At the same time, subsequent waves of the virus, lockdowns, vaccination hesitancy and access challenges, and labour shortages continued to constrain the sector. As of March 2022, Canadian tourism activity was down by 29.1 per cent from March 2019 (Statistics Canada 2022a). By March 2022, governments across the country had started lifting COVID-19 restrictions (Government of Nova Scotia 2022; Jabakhanji and Knope 2022; Government of British Columbia 2022a), and tourism began a more stable recovery, with evidence of the associated economic and social benefits (Statistics Canada 2022p; Zins and Ponocny 2022).

Responses to COVID-19

Tourism industries had better access to government supports during COVID-19 than in previous crises. In 2020–21 the federal government introduced several COVID-19 relief programs that benefited tourism industries, including the Canada Emergency Rent Subsidy (CERS), Business Credit Availability Program, Highly Affected Sectors Credit Availability Program, and Canada Emergency Wage Subsidy (CEWS), which provided over $8 billion to accommodation and food services between March 2020 and October 2021, accounting for more than 10 per cent of the program's total funding distribution (Canada Revenue Agency 2022). Tourism workers also benefited from the Canada Emergency Response Benefit (CERB), with 66.6 per cent of those working in accommodations and food services receiving payments in 2020 (Morissette et al. 2021).

The Government of Canada also allocated 25 per cent of the Regional Relief and Recovery Fund to the Tourism Canada Emergency Business Account and extended its Work-Sharing Program, which helped businesses prevent or reduce staff layoffs during periods of low demand and activity (DC 2021a, 21; Government of Canada 2023c). As of April 2022, emergency government supports amounted to $23 billion in direct funding to the tourism sector (Government of Canada 2022a, 83). The federal government also contributed $1 billion to a recovery package for tourism industries over three years, which included the Tourism Relief Fund (Government of Canada 2021i; 2021l, 200).

Although federal supports for the tourism sector have been among the largest in the country, the challenges for the sector are ongoing. To replace the CEWS and CERS programs, the Government of Canada (2022b) introduced two new programs, the Tourism and Hospitality Recovery Program and the Hardest-Hit Business Recovery Program, in October 2021. In contrast to small tourism businesses and SMEs, Air Canada has benefited from significant support throughout the pandemic. It secured a support package valued at $5.9 billion from the federal government in April 2021. (For further discussion on Air Canada see chapter 11.)

The tourism sector has benefited from sustained media coverage. Some of the coverage was negative. The media occasionally featured those who disregarded public health directives, including several public officials who travelled abroad for the holidays (Somos 2021). There was also coverage of airlines who refused to reimburse customers who had booked holidays in advance of the pandemic (Burke 2020; Benjamin

2020). On balance, however, media coverage was sympathetic towards the popular and devastated sector.

As during the SARS outbreak in Toronto, responses to COVID-19 emphasized a need for collaborative and cooperative policy-making. The introduction of the Atlantic Bubble in July 2020, which permitted travel between the Atlantic Canadian provinces without quarantining and enhanced regional tourism opportunities, required significant policy alignment (Government of Nova Scotia 2020a). The volatility of the Atlantic Bubble also demonstrated the challenges in the sector (Lau 2021). Atlantic Canada's quarantine requirements all but shut out people from outside the region for months and made it extremely difficult for those within the region to travel outside of it.

Ultimately, the tourism sector's responses to the COVID-19 pandemic, including marketing, were initially based on the notion that operations would return to normal in 2021. Following various setbacks, such as new waves of the virus and extended travel advisories, however, tourism industries remained vulnerable. The financial challenges associated with COVID-19 stretched some tourism businesses to their limits, leaving no resources to invest in future projects (Orîndaru et al. 2021, 3–4). Travellers' tastes may also be shifting towards more domestic travel and sustainable tourism (Orîndaru et al. 2021, 5, 16). Europe has responded to these changes in its tourism marketing and planning by focusing more on health and safety and environmental protocols (Orîndaru et al. 2021, 17). In Canada, GreenStep Sustainable Tourism (n.d.) recently introduced a pledge program that encourages destinations and tourism industries to become more sustainable by 2030.

CONCLUSION

Global travel is a feature of modernity (Polat and Arslan 2019; Christou 2022). The tourism business model (Butcher 2020) can enable disease transmission because it often results in many people being concentrated in small spaces, such as planes, trains, boats, buses, hotels, amusement parks, lineups, and live performance venues. The episode is a reminder that aspects of modernity are available to some and not others and are achieved through low-cost labour. Many in the sector work part time for low wages and few benefits and are vulnerable to the whims of the market. While some may see the sector as trivial, it is not. One in ten jobs in Canada and globally depends on this sector.

The context in which COVID-19 emerged called for dramatic action. The effectiveness of border closures remains inconclusive (Shiraef et al. 2022; Emeto, Alele, and Ilesanmi 2021; Bou-Karroum et al. 2021; Kaimann and Tanneberg 2021). The aggressive stance was contrary to the advice that public health had offered during the H1N1 pandemic, but in any event it can be considered a precautionary measure that aligned with the policies of most Western countries and allayed the concerns of an anxious public.

At times, the tourism sector illustrates powerfully the trade-offs implicit in the various restrictions on travel. Cancelling travel plans for months on end is not merely inconvenient; it jeopardizes people's subjective well-being. Recall from chapter 5 and noted in chapter 10 that Canadians' mental health deteriorated to the lowest levels ever recorded by the federal government (Statistics Canada 2020g). Tourism is not a panacea for mental health challenges, of course. Nevertheless, researchers note that there is a correlation between the two (L. Sun, Wang, and Gao 2022; J. Zhang 2023), which can last for about two months after travel (Kwon and Lee 2020). People with disabilities, for example, often at a disadvantage when travelling (McKercher and Darcy 2018; Darcy, McKercher, and Schweinsberg 2020; Moura, Eusébio, and Devile 2023), suffered considerably during extended quarantines and faced additional barriers when trying to travel during the pandemic (Park et al. 2022; Alves et al. 2023; Dadashzadeh et al. 2022). As mental health issues rose dramatically during the pandemic, restricting tourism (including for its most common purpose, to visit and friends and family) almost certainly contributed to the malaise.

The outcome was not strictly a function of government policy; even if there had not been border closures, many still would have chosen not to travel out of fear of contracting the disease. Still, the rationale for the length of time the orders were in place, the specific policies the governments adopted, and the cost of government decisions were not always clear. The Atlantic Bubble, for example, designed to allow people in the region to travel between the Atlantic provinces, effectively prevented people from leaving or entering the region for months on end, limiting their right to travel, unless they were prepared to undergo extended quarantines that were not practical for most people (English and Murphy 2020).

There was a significant economic cost. As happened during much of the pandemic, in the tourism sector the circumstances exacted a heavier price from vulnerable populations, including youth, immigrants, and racialized communities (ILO 2022, 14–15). Almost one in three people in the sector could not find work.

The sector is made up mostly of SMEs and does not have the capacity to prepare for rainy days. The absence of foresight raises significant doubts about the sector's ability to address longer-term societal risks on its own, like those resulting from climate change. As the newly developed Tourism Relief Fund has emphasized, "investing in products and services to facilitate future growth" remains the priority (Government of Canada 2021i, para. 3). The episode underscores the challenges of a volatile labour force. The sector has an insatiable appetite for low-paid service workers, and at present, accommodations, food and beverage industries, and airports have significant staff shortages (Statistics Canada 2022g; K. Campbell 2021b; Zaidi 2022; Atkins and Habibinia 2022). As in the health sector, many of these jobs were filled by unskilled immigrants and TFWs. The pandemic limited the admission of both. The sector also depends for labour on rural workers who are increasingly aging into retirement or moving to cities. The situation provides a glimpse of the labour challenges Canada will face in the future.

There are steps industry can take to improve its strategic stance. The sector needs to organize itself more effectively. National, regional, and local industry associations need strong connections to the grassroots, a solid research function, and the capacity for strategic marketing and lobbying. Many communities lack even basic coordination and information sharing about tourism (Cassia et al. 2020). Tourism representatives must convey to policy-makers the strategic importance of the sector to the national economy not just in creating short-term jobs but in achieving environmental, social, and economic sustainability targets (Sharma, Thomas, and Paul 2021, 6; ILO 2022, 15).

There is also an important role for governments, particularly with stronger regulatory presence in matters of health, environment, and labour. Securing international labour cannot be seen strictly as a way to secure low-cost workers, for example; there has to be a broader and more humane strategy, particularly with the oversight of the TFW program. Universities and colleges need more and serious accredited tourism programs with research capacity and outputs that support students, including international ones (Bascaramurty, Bhatt, and Rana 2021).

Government can incentivize infrastructure investments that consider an aging population and a volatile labour supply. Businesses without a strong online presence suffered more than most throughout the pandemic. Therefore, investing in technology, such as automated services, can help the sector prepare for a future in which governments and tourists are more concerned about disease transmission (WTTC, n.d.b); this is particularly so for an aging population that can be vulnerable to disease yet constitutes a lucrative travel market (Patterson and Balderas 2020, 387–8). Rural communities will have to address these challenges in particular; many of these communities depend on tourists and were the most nervous about welcoming them back.

Based on experience, the sector will face periodic challenges and, in its present form, will be ill prepared to address them short of lockdowns and layoffs. The pandemic will generate changes in consumer preferences and the regulatory environment in Canada and the US; recall that after 9/11 it took six years to implement new passport controls at the border. COVID-19 may pass but border restrictions might grow. Thus, the sector needs better coordination and a closer relationship with the government, particularly the provincial, territorial, and federal orders, to prepare for plausible scenarios and the risks that go with them. The sector is clearly not a government priority, but given its social and economic importance, size, and vulnerability, it should be.

PART FOUR

Regime Context:
Pressures and Explanations

Part 2 of this book described and analyzed the control mechanism of information gathering, standard setting, and behaviour modification at play throughout COVID-19. In this section we will explore the contextual pressures that influenced the control mechanism and shaped governments' responses through three specific lenses.

Chapter 9 tests Hood, Rothstein, and Baldwin's (2001) market failure hypothesis. We examine the role of law and insurance and market dynamics throughout the pandemic. This includes a summary of the market winners and losers and an examination of information and opt-out costs to determine the extent to which market failures explain governments' responses. Next, chapter 10 tests the opinion-responsive hypothesis, primarily through a study of media coverage and popular polling data. We discuss the extent to which these popular contextual pressures align with government intervention. Lastly, the interest group hypothesis is tested in chapter 11. We use Dunleavy's bureau-shaping model to determine the extent to which the government's pandemic response can be attributed to the preferences and behaviours of public health officials prior to the pandemic. We also discuss audits and reports from prior disease outbreaks, the limitations of the precautionary principle, and its susceptibility to being influenced by those with resources and privileged access to decision makers. We use Wilson's interest group typology to examine the relationship between power and the concentration or dispersal of costs and benefits resulting from government policies.

Market Failure Hypothesis:
Market Performance, Information Costs,
and Opt-Out Costs

The market failure hypothesis (MFH) invites us to consider the nature of a risk and the extent to which it is addressed by markets, as well as the extent to which government addresses failures that manifest from a market response. A conventional welfare economics definition of a market failure is an inefficient allocation of resources in the free market, caused by information asymmetries, a natural monopoly, the presence of externalities, or the delivery of public goods (Bator 1958; Pigou 1932). A market failure according to Hood, Rothstein, and Baldwin (2001), which is the concept used in this chapter, incorporates these signposts but is less prescriptive: a market failure is said to occur when a market left to its own devices, coupled with insurance and existing laws, does not achieve desired outcomes. The MFH expects that governments will intervene when there is evidence that these existing mechanisms are insufficient to achieve broad social goals. It also expects that the extent of government action should be proportional to the failure addressed (89).

This chapter examines the extent to which the MFH provides an explanation of government response during the pandemic. It starts with an overview of how the market performed during the pandemic. We highlight who thrived and who was vulnerable. We then examine market failures more closely and recall why health care is generally treated as a market failure. Hood, Rothstein, and Baldwin (2001) examine information and opt-out costs when considering the arguments for market failures and government interventions. The chapter outlines the ways in which government intervention was necessary and appropriate in learning about the pandemic and seeking to contain it.

For Hood, Rothstein, and Baldwin, the MFH is a starting point for analysis; it allows us to examine the extent to which the system was prepared to address the risk and whether interventions could be justified on rational economic grounds. Certainly, existing insurance and legal instruments were tested and showed their potential and limitations in opting out of the risk. While public health insurance ensured that people had access to physicians and hospitals to be treated for COVID-19 if they were infected, the system was placed under immense pressure, and at times its ability to provide service was tested. The focus on COVID-19 disrupted access for other health issues with few viable alternatives. Calls for alternative private-sector provision of health care came to the fore (Speer 2022; Wherry 2022). In reference to the insurance industry more generally, policies did not protect people or businesses from losses throughout the pandemic. In contrast, laws protected most workers, but many were still vulnerable, and laws were not always enforced. Beyond these mechanisms, governments acted to reduce opt-out costs, with mixed success. We conclude by examining the practice of working from home as an example of opt-out strategy, which represented a seismic shift in the economy. The impacts are still being felt.

Beyond questions concerning government readiness and effectiveness at containing the virus's spread, there remains the motivation for the specific approach adopted by government. While basic health and legislative protections were in place to mitigate the effects of a pandemic, the event and response were larger than foreseen in most theoretical exercises (Ogden, AbdelMalik, and Pulliam 2017; Henig 2020). Significant government intervention was required quickly, not only to contain the virus but also to protect the vulnerable, cope with a global economic shutdown, and enable and motivate a market in a national effort to ensure stability. Government and market responses were not dichotomous forces; they were iterative and interdependent. Government interventions themselves – lockdowns, border controls, and CERB, for example – were offered as protections but were also highly disruptive, reducing some risks while increasing others. The response was top-down and largely aligned with the precautionary principle, the concept that actions should be taken to protect against a risk even if it is not fully understood and there is uncertainty over the benefit of interventions (Kriebel et al. 2001, 871). The precautionary principle acknowledges the limits of scientific inquiry to describe complex risks precisely, as well as the need for leaders to act regardless of these limitations (Flood, Thomas, and Wilson 2020, 253).

Although containing the spread of the virus and providing appropriate medical care were governments' central concerns in the early stage, the cascading effects of the aggressive containment strategy were felt across almost every facet of life. While most supported government's ultimate objective of containing the spread of the virus, the cost of the strategy was not fully understood, let alone explained. As time went on and trade-offs became more apparent, and particularly as vaccines and diagnostics became more readily available, any consensus on the broader social goals of government response started to fray. In this sense, an MFH provides important justification for government's containment strategy but struggles to justify its cascading effects and explain what a proportionate response might be in the face of such uncertainty.

SELECTED KEY ECONOMIC INDICATORS IN CANADA

Canada's economy performed similarly to the economy of other members of the G7 and the EU as a whole. In comparison, Canada was in the middle in terms of change in nominal GDP between the second quarter of 2019 and the second quarter of 2020 (–13 per cent) and higher in percentage change in public sector debt (17.2 per cent; OECD, n.d.a). Many European countries tended to offer financial support directly to companies, with conditions, thereby preventing layoffs and bankruptcies (Drahokoupil and Müller 2021). In contrast, the bulk of Canada's support, such as CERB, was paid to laid-off workers (OECD 2020d, 6–7). Early in the pandemic some laid-off staff refused to return to work, sometimes due to health concerns, and instead continued to collect CERB or CESB (CFIB 2020). Though Canada had recovered the three million jobs lost due to COVID-19 by October 2021 (Hagan 2021), labour shortages in certain sectors remained or increased (Statistics Canada 2021f, 3–4).

BANK OF CANADA, INTEREST RATES, AND INFLATION

Following the WHO's (2020i) announcement of a pandemic, the Bank of Canada's policy interest rate, 1.75 per cent, quickly experienced decreases until it reached 0.25 per cent, a historic low. The rate for household borrowers of chartered banks did not drop as drastically, though mortgage rates did eventually become low (Bank of Canada, n.d.b, n.d.c).

Inflation dropped, then surged. Initially the annual inflation rate dropped below the Bank of Canada's inflation-control target of 2.0 per cent (Parkinson 2022) in 2020, hitting 0.7 per cent (World Bank, n.d.a), but later rose steadily, reaching 6.7 per cent in March 2022 – the highest recorded in Canada since 1991 (Evans 2022) – driven largely by the housing market, ongoing labour shortages, higher consumer demand for products, and supply chain disruptions (Parkinson 2022; Sivarajan 2022). Inflation spread across the economy at a rate that outpaced central bank estimates (Parkinson 2022; Varadarajan 2022). Low-income workers lost the most due to the changes (Rauh and Warsh 2022; Shahid 2021; Sivarajan 2022).

Trade

Canada is a trading nation, with sixty international trade agreements in force (Government of Canada 2021n). The Canadian supply chain involves the movement of approximately $1 trillion worth of goods, primarily with the US, China, the UK, Japan, Mexico, and Germany (Observatory of Economic Complexity, n.d.; World Bank 2018). Figure 9.1 captures COVID-19's impact on Canadian trade. This disruption was worldwide due to border controls, factory closures, higher shipping costs, and increased demand for certain products, such as electronics (Armstrong and Mazerolle 2021).

MARKET PERFORMANCE

The rapid spread of COVID-19 in mid-March 2020 (figure 9.2) corresponded with a significant drop in stock prices. In time, the market bounced back, and some sectors prospered.

The weaknesses of supply chains were highlighted as the global economy shut down in March (Shih 2020). Competition for medical supplies and PPE was chaotic, deemed to resemble the "Wild West" and "a world of the *Lord of the Flies*" in April 2020 (M. Walsh and Vanderklippe 2020, para. 2, 16; D. Cochrane and Harris 2020). Health Canada lowered its standard for PPE so that demand could be more easily met (Leo 2020). Even so, procuring supplies was fraught with shipment delays, order shortages, trade restrictions, and defective or contaminated supplies (K. Allen 2020; Rieger 2020a).

Some small businesses retooled their production lines to help with these challenges, which was in the national interest but also was an effort to keep their business afloat. Dozens of small breweries and distilleries shifted to making hand sanitizer (Brend 2020).

Many people lost income, but reduced household spending coupled with federal government programs to support the economically

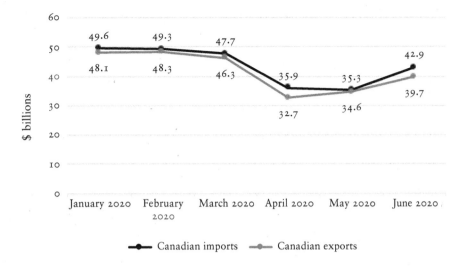

Figure 9.1 | Canadian imports and exports, January–June 2020.
Canadian trade plunged in spring 2020. *Source:* Statistics Canada 2022k.

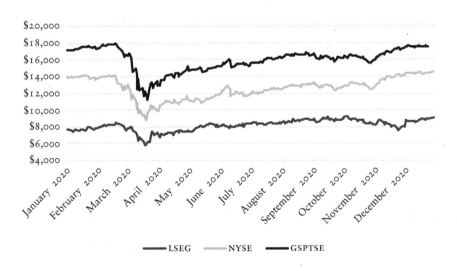

Figure 9.2 | Global stock prices, 1 January–31 December 2020.
Stocks had largely rebounded by the end of 2020. *Sources:* Yahoo Finance
2020f, 2020j, 2020k.

Table 9.1 | Stock prices of pharmaceutical, digital, big-box retail, and food companies, 2020

Company	Closing stock price, 1 January 2020 ($)	Closing stock price, 31 December 2020 ($)	Change (%)
Pharmaceutical			
Novavax, Inc.	4.5	119.0	2,549.2
Moderna, Inc.	19.2	111.1	477.8
Digital			
Amazon	1,898.0	3,285.9	73.1
Zoom	68.7	353.4	414.3
Netflix	329.8	524.6	59.1
Big-Box Retail			
Walmart Inc.	118.8	144.2	13.4
The Home Depot, Inc.	218.4	265.3	21.5
Grocery Stores			
Sobeys/Empire	30.5	35.0	14.9

Some companies prospered in 2020. *Sources:* Yahoo Finance 2020b, 2020d, 2020f–h, 2020k–m.

vulnerable meant that savings increased by an average of $5,800 per person in 2020 (Schembri 2021). Wealthy households tended to see the largest increase, but some in lower income groups also saved extra money (Bank of Canada 2021). Spending patterns shifted away from restaurants, bars, and hotels and, later in the year, towards cars, recreational goods, furniture, and home renovations (Schembri 2021). These savings contributed to increased inflation in the coming years.

Winners, Losers, and Volatile Sectors: Selected Examples

With heavy investment in the development and procurement of an effective COVID-19 vaccine, the pharmaceutical industry generally fared well financially (table 9.1). The success of the vaccine also improved perception of the industry (Merino and Ware 2021).

As in-person shopping functioned at reduced capacity, Amazon capitalized on the surge of online shopping; its workforce increased correspondingly (Wakabayashi et al. 2020). In Canada and the US, Netflix gained six million subscribers (Moody 2021) and acquired $70 billion in market capitalization in 2020 (Pandey 2020). Zoom had more than three hundred million active users on several days in April 2020, an increase from ten million in December 2019. These digital companies saw substantial revenue increases.

Though retail stores had to operate at reduced capacity, big-box stores (table 9.1) had floor space to accommodate social distancing and an ability to sell a variety of items in addition to those deemed "essential," resulting in increased revenue.

Grocery store sales in Canada peaked in March 2020 at $10.4 billion, an increase of about $2 billion from February 2020 (Tighe 2021). This corresponds to the first round of lockdowns, when people anticipating shortages stockpiled some goods. Leading grocery retailers saw increased sales in 2020 (Statista 2021) and, in the case of Sobeys/Empire, a steady increase in stock prices (table 9.1).

Other sectors fared poorly. At the beginning of the pandemic some small businesses pivoted successfully to change how they offered their product or service (Alini 2021); others saw a boost in demand for their original service as people's habits changed (Cowley and Haimerl 2020). Public health orders limiting in-person, non-essential shopping, however, meant that many small retail businesses lost revenue (Tam, Sood, and Johnston 2021a) and took on debt (CFIB 2021). Overall, more businesses closed than opened in 2020 (Statistics Canada 2022n).

The entertainment sector was hit hard. Revenue of Cineplex Inc. fell from $439.2 million in the second quarter of 2019 to $22.0 million in the second quarter of 2020. Stock prices plunged from $32.90 on 4 March 2020 to $8.80 two weeks later (Yahoo Finance 2020c). They did not recover by the end of the year.

With government interventions like border controls and advisories against travel, companies in the travel and tourism industry, such as cruise lines, saw drastic drops in revenue. Air Canada's stock price decreased by 52.2 per cent during 2020; its revenue fell by 85.0 per cent (Yahoo Finance 2020a). For further discussion on the tourism sector and Air Canada, see chapters 8 and 11.

Other sectors of note include energy, manufacturing, and housing. The energy sector directly and indirectly employs about 4.9 per cent of workers across Canada and accounts for 11.1 per cent of nominal GDP (Natural Resources Canada 2018, 8, 12). Global oil demand dropped by an estimated 30 per cent at the start of the pandemic compared to a year earlier because of containment measures and economic disruptions (International Energy Agency 2020); crude oil prices plunged amid declining demand in spring 2020 (Government of Canada 2022l). Overall, demand for oil dropped by 9 per cent during 2020 (Statistics Canada 2022m). Demand had largely rebounded by March 2022 (Statistics Canada 2022d).

The manufacturing sector provides about 9 per cent of total Canadian employment and represents 10 per cent of total GDP (Government of Canada 2021e), while also contributing indirectly to other sectors (Cléroux, n.d.). Supply chain disruptions and new health and safety regulations challenged manufacturing. Early in the pandemic 65 per cent of manufacturers experienced declines in output, but by May 2020, manufacturing sales had increased in most provinces as industries adapted (Adecco 2020).[1]

Before COVID-19, most housing markets in Canada "were operating with shrinking inventories as growth in demand was outpacing supply supported by economic growth, low unemployment rate, and population growth" (Siatchinov, De Champlain, and Verma 2020, para. 1). In response to COVID-19, virtual house tours and digital contract signing became common. Demand for larger houses grew as the number of people working from home increased (Statistics Canada 2020h). While sales dropped by 70.0 per cent in the early stages of the pandemic, benchmark house prices (aggregated) increased by 25.9 per cent between June 2020 and June 2021 as the impact of low mortgage rates took hold, leading to a highly competitive market and a drop in supply (Canadian Real Estate Association, n.d.).[2] Atlantic Canada, with lower prices and less dense populations, became an appealing destination and saw the highest net interprovincial migration to the region in the past sixty years (O'Kane 2020; Parkinson 2021).

In sum, pharmaceutical, digital, and big-box retail sectors did well; small business, entertainment, and travel and tourism generally did poorly, while energy, manufacturing, and housing saw fluctuations.

MARKET FAILURES

To test the MFH, Hood, Rothstein, and Baldwin (2001) measure information costs and opt-out costs. Information costs are faced when one assesses the probability and severity of risks to which individuals are exposed (Hood, Rothstein, and Baldwin 2001, 73). Opt-out costs are incurred when one avoids risk exposure through, among other things,

Table 9.2 | Information and opt-out costs

Information costs	High	Focus on gathering information and sharing it	Extensive government intervention focused on all three components of control
	Low	Minimal government intervention	Focus on modifying behaviour
		Low	High
		Opt-out costs	

Government intervention increases when information and opt-out costs are high.
Source: Adapted from Hood, Rothstein, and Baldwin (2001).

insurance and legal processes (73). Where either information costs or opt-out costs are high, a market failure is said to exist, and the MFH predicts that governments will act to reduce the cost. Maximal regulatory intervention is expected in cases with high information and opt-out costs (table 9.2).

Health Care as a Market Failure

Health care is generally treated as a market failure (Frakt 2011; Mwachofi and Al-Assaf 2011; Barrie 2016). People do not have complete information about the risk that they will require health care, and most lack sufficient knowledge to assess medical treatments, leading to an asymmetry of information between patients and providers (Haas-Wilson 2001, 1032). This context means that people could be taken advantage of by fraudulent treatment and made to carry excessive costs individually, which leads to inefficiencies and inequities (Birch 2019, 291). To intervene in these market failures (Watts and Segal 2009), health care in Canada is characterized by care delivered based on need regardless of an ability to pay, pooled resources, professionalism and ethical training, and regulation of systems and professions, though there is variation across the provinces.

Throughout the pandemic – a high-impact, low-frequency event – government intervention to address market failures was evident. There was widespread effort to lower information costs; government focused on creating standards to limit disease spread. Various ways to opt-out of the risk were modified or introduced, as will be discussed. These interventions led to externalities. For example, widespread vaccination aided by government policy benefited more than just an individual becoming vaccinated. The individual risk of severe illness from COVID-19 was in most cases already low, but the overall gain from vaccination, in the form of reduced disease transmission, higher population immunity, and subsequent effects on hospitals, benefited society overall (Healy 2016). However, vaccine hesitancy or refusal by portions of the population contributed to an overwhelmed health-care system and delayed surgeries (see chapter 6). Government interventions were particularly evident in the collection of data, the communication of health risks, and the setting and enforcing of standards, steps that were necessary because the market on its own was not equipped to do so (Helland and Morrison 2021, 839).

About 70 per cent of health-care costs in Canada are publicly funded; the rest is paid out of pocket or through private insurance (Norris 2020).[3] Throughout the pandemic the system was under immense pressure for prolonged periods, leading to difficult trade-offs. Many health-care providers, including nurses and family doctors (G. Murphy et al. 2022; Canadian Federation of Nurses Unions 2022; McKeen 2022) left or retired from the profession due to exhaustion and excess stress, thereby exacerbating shortages and putting further strain on the system, including emergency departments (Duong 2021). These problems existed prior to the pandemic, but the pressure of the pandemic amplified them. Many non-COVID-19 medical treatments and elective procedures were delayed for extended periods.

Without enough surge capacity in hospitals, many governments, including Manitoba's (Greenslade 2022) and Quebec's (Lacoursière 2021), increased their use of private clinics and private nurse agencies. There was some speculation that this would violate the Canada Health Act (Turnbull 2020). Public objections were muted, and indeed there were also calls to allow people to pay directly for privately offered health care (A. Miller and Shingler 2022; Mertz 2021; Lindsay 2022).

By 2022 many called the system broken; in June the president of the Canadian Medical Association declared that the system was on the verge of collapse (Hassan 2022). Given the significant allocation that health care receives in government budgets, it is difficult to see how much more can be spent as Canada's population ages; the demands for more funding are endless. Concerns about privatization or a public-private system persist, with one research chair calling it a "zombie" option that does not address the underlying problem, has the potential to drain resources from the public system, requires costs to oversee, and makes access more difficult for those less able to pay (Miller and Shingler 2022). The debates were not new, but they raise important questions about the stability of the publicly funded system in a crisis and its aftermath.

COST OF GETTING INFORMATION
ABOUT THE RISK

Information costs measure how difficult it is for individuals to assess risk. Low information costs make it easier to obtain information about a risk, while high information costs may indicate a market failure. Information costs can vary from person to person.

COVID-19 required collaboration among international actors to develop and refine a response to the risk. Information costs were higher at the start of the pandemic. International governing bodies and public health organizations, with financial capacity and support to mobilize resources, helped to generate knowledge about the virus, its symptoms, and how to prevent transmission. These public organizations had credibility in ways that the private and not-for-profit sectors on their own did not. In other words, the market required government intervention to provide people with reliable information about the risk of COVID-19.

In the early stages of the pandemic, updates were hourly. At times, the volume of information was overwhelming. Public health helped to ensure the quality of information during chaotic periods, in which reams of information were constantly available, updated, and interpreted by several reliable and not-so-reliable online sources. Asymptomatic transmission and the benefit of mask-wearing demonstrate how information changed over time and affected policy (R. Zhang et al. 2020, 14859; Ogden et al. 2020, 198).

The pandemic brought to light several information deficiencies at a macro level. We highlight here some particularly salient ones. Some information networks were unreliable (Beaunoyer, Dupéré, and Guitton 2020, 1; see chapter 1 herein). When countries were forthcoming with information, it was not always handled well, as seen in unwarranted travel bans when the Omicron variant was detected in South Africa in November 2021, with implications for countries' willingness to share information in the future (Mendelson et al. 2021, 2212). Managing misinformation and conspiracy theories was an ongoing challenge (E. Thompson 2020; Ormel et al. 2021, 7). Though information about COVID-19 was shared across all forms of media, the prominent use of digital platforms disadvantaged people who lacked access to the Internet, digital devices, or digital literacy (Beaunoyer, Dupéré, and Guitton 2020, 2).

Reliance on digital platforms for shopping, socializing, and working remotely posed cybersecurity threats (Canadian Centre for Cyber Security 2020, 12; Pottie 2021). About four in ten Canadians experienced a cybersecurity incident during the pandemic (Statistics Canada 2021j, 3), including COVID-19–specific fraud (Canadian Centre for Cyber Security 2020, 16; Fraser 2020). The number of reported fraud victims more than doubled in 2020, with COVID-19–specific fraud causing $7.8 million in losses[4] between 6 March 2020 and 31 December 2021 (Canadian Fraud News 2020; Canadian Anti-Fraud Centre 2022).

The absence of race-specific and community-level data led to jurisdictions missing important trends. Some provinces eventually mandated race-based data collection (McKenzie 2020; Government of Ontario 2020a). However, much of what was learned about the disproportionate impacts of COVID-19 on marginalized communities came from comparing maps of COVID-19 cases with known information about racialized communities.

Besides the slowness with which provincial and territorial governments collected race-based data, there remains the question of how information is interpreted. Given the problematic history of how governments have interacted with certain racialized communities, the information that public health offers a community is not necessarily interpreted as intended. Several lenses are used to filter and interpret information (see chapters 2 and 6 for a more complete discussion about the psychology and social construction of risk).

There were also limits to economic information. Governments did not have a complete picture of the economy. For example, the gig economy, a sector characterized by short-term contracts and flexibility for workers (Frazer 2019), has seen growth since 2006 and is now estimated to employ between 8 and 10 per cent of the labour force (Jeon, Lius, and Ostrovsky 2019, 6; Jeon and Ostrovosky 2020). Statistics Canada had difficulty "tracking the gig economy in real time" (Jeon and Ostrovsky 2020, para. 2) and determining the impact of COVID-19 on the sector as data were not recorded according to standard employment indicators. Approximately half of all gig workers in Canada are self-employed, which means they faced challenges in gathering government benefits introduced in response to COVID-19 (K. Campbell 2021a).

Incomplete information about businesses and individuals resulted in challenges administering CERB and CEWS (for more on this, see chapter

4). There was never a reliable way to reconcile the costs and benefits of the government-implemented shutdowns. The focus was on containing the disease, keeping the economy going, and counting the costs later, characteristic of a precautionary stance in a crisis. This was made more difficult by the cyclical nature of the pandemic, with variant-driven waves of the virus peaking at different times. This uncertainty made it difficult for businesses to do any advanced planning. Provincial and territorial governments were constrained in their ability to address these uncertainties, though attempts were made by designing staged levels of reopening.

Misinformation about COVID-19 also spread. This in turn affected vaccination and infection rates, causing, by some estimates, an additional 200,000 cases, 13,000 hospitalizations, 2,800 deaths, and $300 million in hospital expenses over nine months (Council of Canadian Academies 2023).

COST OF OPTING OUT OF THE RISK

A market failure is assumed to exist when opt-out costs are high and require government intervention to lower them (Hood, Rothstein, and Baldwin 2001, 74), or when opt-out costs vary and require intervention to create a balance between people (Aven and Renn 2018, 232–3). Opt-out costs are those associated with removing oneself from risk exposure, often through insurance and legal processes (Hood, Rothstein, and Baldwin 2001, 70). Throughout the pandemic, opt-out costs were high due to the pervasive nature of the risk, and options were more readily available to some than to others. Eventually, vaccination was one way to opt out of the risk of disease, albeit with important limitations (see chapter 6 for more). Insurance policies were generally weak; legal mechanisms to opt out of pandemic-related risks had mixed results.

INSURANCE AND RARE EVENTS

Kunreuther, Pauly, and McMorrow (2013a, 11) describe insurance as "one of man's greatest inventions" for reducing risk and addressing uncertainty. When responding to simple risks, such as car accidents, which are predictable, frequent, consistent, and traceable to one person or place, the insurance industry can set reliable policy premiums, distributing the cost of the risk (Loubergé 2013, 15; Quigley, Bisset, and Mills 2017, 38). High-impact, low-frequency events, however, are difficult to insure against. With less reliable predictive data to estimate the

likelihood and consequences, these events defy the business model of
insurance companies and make it difficult to develop policy premiums.

Before 9/11, for example, losses from acts of terrorism were not
explicitly included or standard in insurance policies (Kunreuther, Pauly,
and McMorrow 2013b, 221). Following 9/11, the US government introduced the Terrorism Risk Insurance Program to provide support for
private insurance companies offering coverage to commercial and P&C
policyholders for certain terrorism-related losses (Federal Insurance
Office 2020). The US government also contributes significant money to
the National Flood Insurance Program, distorting the insurance market. The program provides subsidies to residences in flood-prone areas,
which can benefit wealthy owners of older oceanfront homes (Quigley,
Bissett, and Mills 2017, 150).

Following the 2013 floods in Alberta, which resulted in $2 billion in
insured losses and $6 billion in economic losses, the industry began includ-
ing overland flood coverage in more home-insurance policies (Meckbach
2020d). In 2019, only 39 per cent of Canadians were eligible; many
people in high-risk areas went without coverage due to high premiums
(PS 2020a). In 2020 the Task Force on Flood Insurance and Relocation
was created to improve protection for homeowners (PS 2020a). These
examples underscore the challenges for the insurance industry in establishing policies to cover rare and costly events (Kunreuther, Pauly, and
McMorrow 2013b, 224), which cause cascading failures across systems
and organizations and generate broad social risks (Loubergé 2013, 3). As
we will discuss, business and travel insurance proved inadequate as a way
to opt out of pandemic risk (Hay 2020).

INSURANCE POLICIES AND COVID-19

By the end of the second quarter in 2020, the P&C insurance industry
had experienced millions in underwriting losses due to lower interest
rates, decreased investment income, and lost clients as small businesses
closed (Colaço, Duvinage, and Mahony 2020, 8, 12). Insurance companies started to focus on carrying less risk and lowering their underwriting capacity. Some insurers created COVID-19 exclusions (Colaço,
Duvinage, and Mahony 2020, 8; Hay 2020) to limit revenue losses.

By the end of 2020 the industry had bounced back to underwriting
profit. There were some unintended savings. In 2020, home-insurance
companies in Canada experienced a 10.3 per cent decline in claims and
saved an estimated $1.1 billion, which companies partly attributed to
fewer burglaries, for example, because people were at home more and

therefore break-ins were less common (Adriano 2020). Overall, the P&C insurance industry's net income increased by 54.7 per cent from the year before (Gambrill 2021).

Despite Insurance Bureau of Canada (IBC) companies paying out $1 billion in auto, commercial, and personal insurance to policyholders in 2020, along with $200 million in deferred premiums for personal and business policyholders (IBC 2020a), the lack of clarity about insurance and the growing number of denied business claims challenged the insurance industry's reputation and revealed the difficulty of insuring against rare events. Business-insurance holders discovered that their policies were not very flexible or, put more harshly, "virtually useless for this type of catastrophic event" (Plunkett 2020, 5). Most standard business-insurance policies do not cover closures caused by pandemics. Instead, most business insurance falls under commercial general liability or commercial property insurance. Commercial general liability covers businesses and their employees for accidental injuries, bodily injuries, loss or damage to third parties, personal injuries, property damage, and tenants' legal liability, while commercial property insurance covers physical assets, like equipment, for loss or damage (IBC 2020b, 53).

Businesses can also apply for business-interruption (BI) coverage, which covers expenses for income or profits lost because of disasters and related business closures (IBC 2020b, 53; Top Class Actions 2020). Typically, BI insurance provides coverage for physical damage to a business's property, nearby property, or physical damage caused elsewhere due to the disruption of supplies or to difficulties accessing the business (Dolny, Iqbal, and Rosenstein 2020). The Insurance Institute of Canada, however, stated that BI insurance did not include losses from the pandemic (Dolny, Iqbal, and Rosenstein 2020). This declaration was challenged by businesses that closed because of provincial or territorial orders (Meckbach 2020a). Insurance companies rejected most of these claims because the closures did not result from property damage (Meckbach 2020c). This interpretation was previously used to deny BI coverage claims after a government exclusion order shut down the central business district of Christchurch, New Zealand, following a 2011 earthquake (Lennox 2011; Clement 2020; C. Brown, Seville, and Vargo 2016, 397).

With viral outbreaks not listed specifically in insurance policies, businesses that closed because of COVID-19 public health orders had few options (Top Class Actions 2020; Lafrance-Cooke, Macdonald, and Willox 2020). Legal clauses, such as force majeure or unforeseeable circumstances, could be used by insurance companies to deny claims based on the difficulties associated with predicting and planning for unknown or rare events (Top Class Actions 2020). A lack of clarity between recommendations and mandates by public officials also had an impact on the ability of business owners to collect insurance coverage (Ghoussoub 2020).

Many people and businesses were significantly affected by the industry denying claims, including taxi drivers (Modjeski 2020; Asquith 2020; A. Jones 2020) and dental practices (J. Hall 2020; Ghoussoub 2020). Travel insurance received considerable attention. Before the pandemic there was a lack of interest in and understanding of travel insurance policies (Lahey 2020). By early March 2020, providers had announced they would "no longer reimburse new customers who need[ed] to cancel their trips due to the coronavirus outbreak" (S. Harris 2020, para. 1), as the virus was a "known" issue, demonstrated by government-issued advisories against non-essential travel to certain countries. Some providers also offered an option providing cancellation coverage for a fee (S. Harris 2020, para. 9).

In the final week of March 2020 airlines announced that clients without travel insurance would only receive a travel credit (Marchitelli 2020): airlines began to hold passengers' money (G. MacDonald 2020). Air Canada alone was reported to be holding $2.6 billion in "prepaid passenger income" by the end of the month (Nardi 2020, para. 8); part of its financial support relief package from the federal government a year later had to be used to refund customers whose flights had been cancelled (R. Jones 2021a).

The policy change of receiving travel credits rather than refunds, which the Canadian Transportation Agency approved, frustrated many consumers (G. MacDonald 2020; Marchitelli 2020; Britneff 2020b; Nardi 2020). They could request a refund through their credit card company or small claims court, but success rates were low (Marchitelli 2020).

Although insurance is a traditional market tool used to pool risk and cover losses, it was largely ineffective as an opt-out strategy during the pandemic.

SELECTED LEGAL ISSUES

Emergency Legislation

The Emergencies Act enables the federal government to enact "special temporary measures to ensure safety and security during national emergencies" in which provinces and territories lack the capacity to respond effectively, and/or the situation cannot be handled by other existing laws or authorities (Government of Canada 2022e, 1, 7). There was federal support for provinces and territories in the form of relief programs, distribution of PPE, and, later, vaccines, but the Emergencies Act was not enacted in the early stages of the pandemic (Lang 2021). In January 2021, 70 per cent of Canadians said they wanted the federal government to use the Act to help standardize the response and reallocate PPE (Lang 2021). Most parts of the country were struggling with similar shortages; resource reallocation may not have helped.

The Emergencies Act was invoked for ten days starting on 14 February 2022. Its use did not ensure safety from a public health perspective; rather, it was provoked by extreme reactions to public health measures: a three-week occupation of downtown Ottawa, and blockades at border crossings (C. Tunney 2022b). Two-thirds of Canadians supported the Act's use (Maru Public Opinion 2022), though it was not clear if the measures enabled by the Act were necessary to control the situation. The federal government faced lawsuits from civil liberties associations, which contended that there was no threat to the security of Canada, the measures violated freedom of assembly, and the Act's application set a dangerous precedent (Fine 2022). (For further discussion see chapters 6 and 12.)

The Quarantine Act was also used. The purpose of the federal Quarantine Act is to protect public health by regulating the use of quarantine measures for preventing the transmission of communicable diseases (Government of Canada 2020c, 3). Throughout the pandemic, provinces and territories developed measures that generally reflected and supported the federal act (Gibson 2020), though some measures varied by region.

The emergency component of the pandemic was largely regulated through provincial and territorial emergency and health legislation. At the provincial and territorial level, emergency management legislation gives the government the authority to declare a state of emergency and manage essential supplies (Gibson 2020). All provinces and territories declared either a state of emergency or a public health emergency by 22 March 2020 (Lawson et al. 2022). Provincial and territorial health-protection legislation provides CMOs with significant authority in public health emergencies (Fafard et al. 2018, 588). Health-protection legislation, on the advice of CMOs, was used across Canada in spring 2020 to close public schools and implement self-isolation requirements (Gorman 2020). The legislation provided police and the courts with the authority to enforce rules and issue fines (Gorman 2020). The anonymity of the collection, use, and disclosure of personal health information by public health authorities (OPC 2020a) and the use of digital tools, such as contact-tracing applications, raised privacy concerns (OPC 2020b).

Employment Legislation

While existing laws and legislation provided a structure for balancing the rights of employers and employees and required health and safety protocols, COVID-19 posed additional challenges and demonstrated the limitations of using legal means to opt out of risk. Federal and provincial and territorial occupational health and safety legislation protects workers by outlining employers' duties for maintaining safe and healthy working conditions (Government of Canada 2021d, 103; CCOHS 2019, para. 5, 7). In the case of COVID-19, employers were required to operate workplaces according to public health and safety protocols. Employees were required to inform their employers of positive diagnoses and to stay home (CCOHS 2019). The number of claims regarding lost time due to COVID-19 and COVID-19 injury-related deaths and occupational-disease-related deaths were about 13 per cent and 4 per cent, respectively, of total claims in 2020 (table 9.3; AWCBC 2021a, 2–3, 272–3; 2022).[5]

Occupational-health-and-safety legislation gives employees the right to refuse unsafe work (Boyle 2020). Claims generally require an employee to be able to prove the presence of danger and not just a risk, fear, or anxiety about the situation (Levitt 2020). Work-refusal claims, largely related to a lack of PPE and social distancing, increased at the provincial and territorial level throughout 2020; the number of approved claims did not (Singh 2020; Neustaeter 2020).

Some legal professionals argued that ongoing claim denials highlighted the inadequacies of labour laws for responding to the pandemic, and that individual circumstances, such as pre-existing health conditions or the required use of public transit for commuting, should be sufficient support for the claim (Singh 2020; Wozniak 2020, 18; Roberts 2020, 7). Others argued that refusing to work because of general fears of contracting the virus invalidated the claims (Singh 2020; Bholla 2020).

Under labour-standards codes, employees are eligible for emergency leave if an emergency impedes their ability to work, with some exceptions (Government of Nova Scotia 2021a). By December 2020, seven provinces and the federal government had established new work-leave options offering employees job and benefits protection; however, all were unpaid or left to the employer's discretion (Ma and Popp 2021; Page 2020).

Two-thirds of Canadian companies do not provide employees with paid sick leave, which places Canada among a group of countries with "insufficient" sick-leave policies (Spence 2020, para. 3). Canada, however, introduced the highest number of COVID-19–related paid-leave

Table 9.3 | Workplace injury claims and fatalities, 2019–20

Year	Accepted lost-time injury claims	Number of injury or occupational disease–related fatalities
2019	271,806	925
2020	253,397	924
2020 (COVID-19–specific)	32,742*	39

*This number also includes non-lost-time claims (Tucker and Keefe 2021, 35). The number of lost-time injury claims and fatalities related to COVID-19 made up a small proportion of total workplace injuries and fatalities. *Sources*: AWCBC 2021a, 2022; Tucker and Keefe 2021; CCOHS 2021.

options for workers, with 15 per cent of companies offering paid leave (Väyrynen 2020, 4; Marotta 2020). Considering that 29 per cent of COVID-19 outbreaks in Canada are estimated to have occurred at workplaces, paid-leave options were important for workers and helped slow transmission (Marotta 2020; Woods 2021; Kumar et al. 2012, 134).

The CRSB was introduced in October 2020 and provided $450 after taxes for a one-week period for workers who missed at least 50 per cent of their work week because they were unwell or isolating because of COVID-19 (Government of Canada 2022d). This program was of particular importance for essential workers whose jobs were less likely to have sick-leave benefits (A. Thompson et al. 2021, 3). The CRSB allocated less than a full-time weekly salary at Ontario's minimum wage, and payments could take weeks to reach workers (4).

Some legal professionals contended that temporarily laid-off employees during COVID-19 were entitled to common-law damages. Others argued that temporary layoffs should not be considered terminations or constructive dismissals because employers did not intend to lay off workers and had reasonable expectations that workers would return (Levitt 2020; Lowe 2020). In this situation "employers can request employees to waive their rights to common-law damages in exchange for some consideration" (Lowe 2020, 2), while the federal, provincial, and territorial governments may issue orders to employers that confirm that COVID-19 layoffs are not constructive dismissals. As a result, employers laid off employees without knowing the possible legal risks or financial costs for both parties.

In sum, the law worked to protect the population at large, but in many cases it was unclear or inadequate. Legal protections for workers had to be balanced with the containment of the spread of disease and the maintenance of economic stability. Safety measures at work were recognized, if not always enforced. During some outbreaks, protections for workers were absent, and employees were incentivized to increase their risk exposure by continuing to work, or to continue to work while sick. Existing protections, like dangerous work claims, were rarely recognized; paid sick leave and federal relief programs increased and offered some support, but often fell short. Questions of fairness persisted.

LIMITS TO OPTING OUT: WORK FROM HOME

Throughout the pandemic, governments encouraged organizations to offer work-from-home (WFH) arrangements to employees, as it represented one way in which people could opt out of risks, including exposure to and transmission of the virus, work interruptions, and income losses (Deng, Morissette, and Messacar 2020). Between 2000 and 2018 the number of Canadians working for any amount of time at home grew from 10.0 to 13.0 per cent (Turcotte 2010, 3; Statistics Canada 2018b). By the last week of March 2020, 39.1 per cent of Canadians worked remotely (Deng, Morissette, and Messacar 2020); many continued doing so or worked in a hybrid manner for some time (Messacar, Morissette, and Deng 2020). Employers were still responsible for ensuring that remote employees were safe and healthy (Wozniak 2020, 18). If deemed essential, employees were legally obligated to return to work (CBC News 2020j).

The option to WFH varies by socio-economic characteristics and by sector. Finance and insurance, educational services, and scientific and technical services are among the industries whose workers can most commonly WFH (Deng, Morissette, and Messacar 2020); agriculture and oil and gas industries demonstrate lower WFH capacities.

The option to WFH is positively correlated with the education level of a household's primary income provider (Messacar, Morissette, and Deng 2020) and level of income: households with two sources of income demonstrate greater WFH capacity. WFH capacity also varies by gender, with women having higher rates than men, in both single- and dual-earner households (Messacar, Morissette, and Deng 2020). These differences correspond to the fact that more men work in industries that cannot be remote, like agriculture or construction (Deng, Morissette, and Messacar 2020). WFH capacity also increases with age (Angus Reid

Institute 2020c). Only 20.0 per cent of workers under the age of twenty-five, and 12.7 per cent of those with less than a high school diploma, were able to WFH (Deng, Morissette, and Messacar 2020).

The flexibility associated with working from home reduced worker burnout and sometimes improved productivity, based on survey data (C. Miller 2021). Barriers to productivity included lack of interaction with co-workers, inadequate space, and slow Internet. Long-term remote work may carry fewer productivity benefits (Glaeser and Cutler 2021).

WFH presented other challenges, particularly for caregivers and women in this role (M. Miller 2021). Women are more likely than men to be in caregiver positions, with US data suggesting that females perform 70 per cent of child-care and household duties (P. Cohen and Hsu 2020). In addition to professional challenges, WFH arrangements created numerous domestic responsibilities and stress and contributed to mental health problems of mothers (Grose 2021). Many women simply chose to leave the workforce given the additional domestic pressures (P. Cohen 2021; M. Miller 2021). This loss of women from the workforce, and the potential for this trend to occur in the future, poses financial challenges for women and significantly affects their retirement assets (P. Cohen 2021; M. Miller 2021).

Many Could Not Work from Home

Public Safety Canada (PS 2021) divides the list of essential services and functions by sector, which includes communications, energy, finance, food, government, health, information technology, manufacturing, safety, and transportation. The federal government urged workers in these fields to WFH, but many could not (Deng, Morissette, and Messacar 2020).

Various programs existed at the provincial and territorial level to reward essential workers in grocery stores, health-care facilities, and pharmacies. At the federal level the Essential Services Contingency Reserve, announced in May 2020 and valued at $3 billion, provided provinces and territories with funding to support essential workers (Tumilty 2020). Providing higher wages or "hero pay" was determined by province and territory and varied by sector.

Immigrants and racialized communities made up a significant proportion of this working population that was exposed to risk at work, constituting 34 per cent of Canada's front-line workers before the pandemic (Statistics Canada 2020i, 4). In addition to being

Table 9.4 | The unemployment rate by population group in Canada, August 2020

Population groups	Unemployment rate (%)
Arab	17.9
Black	17.6
Chinese	13.2
Filipino	12.7
Latin American	13.9
Neither a visible minority nor Indigenous	9.4
South Asian	14.9
Southeast Asian	16.6

The unemployment rate varied by population group. *Sources:* Statistics Canada 2020i, 2020j.

disproportionately affected by COVID-19, in that racialized minorities were more likely to get the disease, these populations are also overrepresented in industries most disrupted by COVID-19 that are unable to WFH, including accommodation and food services (Statistics Canada 2020i, 5). The closure of restaurants throughout the year, for example, significantly affected the employment of different populations (table 9.4), which the national unemployment rate did not always capture (Statistics Canada 2020j, 9).

Temporary foreign workers (TFWs) were also not able to WFH; the pandemic revealed vulnerabilities in the program and the labour force. A TFW is "a foreign national engaged in work activity who is authorized, with appropriate documentation, to enter and remain in Canada for a limited period" (Kachulis and Perez-Leclerc 2020, 1). Accounting for about 3.0 per cent of total employment, TFWs make up higher proportions in certain sectors (figure 9.3; Y. Lu 2020). COVID-19 outbreaks at farms and plants brought the mistreatment of TFWs to light (Ayres 2020). Reducing the number of TFWs because of the pandemic revealed the vulnerabilities of using foreign labour to meet domestic-labour needs. Some sectors were never able to secure the needed labour. Industries such as seafood processing had to rely on local workers as young as thirteen years of age to meet the local labour shortage (Y. Lu 2020; C. Smith 2020).

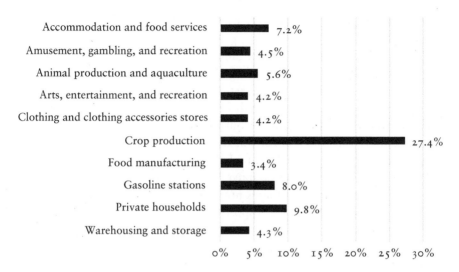

Figure 9.3 | Proportion of temporary foreign workers by industry.
Canada's TFWs are largely concentrated in agriculture. TFWs may be hired
by private households as caregivers for children or people with high medical
needs. Formal roles include child-care provider, live-in caregiver, nanny, registered nurse or registered psychiatric nurse, licensed practical nurse, attendant for persons with disabilities, home support worker, and personal care
attendant (Government of Canada 2023c). *Source:* Y. Lu 2020.

In time, WFH would have unforeseen consequences. Those who
could WFH saved considerably in reduced commuting, clothing, and
eating-out costs (Farooqui 2021). In urban centres like Toronto some
estimate the cost savings to be as high $13,000 per year before taxes
(para. 3). These savings effectively became a significant pay increase
for many (T. Keller 2023). This contributed to inflation and caused
labour disruption as unions sought to formalize WFH arrangements in
collective bargaining (Shingler 2023). Relatedly, with such a drop in
people working downtown, there was an increase in spending in the
suburbs and a decrease in downtown centres, including on commercial
real estate (PricewaterhouseCoopers Canada 2021, 18; Saminather and
Waldersee 2020; Magee 2021). This change could constitute a significant and long-lasting change in metropolitan areas (Wheat et al. 2023;
Lord 2023).

CONCLUSION

The pandemic resulted in market failures that only governments could adequately address. The scope of COVID-19 and the nature of the risk necessitated a fast, large, and accurate information-gathering operation. Government was best suited for this role, with international networks and its ability, credibility, and resources to leverage local research labs and set up testing and contact tracing. Challenges persisted, however, among them a lack of quick and reliable information; projections and directives were always being adapted. Such is the nature of an uncertain risk coupled with a system that is not quite ready to address it. Certain populations were affected disproportionately by the pandemic, including low-income workers and racialized communities. Government information-gathering mechanisms were slow to detect these issues.

The enormity of the event resulted in striking a balance between a variety of competing pressures, including workers' and employers' rights, containing the spread of the disease, and trying to ensure national stability. Traditional market tools such as insurance policies were largely ineffective as an opt-out strategy; most insurance claims were denied throughout the pandemic. In terms of legal protections for workers, much of the population shifted to working from home. If workers had to be present, measures such as providing PPE or mandating social distancing were recognized, if not always enforced. The Quarantine Act had mixed success.[6]

Outbreaks of the virus at workplaces demonstrated the risk exposure that some workers faced due to unsafe working practices. Cargill's meat-packing plant in Alberta had the largest COVID-19 outbreak linked to a single facility in North America (Rieger 2020b; Dryden and Rieger 2020). Protections for workers were severely limited, coupled with incentives to work while sick (K. Baum, Tait, and Grant 2020). No stop-work order was issued to Cargill, though both Alberta's Health Services and Alberta's Occupational Health and Safety had the authority to do so.

The costs of the pandemic and government response were not evenly distributed. Certain sectors were better able to have employees WFH. Some people were better off financially at the end of the pandemic. They often directed their savings to home renovations (Peesker 2020), moved to bigger homes, or speculated on the rebounded stock market. Some businesses thrived. There was an advantage for bigger businesses that sold a variety of goods, had sufficient floor space to allow for social distancing, and had the resources to pay for sick leave and PPE. There were also advantages for digital businesses, like Zoom, that allowed people to stay home more comfortably.

For others, the pandemic and ensuing government regulations had a negative impact. Essential workers who could not WFH were exposed to higher risk. Many were immigrants and racialized minorities (Statistics Canada 2020i, 4; Turcotte and Savage 2020). Businesses based on mobility and face-to-face interactions like the energy sector, small retail, live performance, and tourism were hit hard. Inflation generally affects the less well-off more severely.

While expensive and, according to some economic analyses, at times more generous than required (Morneau 2023; see chapters 4, 10, and the book's conclusion), programs like CERB and CEWS were necessary to protect large numbers who lost jobs overnight due to lockdowns and economic slowdowns. Disruptions, however, affected more than just financial well-being. Lockdowns contributed to a deterioration of people's mental health (Canadian Mental Health Association, n.d., 1). Women were more likely to take on child-care roles at home as schools and daycare centres shut (Deng, Morissette, and Messacar 2020). People living in crowded accommodations could not reduce their risk of exposure by staying home. There were increases in calls related to domestic violence (N. Thompson 2021). Use of food banks rose significantly (Jabakhanji 2020; A. Harvey 2020). Some argue that COVID-19 contributed to rising numbers of unhoused people (Falvo 2020, 7, 43).

Finally, a generally publicly funded and directed health system had limited capacity with few options in the short term to expand that capacity. Many health services were limited or delayed. By 2022, many were describing the system as broken; historic debates about more public money and private options in health care re-emerged.

The market failure hypothesis is helpful because it allows us to focus on the impact of government interventions on gathering and validating information and providing opt-out opportunities for those who need them. Governments placed considerable emphasis on both. Nonetheless, there were significant gaps in information gathering as well as inequalities in ability to opt out. Thus, the MFH does not provide a fully satisfying explanation of government response.

Moreover, these consequences of government interventions leave unanswered questions, not strictly because of the costs but also because of the inability of government to understand and communicate clearly how it struck a balance between risks, and if its interventions were "proportionate to the risk," as Hood, Rothstein, and Baldwin (2001) argue that a market failure response ought to be. Operationalizing a precautionary approach in a bureaucratic context reinforces a heavy-handed response that emphasizes standardization and lacks nuance, an expensive legacy of the pandemic.

Advocates argue that precaution is an essential tool to limit severe damage from public-health, environmental, or other risks (Pinto-Bazurco 2020, 1). It is not meant to provide clarity, but rather to provide flexibility for organizations to make practical decisions under conditions of uncertainty (Pike, Khan, and Amyotte 2020, 159; Resnik 2004, 282); it is also meant to encourage foresight, rather than the reliance solely on reactive policies (Tickner, Kriebel, and Wright 2003, 489). The precautionary principle is designed to promote the values of protection and the prevention of harm, rather than deciding how much harm is acceptable (Schettler and Raffensperger 2004, 66).

By its nature, precaution is a costly approach to risk that often neglects trade-offs (Sunstein 2009). Firms and individuals will not adopt it unless it is in their interest to do so, which is unlikely for a low-probability event; that is why precaution sits in the government's market-failure tool kit. With high uncertainty regarding COVID-19, coupled with potentially catastrophic and irreversible consequences, government was not guided by being proportionate – a nebulous concept, particularly at the start – but by containing the spread of the virus in light of its perceived threat (Sunstein 2005a, 114).

Hood, Rothstein, and Baldwin (2001, 71) note that the MFH is "more useful as a method of analytical benchmarking than as a reliable predictor of regulatory content." However imperfect their response according to the MFH, governments were trying to meet the expectations of an anxious public who demand a significant response from government during crises, a point we explore in chapter 10.

Opinion-Responsive Hypothesis:
Media and Public Opinion Polls

With Hala Nader

The opinion-responsive hypothesis (ORH) considers the extent to which government regulatory policy is in response to public preferences and attitudes as reflected through news media and public opinion (Hood, Rothstein, and Baldwin 2001, 90). The risk-psychology and social-psychology literature are particularly helpful in interrogating this hypothesis.

This chapter has two sections. The first examines media coverage. The media played an indispensable role in communicating risks to the public and holding governments to account. Once the CDC started addressing the issue more seriously and openly in February and early March 2020, media provided extensive coverage; media consumer numbers surged, and non-COVID-19 stories that had received coverage prior to the pandemic were significantly reduced. After the first five months, coverage was significant but trended downwards and did not necessarily correspond to waves or mortality rates. At times, media emphasized conflict that was not representative of overall public opinion or behaviour. Generally, media coverage focused on health issues more than on economic ones by a ratio of three to one. It is difficult to discern whether media coverage had an impact on government response to the pandemic, or whether governments influenced media; it is an iterative and dynamic process. What can be said, however, is that the media's examination of COVID-19 was exhaustive, often anxious, and crucial in framing the story for the public and helping governments achieve various public policy objectives.

The intention of media analysis, according to Hood, Rothstein, and Baldwin (2001), is to understand the flavour of public debate; it is not a definitive account of public views. When referring to media in this chapter, we review traditional media. Generally, we refer to the *Toronto*

Star, *National Post*, and CBC News as our sources, which provide a range of political perspectives. We also compare the volume of coverage of COVID-19 to that of other major crises to appreciate more fully the extent of the COVID-19 coverage. With this in mind, we compared coverage of COVID-19 to that of 9/11 and the financial crisis (2007–09). In these cases, we examined coverage in the *New York Times* (NYT), which included extensive local, national, and international coverage of these other events. The sources of all graphs are indicated.

The second section examines polling data. There was variation in the attitudes of different demographic groups regarding the threat of COVID-19, government interventions, and the use of vaccines. Generally, people were aware of the threat, accepted restrictions, and felt they abided by them, even if at times they did not. Interventions may not have been popular, but governments' actions were never far from the majority view. Their interventions aligned with an apprehensive public; it is also true, however, that governments invoked deliberate and intense strategies to shape public opinion on the issue. While trust in public health officials and satisfaction with elected governments were generally high, they trended downwards throughout the pandemic. While the public was anxious about the pandemic, many also believed that media reporting could be selective and exaggerated when it came to COVID-19 and its consequences. Our polling data in this chapter came largely from national polling institutes, such as Leger. (For further discussion of our research method with respect to media analysis and polling data, see the "Methods" section in appendix 1.)

MEDIA ANALYSIS

Despite claims of the growing role of social media, which we will discuss, our analysis is anchored by traditional media. There are still many people who trust and refer to traditional news sources. Based on a global study, most people regardless of age ranked traditional media outlets (newspapers, television, and radio) and the social media accounts belonging to these outlets as their primary sources of information during COVID-19 (Hess et al. 2021).

The pandemic actually resulted in an increase in demand for traditional media. In Canada an April 2020 survey found that less than 10 per cent of respondents relied on social media as their main source of information; 51 per cent relied on local, national, and international news outlets, and 30 per cent relied on daily briefings from public health agencies and political leaders (Statistics Canada 2020c). In fact, the pandemic resulted in increased ratings for news programs and increased online news traffic as all major daily television news programs nearly doubled their year-to-date average minute audience; online traffic increased by 19 per cent in Canada at the beginning of the pandemic (Briggs 2020; Brioux 2020).

Volume of Media Coverage of COVID-19

Normally, high-impact, low-frequency events generate high-volume media coverage for a short time, spiking soon after the event occurs and decreasing over time. Different types of events generate different volumes and patterns of coverage; the coverage also has a different tone, depending on the type of event, and describes governments' performances differently. Notwithstanding recent climate-change debates, natural disasters, for example, are generally described as "acts of God" and are seen as no one's fault. This blamelessness makes it difficult to hold people to account for planning decisions made years earlier that make communities vulnerable to certain natural disasters. For industrial failures, like bridge collapses and train derailments, there is usually a narrow and somewhat ruthless hunt for accountability (Quigley, Bisset, and Mills 2017).

Pandemics have their own patterns; like the disease itself, media coverage starts slowly, increases, and stays in the media for a longer time than other crises. Such was the case with COVID-19 but on a much larger scale than any other pandemic. COVID-19 overshadowed all other events in 2020 in what is being called a "media eclipse," defined as the concentration of coverage on a single story that typically occupies over 20 per cent of media space, significantly reducing the amount left to cover other issues (Lalancette and Lamy 2020). Prior to the COVID-19 pandemic, the last global media eclipse was 9/11.

To place the media coverage of the pandemic in perspective, we compared the number of articles published in the front sections of the NYT in the first six months of the pandemic to those published in the first six months following 9/11 and during the peak of the financial crisis (2007–09) and its aftermath. The comparison can be somewhat misleading; the growth in digital media since 2001 and 2007–09 has lowered the cost of media. Still, the difference in media coverage of the three events is considerable.

The data show that the coverage of COVID-19 dwarfed that of both 9/11 and the financial crisis (figure 10.1). In the first six months of the pandemic, COVID-19 received twice the coverage that terrorism did in the six months after 9/11, and four times the coverage that the

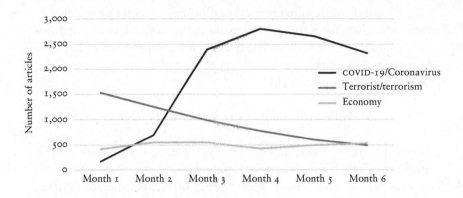

Figure 10.1 | The first six months of media coverage.
The NYT's coverage of COVID-19 was greater than that of 9/11 and at the
peak of the financial crisis (2007–09). *Sources: New York Times*, September
2001–February 2002, September 2008–February 2009, January–June 2020.

economy received during the peak of the financial crisis (2007–09)
and its aftermath. Not only did the pandemic receive a high volume of
media attention, but also the coverage grew in the first four months and
continued to have a high profile for several months afterwards.

In Canada, much like in the US, coverage of the virus increased as
it began to spread, but the news story remained a low-yield one until
the end of February, beginning of March 2020, when governments
began speaking more frequently and publicly about it. The second
week of March saw a rapid increase in references to the coronavirus
as the federal, provincial, and territorial governments began declaring
states of emergency and introducing restrictions to limit the spread of
the virus as cases were increasing throughout the country (Dawson
2020). Although the media's focus on the virus persisted, coverage of
the pandemic started a downward trend after the first four months; in
April 2021, 50 per cent fewer articles were published about the virus
compared to April 2020. By April 2022, coverage had decreased by
50 per cent compared to April 2021. When looking at the correlation
between the number of deaths in Canada and the amount of coverage
COVID-19 received (figure 10.2), we see that after an overwhelming
amount of coverage for the first five months of the pandemic, the number of published articles steadily decreased between May 2020 and
June 2022, increasing slightly when the number of deaths was high in
January 2021.

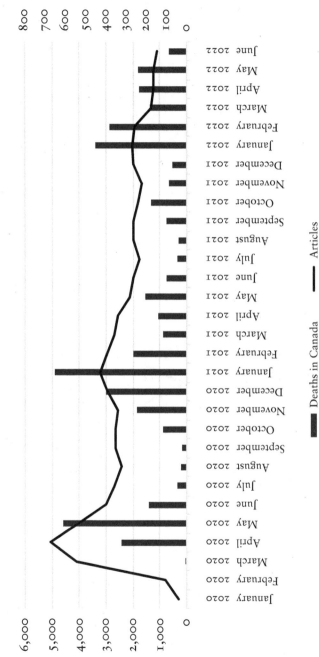

Figure 10.2 | COVID-19 deaths in Canada versus articles published, 2020–22. Initial coverage was massive but steadily decreased over time, irrespective of the death count.

Number of articles

Number of deaths

——— Deaths in Canada   ——— Articles

Sources: Government of Canada 2022i; CBC News 2020–22.

Figure 10.3 | Health and economic coverage compared, 2020–22. Articles highlighting health outnumbered those on the economy by a ratio of 3:1.

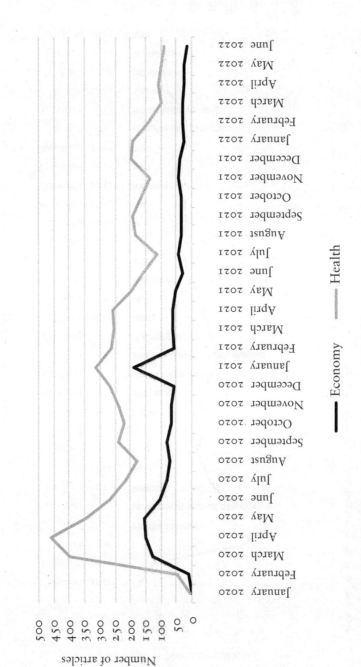

Sources: CBC News, January 2020–June 2022.

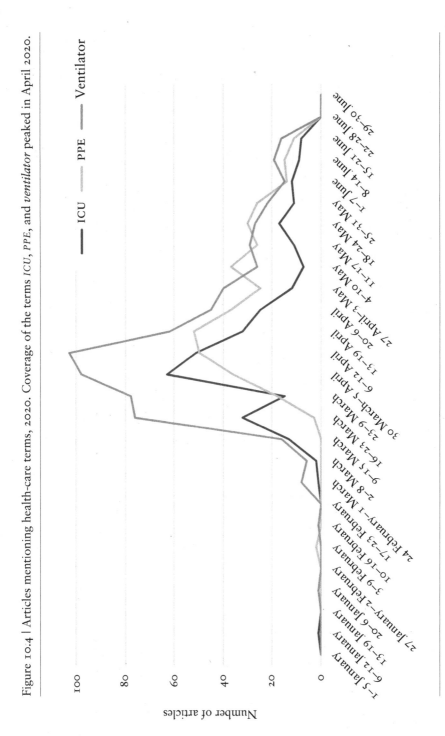

Figure 10.4 | Articles mentioning health-care terms, 2020. Coverage of the terms *ICU*, *PPE*, and *ventilator* peaked in April 2020.

Sources: Toronto Star, National Post, and CBC News, January–June 2020.

Health Coverage throughout the Pandemic

Between January 2020 and June 2022, media coverage referred to health three times more often than it did to the economy (figure 10.3). This pattern was generally consistent throughout the time frame, except for Christmas 2020, a key economic period for retail.

The media primarily focused on two types of health issues: the health-care system's ability to manage the pandemic, and how to avoid contracting the virus. Reporting on hospital capacity and the system's capability to deal with the crisis (measured by tracking references to ICU, PPE, and *ventilator*) began in March 2020 and peaked in the second week of April (figure 10.4).

At the same time, media references to interventions that limit the spread of COVID-19, such as *masks* and *social distancing* (figure 10.5), began and outnumbered those that referenced ICU, PPE, and *ventilator*. The WHO Emergency Committee began promoting these measures at the end of January 2020 (WHO 2021e); the Government of Canada started publicly discussing social-distancing measures (among others) at the end of February, and provincial and territorial governments implemented them in March (Staples 2020b). Despite the federal, provincial, and territorial governments recommending (and later mandating) the wearing of masks in public on 20 May 2020, media references to masks peaked in the first week of April, prior to that announcement (K. Harris 2020b; Shukman 2020). Mentions of the term changed as the pandemic evolved, particularly as anti-mask protests became more pronounced across Canada (Bogart 2020; Browne 2021).

References to COVID-19 vaccination grew throughout the first year of the pandemic, peaking in April 2021 (figure 10.6). At its media-coverage peak, the 841 articles mentioning *vaccine* outnumbered the peaks of the other related terms, including ICU, PPE, *ventilator*, *mask*, and *social distancing*.

A Change in the National Discourse

The emergence of COVID-19 changed Canada's national policy discourse. To examine the extent to which the media's focus was affected by COVID-19, we looked at the issues being covered during the last six months of 2019 – which included the 2019 Canadian federal election held in October and ostensibly discussions about national priorities – and how that coverage changed during the first six months of 2020.

Figure 10.5 | Number of articles mentioning the terms *mask* and *social distancing*, 2020. Media coverage of terms peaked in early April and late March, respectively.

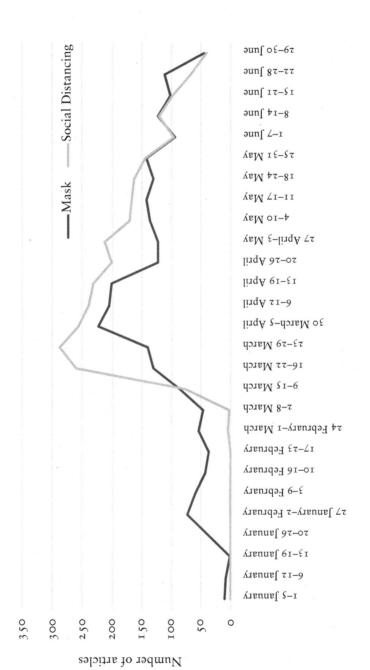

Sources: Toronto Star, National Post, and CBC News, January–June 2020.

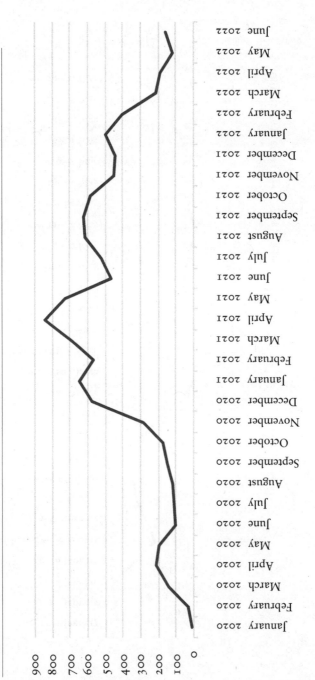

Figure 10.6 | Number of articles mentioning *vaccine*, 2020–22. Media coverage of vaccines peaked in April 2021.

Sources: Toronto Star, National Post, and CBC News, January 2020–June 2022.

Table 10.1 | Number of articles mentioning health and economic terms, 2019 versus 2020

Key terms	July–December 2019	January–June 2020	Change (%)	Peak month, 2019	Peak month, 2020
		Selected Health Terms			
Healthcare	1,169	2,941	152	September (251)	April (912)
LTC	227	1,398	516	December (44)	April (510)
Mental health	1,540	1,557	1	August (265)	May (381)
		Selected Economic Terms			
Small business	233	598	157	September (54)	March (181)
Stock market	67	232	246	August (24)	March (115)
Unemployment	210	511	143	October (48)	April (121)

LTC coverage was up by 516 per cent in 2020. *Sources: Toronto Star, National Post*, and CBC News, July 2019–June 2020.

The onset of COVID-19 led to increased coverage of several health issues (table 10.1). Discussions regarding health care and LTC experienced the most growth; articles focusing on health care increased by 150 per cent in 2020, peaking in April.[1] Eighty-five per cent of Canadians with a senior relative living in an LTC facility were concerned about their well-being because of the reported conditions in these facilities (Leger and Association for Canadian Studies [ACS] 2020b). A study released by the Canadian Institute for Health Information (CIHI) revealed that as of 25 May 2020, LTC residents accounted for over 80 per cent of COVID-19 deaths in Canada, the highest among all countries studied (CIHI 2020d; Szklarski 2020). LTC outbreaks contributed to an 8 per cent COVID-19 fatality rate in May, several percentage points higher than predicted. While mainly a provincial and territorial responsibility, health care is frequently debated during federal elections. LTC received little attention during the 2019 election, but the number of articles mentioning it increased by over 500 per cent in the first six months of 2020. Although mentions of the terms *healthcare* and *long-term care* or LTC largely stabilized throughout 2021, there was a small increase in mentions leading up to the September 2021 federal election. (For further discussion on LTC and COVID-19 see chapter 7.)

The media focus on mental health increased slightly as discussions about anxiety and stress surfaced after governments began imposing lockdowns and social-distancing rules (Hiremath et al. 2020, 1); between April and August 2020, 55 to 65 per cent of Canadians indicated that their mental health was suffering because of the COVID-19 crisis (Leger and ACS 2020d). The pandemic led to the lowest levels of life satisfaction in Canada since the federal government began measuring it in 2003 (Statistics Canada 2020g).

The economic discourse also changed between the last half of 2019 and the first half of 2020. The focus on unemployment and economic vulnerability increased in mid-March and began decreasing when the federal government introduced the CERB and CESB. Affordability and cost of living were salient topics in the run-up to the federal election; however, their coverage decreased considerably in 2020 as COVID-19 issues emerged or were reframed in the context of a crisis. Media references to oil remained relatively stable between July 2019 and July 2020.

Coverage of the Freedom Convoy was also a notable change in Canadian media. The coverage surged between January and March 2022, with nearly 600 articles published across the *Toronto Star*, *National Post*, and CBC News. References to the convoy peaked in February 2022 but dropped quickly following the federal government's enactment of the Emergencies Act. (For further discussion on the Freedom Convoy see chapter 6.)

What Dropped Off the Radar?

With the media's focus on the pandemic, coverage of some issues that were especially important in the latter part of 2019 fell away. Climate change, taxes, immigration, and pharmacare were all important topics in the 2019 federal election (Bricker 2019; Turner 2019). In a survey conducted by Ipsos leading up to the election, health care (35 per cent), affordability and the cost of living (27 per cent), and climate change (25 per cent) were the top issues on voters' minds, followed by the economy (24 per cent) and taxes (22 per cent) (Bricker 2019). In 2020, except for health care, media coverage of these topics dropped by over

Table 10.2 | Number of articles containing the terms *climate change,*
immigration, pharmacare, tax, and *debt,* 2019 versus 2020

Key terms	June–December 2019	January–June 2020	Change (%)	Peak month, 2019	Peak month, 2020
Climate change	1,774	817	–54	October (503)	February (239)
Immigration	1,029	501	–51	October (269)	June (103)
Pharmacare	331	50	–85	October (120)	January (17)
Tax	2,411	1,442	–40	October (638)	March (446)
Debt	966	908	–6	October (231)	May (248)

Media coverage of terms decreased in the first six months of 2020.
Sources: Toronto Star, National Post, and CBC News, July 2019–June 2020.

40 per cent. There was decidedly less concern about taxes and more
concern about unemployment. Climate change received a bump during
the Wet'suwet'en protests in early 2020 but dropped again at the start
of the pandemic (table 10.2).

Vulnerable Populations

Homelessness and food banks were receiving increased coverage by
April and May 2020. The media's focus on homelessness increased by 70
per cent in 2020, peaking in April as the news outlets covered the effects
of COVID-19 on people experiencing uncertain and unstable shelter;
the same was observed for media coverage of food banks. These discussions coincided with the media reporting on increased unemployment
in Canada due to the pandemic. By mid-April the use of food banks
had increased by 20 per cent throughout the country, with Food Banks
Canada's chief executive officer, Chris Hatch, expecting the increase to
reach 40 per cent (or a total of 1.1 million visits a month) as the virus
spread (Britneff 2020a). Though significant, these increases remain low

Table 10.3 | Number of articles relating to vulnerable populations,
2019 versus 2020

Key terms	June–December 2019	January–June 2020	Change (%)	Peak month, 2019	Peak month, 2020
Disability	348	334	−4	September (77)	April (85)
Special needs	113	120	6	September (27)	January and June (25)
LGBTQ	491	311	−37	October (105)	February (69)
Gig economy	39	51	31	August (10)	March (17)
Food bank	73	178	144	September (19)	April (64)
Universal basic income	10	43	330	August and September (3)	May (17)
Homeless	198	331	67	August (39)	April (105)
Affordable housing	309	160	−48	October (104)	February (42)

Media coverage of terms related to vulnerable populations varied considerably in 2020. *Sources: Toronto Star, National Post,* and CBC News, July 2019–June 2020.

compared to that seen for the other issues noted. Despite an increase in articles referencing homelessness, those discussing affordable housing, somewhat ironically, decreased by almost half in 2020 after peaking in October 2019 when it was an important part of various party platforms (Watters 2019).

Overall, there was some increased concern for vulnerable populations (table 10.3). As the COVID-19 story progressed, media references to disability and special needs remained unchanged between 2019 and 2020; references to LGBTQ dropped.[2] Media focus on universal basic income and the gig economy, which have a disproportionate effect on low-income populations, received some increased attention but remained relatively low.[3]

Despite the disproportionate impact of the pandemic on racialized minorities, references to topics such as racism were inconsistent and generally low at the start of the pandemic. There was consistent referencing of the terms *Indigenous* and *racism* in the media in 2019, with a small spike in the run-up to the 2019 federal election when coverage of the United Nations Declaration on the Rights of Indigenous Peoples, the Indian Act, the economic development of Indigenous communities, and the Justin Trudeau blackface incidents resurfaced. Another spike in articles occurred in February due to reporting on the Wet'suwet'en blockades and protests. When COVID-19 became the dominant story, these references disappeared and only re-emerged in June 2020 in response to the killing of George Floyd, which sparked protests against police brutality and racism throughout North America and Europe (Dunn 2020).

Social Media and Information Hygiene

In the age of COVID-19, the spread of false information is termed *an infodemic* – a global spread of misinformation that causes problems for public health because it affects transmission patterns and, consequently, the scale and lethality of a pandemic by influencing behaviour (Bridgman et al. 2020, 2; Cinelli et al. 2020, 1). Although misinformation can spread through any medium, the role that social media plays in the sharing of misleading information is concerning. Increasingly, social media is an important and primary source of news (Bridgman et al. 2020, 2; Hussain 2020, 59). Platforms such as Facebook and Twitter (now X) have been shown to have high levels of misinformation compared to other media sources even though misinformation makes up a low percentage of overall discussion on social media (Fung et al. 2016, 471; Del Vicario et al. 2016, 558). Around 60 per cent of people surveyed were aware of COVID-19–related misinformation, and 35 per cent claimed to ignore the false information they came across. They did not, however, counter the false information, which arguably contributes to its spread (Hess et al. 2021). Importantly, it was found that the longer one spends on social media, the more likely one is to encounter misinformation, and the more likely one's attitudes towards certain topics will change as cumulative exposure to misinformation (familiarity) leads to a reinforcement of certain beliefs. In fact, it was found that being exposed to traditional news media was associated with higher compliance with social-distancing measures, whereas social media exposure was associated with more misperceptions and less adherence to social distancing (Bridgman et al. 2020, 5–6).

Edelman (2021) identifies good information hygiene as a mitigation strategy to the spread of misinformation, which includes engaging with news, verifying information before sharing it, and "avoiding information echo chambers" (53). Poor information hygiene was linked to vaccine hesitancy: 73 per cent of individuals with good information hygiene were willing to get vaccinated within a year; that number dropped to 59 per cent for those with poor information hygiene.

The role of media in conveying misleading information is more complex than simply focusing on non-traditional social-media channels. Mainstream media also regularly featured compelling personal testimonies from ICU doctors and nurses as well as caregivers who at times were subjected to traumatic events during COVID-19. In the early stages of the pandemic the coverage arguably met the moment: people were dying, and the ICUs were close to capacity. As the third wave started, however, many people had been vaccinated; unvaccinated younger people were more likely to be in hospital or in an ICU, but the death rate had dropped considerably. As young people filmed themselves with hand-held devices describing their illness and fear of dying, given what had come before, one might suggest the media engaged with what risk psychologists call probability neglect or identifiable victim effect (Sunstein 2002b, 63; Jenni and Loewenstein 1997, 236), which focuses on the victim and consequence but downplays the probability of these events. By the third wave, these types of personal testimonies were common in the mainstream media but were not always accompanied by appropriate probability data.

Finally, given the insatiable demand for COVID-19 stories and the nearly endless number of angles one could adopt to frame a story, the mainstream media frequently looked to experts, often academics, as quick and reliable sources for stories. In such circumstances, however, expert opinions were not subject to the normal peer-review process required before publishing in an academic journal; at times, expert opinions were speculative, underpinned by epistemological and ideological biases, and would ultimately prove to be inaccurate (Weber 2020; Chirico, Teixeira da Silva, and Magnavita 2020; Sridhar 2022; A. Miller 2021a). Relatedly, experts had to communicate their message in simple and clear terms, which is not always easy in considering a complex, uncertain or ambiguous risk, and especially for those not expert in risk communication. When the chair of NACI, Dr Caroline

Quach-Thanh, noted that she would not necessarily advise a loved one to get the PHAC-approved AstraZeneca vaccine due to increased risk of blood clots, she left risk-communications experts "cringing" (Kirkey 2021, para. 1). Thereafter, as noted in chapter 6, NACI's public-facing role was significantly curtailed.

POLLING DATA

It is difficult to know whether media coverage of the pandemic reflected the views of civil society. Just as there are important limitations to media coverage, there are important limitations to polling data. The quality of polling data has deteriorated; online media make it very easy to conduct snap polls on different issues, but they are rarely reliable or insightful (Quigley, Bisset, and Mills 2017, 165). Moreover, different polls report different results, indicating that opinion is diverse and unstable and depends on the sample and time the poll was completed. Risk issues present specific challenges. Risk psychologists, for example, note that people will state different preferences if the same situation is expressed in different ways; this is called the framing effect, defined as a cognitive bias that results in people being less likely to accept risks if they are framed as losses rather than gains (Hameleers 2020; Tversky and Kahneman 1981, 456). Issue salience can also influence public perceptions (Halpin, Fraussen, and Nownes 2017, 220).

Notwithstanding these caveats, polling data can give us insight into people's concerns, priorities, and opinions at particular moments in time throughout the pandemic. Almost a year into the pandemic, fear of the virus throughout the Canadian population had been quite steady since March 2020, with 60 per cent of people indicating they were afraid of catching COVID-19 (Leger, the Canadian Press, and ACS 2021a). By 2022 this fear was trending downward, with 44 per cent of Canadians indicating that they were worried about contracting the virus (Leger, the Canadian press, and ACS 2022a). Generally, people may not have liked the restrictive health measures, but they accepted and supported them. At the beginning of the pandemic the majority indicated they were in favour of government restrictions that limited public gatherings and interactions; around 70 per cent supported closing non-essential businesses (Dunham 2020). A survey in January 2021 reported that 79 per cent supported gathering limits for weddings and funerals, 78 per cent supported closing restaurants, 66 per cent supported closing all retail outlets except pharmacies and grocery stores, and 89 per cent believed that the federal government should ban all international travel until COVID-19 was controlled (Maru Blue 2021, 1–2). Two years after the start of the pandemic 58 per cent of Canadians were against the lifting of restrictions by federal, provincial, and territorial governments (Leger, the Canadian Press, and ACS 2022b).

In a May 2020 poll over 95 per cent of people indicated that they socially distanced, and 42 per cent said they were wearing masks (E. Chung 2020; Leger and ACS 2020e). When asked about their 2021 spring-break plans, 90 per cent indicated their intention not to travel (Leger, the Canadian Press, and ACS 2021b). These numbers indicate there was a high level of awareness of public health recommendations. Whether they were respected is a different matter; 39 per cent admitted they did not follow all guidelines, and a report published by Ipsos in January 2021 indicated that 48 per cent admitted gathering outside their household during the holidays despite public health officials across the country urging people not to do so (Connolly 2021; Leger, the Canadian Press, and ACS 2021a). Perhaps as an indication of optimism bias (Sharot 2011, 41), those who did not follow all guidelines believed that their actions did not have an impact on the spread of the virus despite the uptick in cases following the holidays.

Writing about the general population has limitations; it obscures the difference in risk tolerance by subgroups. Risk-psychology literature brings to our attention that different groups perceive and act on risk differently (Olofsson et al. 2014, 420); perceptions of COVID-19 are no exception (table 10.4). For example, in a Canadian poll conducted in January 2021, 82 per cent of women supported closing restaurants, cafés, bars, and pubs, compared to 74 per cent of men; 94 per cent of individuals aged fifty-five and above supported banning international flights, compared to 85 per cent of those aged eighteen to thirty-four; and 70 per cent of those with an income of less than $50,000 supported closing all stores (except pharmacies and grocery stores), compared to 59 per cent of those making over $100,000.

These numbers also differed depending on the state of the virus in each province or territory, with residents of Ontario and Quebec more likely to support restrictions than were the residents of other provinces. Generally, older people, women, lower-income individuals, and university graduates were more likely to support restrictions.

Despite the extensive media coverage of the Freedom Convoy in early 2022, most Canadians supported government directives, although there is some ambiguity. A February poll indicated that 64 per cent of

Table 10.4 | Percentage of respondents in support of various public health measures, disaggregated by age, sex, income, and education, 2021

	In support of gathering limits for weddings and funerals (%)	In support of closing restaurants, cafés, bars, and pubs (%)	In support of closing retail stores except pharmacies and grocery stores (%)	In support of banning international flights (%)
18–34 years old	79	78	68	85
35–54 years old	75	75	61	87
55+ years old	82	82	70	94
Women	79	82	70	91
Men	79	74	62	87
Income <$50,000	81	80	70	88
Income <$50,000–$99,000	77	78	66	89
Income >$100,000	79	74	59	88
≤ High school	78	77	64	90
Post-secondary	77	77	67	88
University grad	82	81	69	89
Average	79	78	66	89

On average, older and more highly educated individuals and women were more likely to support public health measures. *Source:* Maru Blue 2021.

Canadians opposed the demand to end all pandemic restrictions, and 70 per cent opposed the protesters' approach and behaviour (Angus Reid Institute 2022). There were, however, important nuances. Another poll indicated that 46 per cent of Canadians believed the protesters' frustration was legitimate and worthy of some sympathy (*Economist* 2022). After nearly two years of restrictions, many were getting fed up.

Trust

Trust in medical science, and CMOs in particular, was an important ingredient in the early stages of the pandemic. It was a deliberate strategy by almost all governments to have the premier or prime minister sit alongside CMOs to convey health messages to the public. In fact, elected officials often deferred to advice from CMOs and emphasized that government policies would be determined by health sciences. Doctors generally, and CMOs in this case, are highly trusted in ways that politicians are not; doctors typically fulfill the three dimensions that people tend to look for to develop trust: honesty, expertise, and concern (Peters, Covello, and McCallum 1997, 43). This led to the characterization that government policy followed the science. Again, the reality was more nuanced. Different approaches to dealing with the pandemic were being put forward by scientists all over the world, based on models that were in turn based on assumptions and interpretations of data and varied from expert to expert; these models needed to be tested to be assessed (Stevens 2020). Moreover, the science being followed was largely limited to the health sciences; other important disciplines that could have been considered more seriously when making scientific policy decisions, such as economics, sociology, and the behavioural sciences, were arguably less influential in the framing of the challenges (Mercuri 2020, 1576).

This public perception of governments following the science had several implications. First, it obscured the uncertainty and ambiguity, whether the scientists intended it or not. Scientists armed with graphs convey a powerful message in the media that papers over complexity (C. Jaeger et al. 2001; Jasanoff 1990). Second, it seemed to shift accountability to the scientific community and to (unelected) CMOs because provincial and territorial governments appeared to be following their advice, when in fact elected officials were always in charge and there was always a political calculation in decisions; there is a history of politicians using scientists for cover when necessary (C. Jaeger et al. 2001; Mercuri 2020), and we saw it here. Finally, it suggested that policy changes were the result of new evidence. In the UK the virus was downgraded from being labelled a "high consequence infectious disease" – not because of new scientific discoveries but because the country was running low on PPE, and downgrading the virus allowed ministers to avoid providing high-grade PPE (Mercuri 2020, 1575). In short, science, policy, politics, and management were always interacting in a highly fluid manner. Media coverage was not always effective at conveying the balance and trade-offs between them.

Table 10.5 | Percentage of Canadians dissatisfied with provincial COVID-19 measures, 2020 versus 2021

	Atlantic	QC	ON	MB	SK	AB	BC	*Average*
Respondents dissatisfied with COVID-19 measures (%) (13 April 2020)	8	5	14	24	19	22	14	*15*
Respondents dissatisfied with COVID-19 measures (%) (12 April 2021)	22	28	59	49	48	68	41	*45*

The Prairie provinces were among the most dissatisfied with provincial COVID-19 measures. *Sources*: Leger and ACS 2020a; Leger, the Canadian Press, and ACS 2021a.

Although trust in experts remained high a year into the pandemic, it then began to decrease; compared to the survey conducted at the start of the crisis, trust in scientists went down by 7 per cent (to 73 per cent) and trust in academics dropped by 8 per cent (to 57 per cent) in 2021 (Edelman 2021, 22). Fifty-nine per cent of people believed that journalists were misleading the public by reporting things they knew were exaggerations; 61 per cent believed that the media were not being objective or non-partisan in their reporting (Edelman 2021, 25). Trust in all orders of government – federal, provincial, territorial, and municipal – and satisfaction with the measures put in place to contain COVID-19 also decreased, by over 15 per cent in April 2021 when compared to the beginning of the pandemic (Leger, the Canadian Press, and ACS 2021a). This dissatisfaction became worse as the third-wave variants spiked in spring 2021 (table 10.5), which accompanied an increase in negative perceptions of provincial governments' overall COVID-19 response from 11 per cent in 2020 to 34 per cent in 2021 (Pew Research Center 2021, 6).

Polling was somewhat volatile. After governments experienced popular support for most of 2020, their popularity trended downwards, particularly as the third-wave variants emerged.

Many provinces and territories held elections during the first two years of the pandemic, and in the early and middle stages all the sitting governments were re-elected. New Brunswick, British Columbia, Saskatchewan, Newfoundland and Labrador, and Yukon all held elections between September 2020 and April 2021, and, in each case, citizens chose to keep their existing leadership. The Nova Scotia 2021 election was a turning point. Despite having a thirty-point lead in the polls in May 2021, driven largely by what was seen as a very successful response to the pandemic, the Liberals fell to the Progressive Conservatives in the August 2021 election. The election underscored a change: that a good job on the pandemic no longer guaranteed re-election; after sixteen months of hard times economically, socially, and in health care, people wanted change. Also, the central issue was no longer the pandemic but rather life after the pandemic. The federal election in October 2021 also failed to reward the incumbent Liberals; while the government did not fall, the election barely changed the seat count of the parties.

COVID-19 Vaccinations

By spring 2021, COVID-19 vaccination had begun to dominate media coverage in Canada; polling data on vaccination hesitancy had grown. Attitudes towards the vaccine also changed.

Among those with high school education or less, people who identified politically as right of centre, people aged thirty to forty-four, and residents of Alberta showed greater than average vaccine hesitancy (B. Anderson 2021). The populations most likely to be vaccinated or willing to be vaccinated as soon as possible had university education, identified as left of centre, were over the age of sixty, and lived in British Columbia (table 10.6).

Women are a key target group for public health messages. A February 2021 survey revealed that Canadian women reported higher rates of vaccine hesitancy (29 per cent) than men did (20 per cent). Women assume many health-care responsibilities, including on behalf of children, partners, and elderly relatives, and have influence over their family's health-care decisions, including the decision to be vaccinated. Ultimately, women were more likely to be vaccinated than men. As of 20 March 2022, 82 per cent of women and 80 per cent of men were fully vaccinated (Government of Canada 2022k).

Ethnic or racial identity was somewhat of a factor in determining support for vaccinations in Canada. For some, not getting vaccinated seemed like a rational decision; the risk was low, particularly for young

Table 10.6 | COVID-19 vaccine hesitancy in Canada, 2020–21

	Were vaccinated/ would get vaccinated as soon as possible (%)	Would rather wait and prefer not to get vaccinated (%)	Would never take the vaccine (%)
Province			
BC	68	24	8
Atlantic Canada	65	22	9
The Prairies	65	27	8
ON	65	29	6
QC	65	23	12
Canada	64	28	8
AB	56	36	8
Political ideology			
Left	76	20	4
Centre	60	32	8
Right	61	24	15
Age			
18–29	60	30	10
30–44	52	38	10
45–59	62	30	8
60+	72	23	5
Education level			
High school or less	57	32	11
College	66	26	8
University	72	23	5
Month			
November 2020	33	56	11
24 March 2021	62	29	9
14 April 2021	64	28	8

Vaccine hesitancy decreased with age, education level, and time.

Source: B. Anderson 2021.

Table 10.7 | Percentage of those willing to receive the COVID-19 vaccine, 2021

Population group	Very or somewhat willing to receive the COVID-19 vaccine (%)
Canada (excluding the territories)	76.9
Visible minority populations	74.8
South Asian	82.5
Chinese	79.4
Black	56.4
Filipino	75.0
Latin American	65.6
Arab	68.0
Southeast Asian	78.2
West Asian	78.9
Korean	85.4
Japanese	86.7
Additional visible minorities	79.0
Non-visible minority	77.7
Canadian-born	77.8
Immigrant (non-permanent resident)	74.6
First Nations, Inuit, and Métis peoples	71.9
First Nations people (living off reserve)	74.4
Métis	67.8
Inuit	73.2
Non-Indigenous people	77.1

Canadians' willingness to receive the vaccine varied by population group.
Source: Statistics Canada 2021c.

people. As the vaccine rollout continued, many of the vaccine-resistant were White men earning moderate to high incomes (Ibbitson 2021). This type of argument – that the pandemic carried low risk for some – was given little attention in the mainstream media as coverage amplified the most tragic stories.

Generally, Canadians of South or Southeast Asian, Chinese, Filipino, Japanese, and Korean descent, for example, were supportive of COVID-19 vaccinations. Seventy-five per cent of immigrants were willing to receive a COVID-19 vaccine, compared to 78 per cent of the Canadian-born population. Participation rates among immigrants varied; immigrants from South or Southeast Asia, for example, had particularly high participation rates. Vaccine hesitancy was higher among Black Canadians, followed by Latin American, Arab, and Indigenous peoples, especially Métis respondents, compared to the general population (table 10.7). Some of the reasons cited for not getting vaccinated related to access issues, such as reliable transportation and child care, especially for Black Canadians (Parkin et al. 2021; Government of Canada 2021a; A. Miller 2021a).

It is a powerful irony that people who were most vulnerable to contracting COVID-19 and at times paid the highest price throughout the pandemic, in health and wealth, were often the least likely to get the vaccine. This is particularly so for Black and Indigenous groups. That they would act against their personal interests by failing to get vaccinated reinforces the notion that the system does not connect with them or their lived experience well. Medical racism and experimentation perpetrated on Black and Indigenous people in Canada and the US arguably contributed to distrust of the system by many in these communities.

Overcoming the racial gap in vaccine uptake took deliberate effort (Burch and Schoenfeld Walker 2021; Wiafe and Smith 2021; Nuriddin, Mooney, and White 2020, 950; CPHA 2018, 3). Indeed, after targeted efforts, vaccine support among many First Nations, Inuit, and Métis people increased (Parkin et al. 2021).

COVID-19 Response and the Way Forward

Even though media coverage of health concerns outweighed that of economic concerns, public opinion suggested that people were concerned about both. In March 2020, 92 per cent of Canadians saw the COVID-19 outbreak as a major threat to the economy of the country, and 77 per cent saw it as a threat to the health of the population (Leger and ACS 2020a). With a nearly infinite debt capacity (Barrett 2018), the response of the federal government was to avoid more controversial and immediate trade-offs by increasing borrowing, and thereby transferring the consequences of policy decisions to future periods. In July 2020 the federal government announced that the deficit for that year would exceed $343 billion, the largest deficit ever recorded by a Canadian government (Aiello 2020).

Table 10.8 | Percentage of Canadians in support of policies to reduce deficit,
July 2020

	In support of raising taxes (%)	In support of reducing government spending (%)	In support of immediately reducing pandemic support program (%)
18–34 years old	26	57	37
35–54 years old	19	60	40
55+ years old	17	63	45
Average	21	60	41

Canadians under thirty-five were most likely to support raising taxes and least
likely to support reducing pandemic supports. *Source:* Leger and ACS 2020e.

Despite the concern, Canadians were divided about the best way forward (table 10.8). In July 2020, 78 per cent were worried about the
increased deficit. To reduce it, 21 per cent were in favour of raising
taxes, and 60 per cent favoured reducing government-program spending. Canadians were divided on whether the federal government should
immediately scale back COVID-19 pandemic support programs and
payments, with 41 per cent in favour (Leger and ACS 2020f). While the
difference between age groups was not pronounced, the survey showed
that the older the respondents, the more likely they were opposed to
raising taxes and in favour of reducing government spending.

At times, people seemed as concerned about climate change as about
the pandemic, though their commitment was somewhat tepid. In July
2020, 64 per cent of Canadians thought that in the long term, climate
change would be as serious an issue as COVID-19, and 60 per cent
believed the federal government's economic recovery plan from COVID-
19 should prioritize this issue, noting that if the government did not
act to combat climate change, it would be failing Canadians (McLeod
Macey 2020). These views may have been propped up partly due to
the upcoming UN COP26 conference on climate change and the fact
that during the summer the pandemic case count was low. Nevertheless,
the same poll that showed an increased commitment by Canadians to

combatting climate change also indicated that despite wanting the government to act on the issue, only 38 per cent were willing to change their own habits to do so (McLeod Macey 2020); only 68 per cent supported the federal government's goal to achieve net-zero carbon emissions by 2050, and 53 per cent supported the prospect of paying more for gasoline, diesel, and heating fuel as part of the plan to achieve net-zero (Leger, the Canadian Press, and ACS 2021d).

Despite the disproportionate impact of the pandemic on racialized minorities, polling data on racism published in July 2020 suggested that not everyone felt that governments should do more to combat it. In 2020, 60 per cent of Canadians saw racism as a problem in the country, but only 50 per cent felt that governments should do more to fight racism. Like climate change, this suggests a disconnect between recognizing the existence of racism and supporting government action to end it (Bricker 2020).

With a COVID-19 lens, the effects of systemic racism and how it might be reflected in COVID-19–related health outcomes were at times overlooked by governments; immigrants and racialized communities were more likely to be front-line or essential service workers and therefore disproportionately at greater risk of being exposed to COVID-19 (Statistics Canada 2020i). In Ontario the province's science advisors recommended that vaccination should target hot spots such as areas with high-rise buildings, which were more likely to be inhabited by racialized workers. This recommendation was disregarded for months and was only implemented in mid-April 2021 by the chair of Ontario's COVID-19 vaccine-distribution task force, Dr Homer Tien, immediately after he replaced retired General Rick Hillier when his term had ended (Crawley 2021c).

CONCLUSION

Media coverage was indispensable for three reasons. First, the media communicated important health information to the public. Second, the media highlighted the struggles of vulnerable communities affected by the pandemic when non-governmental organizations (NGOs) that typically addressed such issues were struggling themselves. Almost half of charities and NGOs received no support from permanent donors during the pandemic (Charities Aid Foundation 2021). Finally, the media played an important role in supporting democratic accountability and acting as a check on government actions and spending when Parliament and legislatures were much less active.

Despite these important roles, there were limitations to the effectiveness of the media coverage. While one could say that governments did not act quickly enough to prevent the spread of the virus, the media did not prompt governments to act earlier than they did (McLaughlin 2020). Once coverage of the pandemic had begun in earnest, the media focused on the story often to the exclusion of other news. It reveals a cognitive bias in the way we process risk information. We are limited in our ability to compare risks; rather, we want to know what governments are doing to address specific risks that have our attention without reference to other risks and trade-offs implicit in their actions (Renn et al. 1992; Kasperson and Kasperson 1996; Rothstein 2003; Kasperson, Jhaveri, and Kasperson 2005; Fjaeran and Aven 2021).

Media exploited cognitive biases, as they often do. According to risk psychologists, people are typically more concerned about risks that are unknown and have high dread (Slovic, Fischhoff, and Lichtenstein 1982; for further discussion on unknown risks see chapter 2). A pandemic has many of these characteristics, which made it fertile ground for sustained and, at times, sensationalized coverage, focusing on conflict and emotion, excluding probability data, oversimplifying complex matters, and vilifying those who went against the grain.

Despite the frequent claims to "follow the science" that featured so prominently in the media, US research showed that coverage of the pandemic by American publications with a national audience tended to be more negative than the coverage by scientific journals, international publications, and regional media. In 2020, 87 per cent of COVID-19 coverage in US media was deemed negative, emphasizing bad news and amplifying conflict and disagreement over government policies, whether different voices represented a small minority or a sizeable amount of the population (Leonhardt 2021a). In Canada, media often reported on anti-masking and anti-vaccination protests and on individuals lamenting the restrictions imposed by governments. Although these individuals and groups existed, public opinion was not as polarized as depicted in the media throughout the pandemic, according to most polls.

Psychologists refer to identifiable victim effect or probability neglect when people focus on individuals and consequences and omit probability data. COVID-19 coverage was particularly susceptible to this problem because precise and reliable probability data was not always available. The media focused on individual stories without always situating the story with appropriate probability data and being specific about the threat. In hindsight we know that between March 2020 and May 2021, 52 per cent of those who died of COVID-19 were over eighty-five

(Statistics Canada 2021e). Approximately 89 per cent of those who died from COVID-19 in 2020 also had one or more co-morbidities, and 80 per cent lived in LTC (Statistics Canada 2021h; Government of Canada 2021g). Although the excess death rate increased by approximately 6 per cent in 2020, and each death represents loss and suffering, the additional data helps to clarify the threat. The media's amplification of the risk was at times overwhelming, such that it was as alarming as it was informing. Even among those with loved ones in LTC, over 78 per cent commented that they were satisfied with the service of the LTC facility (Angus Reid Institute 2021a), a fact that was virtually unobtainable if one depended solely on popular media for information. During the third wave the media ran stories about Canadian children becoming seriously ill even though youth made up only 2 per cent of hospitalizations (Pelley 2021). While it is true that stories about sick kids are newsworthy, they can also be sensationalist and exploitative (Ayre 2001; J. Kearney 2013; Quigley, Macdonald, and Quigley 2016). After over a year of COVID-19 stories and high death counts, at times it was difficult to distinguish between lower-probability and higher-probability cases, which is a fundamental and crucial characteristic of any risk problem.

The media also tended to vilify young people when they broke public health orders and gathering limits (Abraham and Plowman 2021). Despite being at low risk throughout the pandemic, young people paid a very heavy price for governments' responses. One study found that younger adults had to implement more behavioural changes than older individuals did to comply with COVID-19 restrictions (Klaiber et al. 2021, 30). Younger people also experienced more unemployment (Government of Canada 2021h) and mental health issues (Czeisler et al. 2020, 1053). Social outlets like schools, bars, and clubs were closed. People delayed getting married and having kids. Young parents had to home-school their young ones. Their political priorities, including environment, housing, social justice, and economy, were also sidelined to pandemic health issues. Despite the media coverage of after-hours' parties, young people were only marginally more likely to break the rules than older Canadians were (Canadian Hub for Applied and Social Research 2021).

The ORH provides important insights into government response: media coverage was extensive, the public was anxious, and government response was robust. In this sense, all three were generally aligned, but there were important nuances that challenge the hypothesis. The public was highly anxious, not just about the health risks but also about the economic consequences of government health directives, perhaps more so than the media coverage would suggest. Various demographic groups held different opinions about health directives and economic programs, a difference that governments could not always address and that underscores a vulnerability in government response. While some people would never be vaccinated, many had to be persuaded, which took time for governments to appreciate; targeted efforts to reach some groups made a difference (Parkin et al. 2021). Other non-COVID-19 issues, important to many, were sidelined.

In his book former federal minister of finance Bill Morneau commented on how focused the prime minister's office was on media coverage, and how often decisions were made by the office in light of how they would be received by the media and the public, and not according to any economic analysis as conducted by the Department of Finance (Morneau 2023). In many respects, governments sought to shape public opinion, not just follow it. By March 2020, government and media had engaged with the issue of COVID-19 in what became a highly interactive and iterative dynamic between the two. Government had an aggressive and high-profile communications plan, enacted daily and directed from its highest levels; it needed the public to accept the seriousness of the issue and follow largely voluntarily what would become highly disruptive public health directives. The extensive borrowing that governments did to pay for their containment strategies allowed them (to an extent) to defer some of the tough questions about who was paying for the strategy, but it did not avoid these questions or the related consequences altogether, as time would tell.

Interest Group Hypothesis: Bureau-Shapers and Organized Interests

With Noel Guscott

This chapter uses two lenses – internal interests and external ones – to examine interests at play throughout the pandemic and how these interests engaged with governments and influenced policy and operations. Scholars have examined a multitude of interests that have an influence on shaping care (J. Simpson 2012; Contandriopoulos 2011), such as the pharmaceutical industry (Lexchin 1993, 2016; Batt 2017), doctors (M. Taylor 1960; Contandriopoulos et al. 2018), nurses' unions (J. MacDonald et al. 2012; Chiu, Duncan, and Whyte 2020), and hospital associations (Fulton and Stanbury 1985).

Similarly, there are various theoretical concepts that can be used to examine interests at play during COVID-19, among them network governance (C. Jones, Hesterly, and Borgatti 1997; Daugbjerg and Fawcett 2017), focusing events (Kingdon 1984; Cobb and Elder 1983; Birkland 1998), agenda setting (B. Jones and Baumgartner 2005; Halpin and Fraussen 2019), policy windows (Kingdon 1984; Tarrow 1988; Austen-Smith and Wright 1994), and issue salience (Baumgartner and Jones 1993; Rasmussen, Carroll, and Lowery 2014; Halpin, Fraussen, and Nownes 2017).

As public administration scholars, we are interested in examining the role of public servants, particularly those in public health. Private interests are still at play in public service; questions about accountability, transparency, and incentives in public agencies are important to consider. This chapter will primarily use the bureau-shaping model (Dunleavy 1991) from the public choice literature as the organizing concept to examine the role of public servants in shaping health-agency policy and outcomes. Bureau-shaping assumes that public servants are rational utility maximizers who work within public agencies to satisfy self-interest and divest themselves of operational responsibility. They prefer working on policy in small elite groups, close to the political centre and sheltered from public scrutiny.

Bureau-shaping allows us to examine trends in public institutions in the last three decades, at times specifically within PHAC. Despite the theory's role in explaining the rapid separation of policy and operations in the UK in the 1980s and 1990s (referred to as "agencification"), this theory has rarely been used to understand public-sector reform and the creation of agencies in Canada, which occurred shortly after the UK reforms and ostensibly with similar intentions. Thus, we are adopting the theory to examine public health reforms and to test the extent to which the theory provides insights into why this agencification happened and whether it created problems for public health, specifically in the way it addressed COVID-19. Public health was lauded as a hero in Canada's response to COVID-19 (Porter 2020), and praise has largely overshadowed the short-comings in emergency management that were present despite several prior indications of poor performance and lack of preparation in this area.

The second half of this chapter examines the external interests during the early stages of COVID-19. It discusses how the ambiguity of the precautionary principle, a concept that was frequently used by policy leaders to frame government response early in the pandemic, opened the door to lobbying (Renn 2008b; J. Tait 2008). For the most part, those with access and resources received preferential treatment in the first year of the pandemic. Like Hood, Rothstein, and Baldwin (2001), we use the J.Q. Wilson (1980) typology of interest group configurations to examine the different regulatory dynamics at play and to show who benefited from, and who paid, for governments' interventions.

While Dunleavy's bureau-shaping model and Wilson's interest group typology are the central organizing concepts of the chapter, we also include references to other relevant concepts in interest group theory to enhance the analysis.

INTERNAL INTERESTS: PUBLIC CHOICE THEORY

Despite the necessary and important role of public institutions during the pandemic, and increased trust in them in spring 2020, that trust then declined steadily (Edelman 2021, 2022, 2023). There has been a rise in anti-government rhetoric and suspicion about public institutions in many Western countries, Canada included, and some advocates can be characterized as holding extreme right of centre views (Carr 2022; McLeod 2022).

Suspicions about the state and public service are not new. In the field of public administration this distrust can be traced to, for example, arguments by Jeremy Bentham in the 1820s about the importance of an appropriate incentive structure in public service. Bentham (1824) argued that private interests and public duty should be aligned to achieve effective public service (Schofield 1996).

Public choice literature of the 1970s, and public management reforms in the decades that followed, share a skepticism, if not distrust, of the public service and a general concern about the erosion of democracy (F. Kramer 1983; Knight and Johnson 1999; Ferlie 2010). However inconsistent some of these arguments may be (Aucoin 1990), there are valid questions about incentives, accountability, transparency, and performance to examine. Public choice theory allows us to do so effectively, albeit with some assumptions in place.

Public choice theory is broadly defined as the application of economics to political science (Buchanan and Tullock 1999; Mueller 1976, 395; Riker 1995, 24). The underlying assumptions of public choice are that individuals are rational utility maximizers (Orchard and Stretton 1997, 409) and are motivated by self-interest or the fulfillment of personal goals or preferences (Petracca 1991, 289). Public choice is not a conventional application of economics to market dynamics; it recognizes that public servants are constrained by the rules of the bureaucracy and the political ambitions of the political overseers, and public servants must work within those parameters. Analysis of bureaucracy using public choice theory assumes that the goals of bureaucrats are to expand their authority within bureaucratic and political systems (Blais and Dion 1990, 673; Dunleavy 1986, 13; Niskanen 1968, 293; H. Schwartz 1994, 53; James 1995, 617). The budget-maximization model (Niskanen 1968, 293–4) is one of the most noted public choice theories applied to public administration and has had considerable influence in public management institutional reforms over the last five decades (Simard 2004); the model assumes that bureaucrats try to maximize their budgets and impose their preferences on non-bureaucratic political actors (Niskanen 1994).

In contrast to budget maximization, Dunleavy (1991) proposes the bureau-shaping model, which contends that senior civil servants desire working environments that facilitate a policy-advisory role, rather than maximize organizational budgets or resources (Marsh, Smith, and Richards 2000, 467–8). This role would take the form of a small and elite-led organization close to the centre of political power with few or no management responsibilities (Gains and John 2010, 456). If budget or staff increases are sought, it is to shape the bureau to optimize these arrangements. Dunleavy (1991) argues that senior officials shape their bureau by using strategies such as initiating internal restructuring, redefining relationships with external stakeholders, promoting competition between bureaus, transforming internal work practices, and outsourcing or shifting contract or low-level work to others.

The bureau-shaping model has its critics. Marsh, Smith, and Richards (2000) note that it fails to take full account of the overarching political context constraining the bureaucrats' ability to shape the environment, it marginalizes any sense of a public service ethos, it focuses on the distinction between policy and management when in fact the two cannot be easily distinguished in practice, and it overestimates the time spent by executive public servants on policy. Cope (2000) argues that the model needs to be proven more systematically and notes that it oversimplifies the dynamics of public service. Finally, the model, like most rational choice models, overlooks the role of culture (Hood 1998) and other important contributions to public administration theory, such as institutionalism (Timney 1996; Ferris and Tang 1993).

Nevertheless, Marsh, Smith, and Richards (2000) and Dunsire (1995) note that the model represents a significant advance in public administration theory; it provides a far more nuanced understanding of the preferences of administrators than Niskanen's budget maximization model does and a greater understanding of the powerful role administrators play in shaping reforms. Indeed, while political overseers create parameters for reform, there continues to be considerable room for bureaucrats to shape those reforms according to their own strategic preferences. The theory is particularly helpful in understanding agencification, the administrative process of separating policy from operations that swept across the UK in the 1980s and 1990s (Sześciło 2020). A similar trend took hold in Canada in the late 1990s and 2000s, including the period that saw the creation of PHAC as a response to SARS (Bernier, Juillet, and Deschamps 2022; Vining, Laurin, and Weimer 2015); the bureau-shaping model has rarely been applied in a Canadian context to examine these changes. Ostensibly, they occurred at the behest of political overseers with an eye to increasing efficiency, improving government service for ordinary citizens, and, perhaps more ideologically, distinguishing the policy domain led largely by politicians and the operations domain led largely by professional public servants. Recalling the bureau-shaping model helps us examine the role public servants played in shaping these reforms. In most cases, the new agency, such the Canada Revenue Agency in the

Canadian case, became responsible largely for operations like tax collection, and the traditional government departments, such as Finance, retained responsibility for tax policy; in the case of PHAC, the change was slightly different. The agency became responsible for policy advice with some operational programs.

PREFERENCE FOR HEALTH-PROMOTION POLICY

Public health is jurisdictionally complex, with responsibility residing mostly with the provinces. In general, PHAC does not dictate how the provinces address or control chronic disease, infectious disease, or other public health issues. Federal public health officials produce expert advice and plans for intervention with relatively few opportunities to operationalize these plans. In contrast to the role of the provinces, that of federal public health has traditionally been coordination and facilitation (PHAC 2005, 6). It is also responsible for emergency management, providing information and guidance for quarantine and control of borders, purchase of vaccines, and response coordination (6).

Public health has increasingly focused on promoting population health, which often reduces health-care costs (Abdullah et al. 2017, 794; CPHA, n.d.; Craven et al. 2020; WHO 2014, 11). It achieves this, in part, by building "healthy public policy," which means putting "health on the agenda of policy makers" and "directing them to be aware of the health consequences of their decisions" (WHO 1986, 2). This language makes it clear: health promoters are often not decision makers but experts providing advice.[1] This tendency aligns with neoliberal preferences towards more individual responsibility that have become increasingly common in public sector risk management since the rise of New Public Management in the 1980s and 1990s (Hood 1991); though the public is given information to help the individual, policy-makers' direct responsibility and accountability are reduced (B. Brown and Baker 2012).

Public health's move towards cost reduction by optimizing population health does not align with the budget-maximization argument. Under this model it would be in the interest of bureaucrats to argue that increased budgets are needed to address population health concerns. Yet Canadian public health budgets represent a relatively small portion of Canada's health budgets and have not increased alongside investments in clinical care (Hoffman et al. 2019, 271). Provincial and territorial government public health expenditures make up a low percentage, 5.4 per cent, of all health spending (CIHI 2020c).[2]

Institutional changes to federal public health reinforce the bureau-shaping argument. SARS, which infected 438 and killed 44 in Canada in 2003, acted as focusing event at the time of agencification; the post-mortem inquiry report created a policy window for change (Kingdon 1984). According to the subsequent Naylor report, public health was inefficiently administered by Health Canada, and the department had to manage competing political priorities (National Advisory Committee on SARS and Public Health 2003, 4). The report recommended transferring public health responsibilities from Health Canada to an arm's-length agency to enhance its credibility, operations, and independence (4). As a result, PHAC was established in 2004 and formally confirmed as a legal entity in 2006, breaking from the operational and political issues at Health Canada.

Today the core responsibilities of PHAC are infectious-disease prevention and control, health promotion and chronic-disease prevention, and health security (PHAC 2020h, 7). Emergency preparedness and response, biosecurity, and border health security are considered subsections of health security (24–6). The prominent use of information rather than compulsion reinforces the bureau-shaping argument of delegating responsibility without operationalizing significant activities. PHAC produces outputs such as public policy, programs, and services encouraging positive health outcomes through persuasion, nudging, and various acts of control (CPHA 2021; PHAC 2011b). Some examples include the Healthy Living Fund, the Canada Prenatal Nutrition Program, and the Immunization Partnership Fund. Most strategies, policies, and programs are in the health promotion and chronic-disease-prevention portfolio and are guided by a population health approach (PHAC 2012). There is clear benefit from this from the standpoint of fighting a pandemic: a healthy population, which is what health promotion aims to achieve, is the best defence against a pandemic. Most deaths caused by COVID-19 have been the result of co-morbidities, such as dementia, diabetes, or respiratory diseases.

Health promotion has seen growth in recent years. While the total PHAC budget was relatively stable, federal spending in health-promotion portfolios trended up during 2007–20 (see figure 11.1) and, in recent years, often makes up more than 50 per cent of PHAC's total spending. Ironically, health promotion is a difficult political sell. It is the "process of empowering people to increase control over their health and its determinants through health literacy efforts and multisectoral action to increase healthy behaviors" (WHO 2021a, para. 6). The results of effective prevention are not observable by the

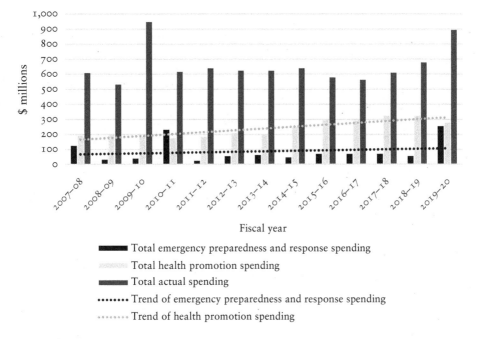

$ millions

1,000
900
800
700
600
500
400
300
200
100
0

Fiscal year

▬▬▬ Total emergency preparedness and response spending
░░░░░ Total health promotion spending
▬▬▬ Total actual spending
•••••••• Trend of emergency preparedness and response spending
·········· Trend of health promotion spending

Figure 11.1 | Public Health Agency of Canada's spending per fiscal year, 2007–20. Spending on emergency management is consistently low compared to that of health promotion. Spending on emergency management is structured differently year to year in departmental results reports. From 2007–08 to 2009–10, it was tracked as Emergency Preparedness and Response; from 2010–11 to 2011–12, as Regulatory Enforcement and Emergency Response; and, most recently, as part of Health Security, amalgamated with other subcategories. Starting in 2015–16, only the total spending for Health Security is identified, not the emergency management spending. This makes spending levels difficult to compare. Health promotion spending was tracked as its own category until 2012–13. It was then amalgamated with Health Promotion and Disease Prevention, with a spending on each subcategory available. In this figure, the spending for Conditions for Healthy Living is used for 2012–13 to 2014–15. Starting in 2015–16, only the total spending for Health Promotion and Disease Prevention is identified, not the health promotion spending. *Sources:* PHAC 2016, 2019, 2020g, 2020h.

population, benefits are difficult to communicate to voters, interventions often require long-term campaigns that have little value in short democratic election cycles, and the measurement of effectiveness is methodologically and rhetorically difficult (Hoffman et al. 2019, 271).

In contrast to measurement of conventional clinical health care, which can evaluate success through clearer and immediate metrics such as treatments administered, measurement of the impact of health-promotion interventions is an arguably more complex task, underpinned by competing world views and ideologies, and often requires much longer time horizons.

Through a bureau-shaping lens, this is an advantage: performance metrics measure the activities and outcomes with which the department has only a tenuous relationship and accountability is blurred. In annual departmental results reports, PHAC's performance in health promotion is measured by a variety of indicators with targets and dates to achieve them. Examples of result indicators are "% of population who have high psychological well-being," and "% increase in average minutes/day of physical activity among adults" (PHAC 2020g, 18). Some indicators are missing data for several years. Performance indicators also change after several years; in previous annual reports, for example, rates of key infectious diseases were indicators.

NEGLECT OF EMERGENCY MANAGEMENT

Direct spending on emergency management, in contrast to health promotion, is consistently less than 15 per cent of PHAC's total spending (see figure 11.1).[3] In 2018–19, spending on health security – a core responsibility of PHAC that encompasses emergency preparedness and response, biosecurity, and border and travel health – was $55.5 million, a drift downward from $67.9 million in 2015–16 (PHAC 2019, 32; 2016, 30). Planned spending on health security in 2019–20 was $52.3 million; the response to COVID-19 ballooned actual spending to $248.5 million (PHAC 2020g, 51).

PHAC's reports do not emphasize emergency management. Between 2008 and 2019, the chief public health officer issued fifteen reports on health priorities for Canadians. None explicitly addresses emergency or pandemic response. One explicitly addresses infectious disease, though pandemic response is discussed by recognizing the threat: "We must remain vigilant" (PHAC 2013a, 73).

With respect to emergency response, departmental result indicators include "% of provincial and territorial requests for assistance responded to within negotiated timelines," for which PHAC scored 100 per cent, and "Canada's readiness to respond to public health events and emergencies as assessed independently by the World Health

Organization," which is rated out of five, and for which PHAC scored a 4.5 (PHAC 2020g, 42). (The latter result was based on a 2018–19 assessment. Data are collected every five years.)

Organizational restructuring of PHAC in 2014 distanced research and policy advice from operations and management, leaving the former to public health officials and the latter to generalist public servants. After the redesign, the CMO was no longer the leading public servant in the department, instead taking an advisory role. Media and public health commentators were critical; they argued that if the CMO lost responsibility for the staff and budget, then the CMO would lose control over the agenda (Bendaoud 2020; Zahariadis 2016). Minister of Health Rona Ambrose disagreed. She noted that changes to the organizational design had come at the request of the department itself and that the changes freed the CMO to focus on providing advice to the government and health messages to Canadians and participating in interjurisdictional committees. The change would free the CMO from day-to-day management responsibilities. This mirrors the existing structure in the public health offices of most provinces (K. Grant 2014).

There are few political or bureaucratic incentives for operational emergency management planning for low probability, "what-if" scenarios. Grand responses to major crises, which have clearer performance metrics, can be a major political boon (Boin et al. 2016). In Canada many provincial, territorial, and federal leaders enjoyed high approval ratings during the first year of the pandemic and won majority governments (Grenier 2021; McPhail 2020; Schmunk 2020). Indeed, there is a history of turning crisis response into political and bureaucratic success (Lalancette and Raynauld 2020; Grenier 2020a).

PHAC departmental reports show that health security and infectious-disease management receive less attention until a crisis occurs, at which time political and bureaucratic attention becomes focused (Halpin, Fraussen, and Nownes 2017). Total authorities available for use increased significantly during the H1N1 and COVID-19 pandemics, when PHAC suddenly had major operational responsibilities (see 2010–11 and 2019–20, figure 11.2). In 2020–21, total spending increased nearly tenfold to $8.76 billion (PHAC 2022b, 71). Planned spending in 2021–22 was similar, over $8 billion, before returning to about pre-COVID levels in the following years (PHAC 2021a). No reasonable person would expect PHAC to spend vast sums on "what-if" scenarios. However, given that the cost of pandemics is so significant, it raises questions about how much time and resources PHAC should dedicate

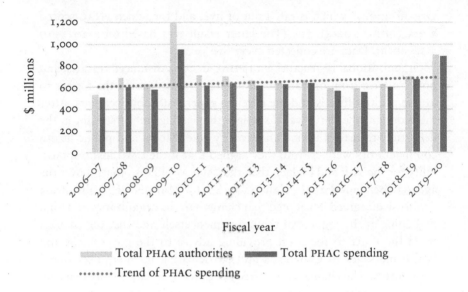

Fiscal year

▩▩▩ Total PHAC authorities   ▬▬ Total PHAC spending

•••••••• Trend of PHAC spending

Figure 11.2 | Public Heath Agency of Canada's authorities (money available for use) versus actual spending, 2006–20. Spending increases substantially during crises. Lower spending in 2015–16 is primarily due to PHAC making final payments for the Hepatitis C Health Care Services Program in the previous year, and the introduction and sunsetting of temporary programs including an Ebola preparedness and response initiative. The lower budget may also be the result of the Harper government's Strategic and Operating Review in 2011–12, which reviewed all departmental spending as part of efforts to reduce the deficit (Government of Canada 2011b). Changes from this review were likely not implemented until the end of the Harper administration. *Sources:* PHAC 2016, 2019, 2020g, 2020h.

to preparing for events that are likely to occur periodically and with varying degrees of impact.

While salient issues can generate organizational attention and action, the absence of profile for certain issues can result in neglect. Post-crisis reports illustrate that a consistent lack of pre-event planning resulted in deficits in execution. There was plenty of blame to go around. In 2003, Canadian governments were criticized for being inadequately prepared to respond to SARS, despite having had regularly updated pandemic plans since 1988 (National Advisory Committee on SARS and Public Health 2003; Expert Panel on SARS and Infectious Disease

Control [Walker] 2003; A. Campbell 2004). Three commissions noted weaknesses in all areas of cybernetics: poorly maintained and operated health-surveillance systems, a lack of information-sharing infrastructure, poor data quality and reporting standards, poor emergency response coordination, disagreement on a common list of notifiable or reportable diseases across jurisdictions, and unclear lines of accountability and transparency to aid in behaviour modification (National Advisory Committee on SARS and Public Health 2003; OAG 2008). The Naylor report concluded that Health Canada's Population and Public Health Branch was not fulfilling its health protection and emergency management responsibilities (National Advisory Committee on SARS and Public Health 2003).

Health protection, emergency management, and practical epidemiological activities are major operational challenges. A. Yu et al. (2020) note that pandemics are uncertain risks requiring significant planning, coordination, and oversight for successful preparedness and response. The *Lessons Learned Review* for H1N1, which examined the response of PHAC and Health Canada to H1N1, identified thirty-four areas for improvement in pandemic response (PHAC 2010, 9), many of which are similar to issues raised following SARS, thereby underscoring a lack of progress. Notable items included a flawed pandemic-emergency-response plan (89), a lack of regular emergency management planning and training (90), a vaccination program that was late in starting and poorly administered (Eggleton and Ogilvie 2010, 28, 33), and concerns with interjurisdictional communication (PHAC 2010, 89–91). A follow-up audit three years later noted ongoing problems, including an ambiguous renewal of the NESS's management and operational functions (PHAC 2013b).

In sum, while health policy promotion has limited political payoff, the growth in the health policy advisory role that has been focused on health promotion at PHAC over the past two decades suggests bureau-shaping strategies that privilege policy over operations, particularly in emergency management. Although health promotion and emergency management are not mutually exclusive, the preference to work in health promotion, with some responsibility devolved to the individual, coupled with limited budget growth and reduced operational responsibilities, has coincided with reduced attention to emergency management portfolios, which require stronger operational action and accountability. Emergency management secures funds and political profile easily during a crisis, which creates incentives to neglect emergency management preparation in the absence of an emergency. Despite shortcomings identified in multiple audits, these issues persisted and left public health vulnerable to an inadequate operational response to COVID-19.

PUBLIC HEALTH'S EARLY RESPONSE TO COVID-19

In 2019, Canada was ranked as the fifth-best country in terms of pandemic preparedness (Johns Hopkins Center for Health Security and the Nuclear Threat Initiative 2019, 20).[4] Significant gaps in Canada's public health pandemic response and preparedness, however, were evident in the "decentralized, uncoordinated, and slow" response to COVID-19 from January until March 2020 (Hansen and Cyr 2020, 1). According to one of the authors of a post-SARS report, recommendations like structural changes to federal public health were implemented, while other issues like hospital surge capacity, a provincial and territorial responsibility, were not addressed and caused severe strain throughout COVID-19 (Watters 2022, 6). Audits have since found that the federal government's pandemic plans were not regularly updated or tested, long-standing issues with health surveillance information had gone unresolved, and recommendations by previous auditors general on data-sharing agreements and privacy had not been implemented.

PHAC's risk assessments in the first three months of 2020 downplayed the risk of the virus. They were also founded on limited information, with no information from an intelligence branch in Canada's military that had begun producing warnings about COVID-19 in early January 2020 (Brewster 2021b). Federal health officials relied almost entirely on the WHO, which in turn relied on information disclosed by China (Brewster 2021b). Infection and mortality rates were downplayed in the Chinese government's official records; key details about how the virus spread were also withheld (Robertson 2021c). Some within PHAC believe that senior officials should have been aware that this information was unreliable (Robertson 2021c). A 2015 decision to remove a Canadian doctor who served as a direct point of connection to health officials in Beijing did not help (M. MacKinnon, Vanderklippe, and Robertson 2020).[5]

The methodology used to determine the risk that COVID-19 posed to Canada was flawed because it focused only on Canada at one moment in time. It did not take into account international data or projections of danger (Robertson and Walsh 2021). Between 2 February and 28 February 2020, Ottawa did not update its risk assessment despite a worsening international situation. From January to early March, PHAC repeatedly issued statements or mild warnings indicating that the virus posed a low risk to the public (S. Maher 2021). On 15 January, PHAC triggered the Public Health Response Plan for Biological Events, which was intended to facilitate efficient and coordinated approaches across all jurisdictions, and activated the Health Portfolio Operations Centre, which acted as a point of contact for communications and emergency-management-governance support (Hansen and Cyr 2020, 2). A coordinated provincial and territorial response did not follow. Particularly during Canada's first one hundred cases of COVID-19, similar public health actions taken by provinces and territories were initiated on different dates over a span of weeks, if at all (Hansen and Cyr 2020); communications lacked uniformity (J. Ling 2020).

By 22 January, screening of passengers from Wuhan had begun at three Canadian airports (S. Maher 2021). A special advisory committee on COVID-19 was formed at the end of January, co-chaired by the chief public health officer of Canada and the chief medical officer of health for New Brunswick. PHAC reiterated several times after this point that the virus remained a low risk. Communications suddenly changed on 16 March, five days after the WHO had declared a global pandemic and three days after the US had declared a national emergency. COVID-19 was declared a high risk to Canada (Robertson and Walsh 2021; PHAC 2021m, 34). This change was not incorporated into the daily situation reports from the agency that were distributed throughout the government for the remainder of March – further evidence of poor coordination (Robertson and Walsh 2021).

Historically, Canada was equipped with a robust early-warning system for the purpose of identifying epidemiological risks, which had international value in tracking outbreaks including SARS, Ebola, and H1N1 (Robertson 2021b; see chapter 1). The Global Public Health Intelligence Network (GPHIN) was built to scan the Internet for signs of disease outbreaks. However, PHAC limited key parts of GPHIN's operations in 2018, and the system experienced a turnover in critical staff (Brewster 2021a). The function to produce international alerts was silenced in May 2019 (para. 9). When it did detect the COVID-19 outbreak in China on 30 December 2019, no warning was issued (Robertson 2021b). Comprehensive risk assessments of COVID-19 were not conducted by the network.

These problems and others, such as serious gaps in the NESS, were neglected and repeatedly detailed in internal audits (Bloodworth,

Table 11.1 | Selected findings from federal reports about COVID-19 response, 2021

Federal report	Weaknesses in information gathering	Weaknesses in standard setting	Weaknesses in behaviour modification
Signals: The Global Public Health Intelligence Network (GPHIN) Independent Review Panel Final Report, by Margaret Bloodworth, Mylaine Breton, and Dr Paul Gully	GPHIN understaffed when COVID-19 was recognized as a global health threat	Did not address audits that found gaps in the NESS Important position with GPHIN left vacant	Lack of timely and relevant management information to coordinate pandemic response
Report 8 – Pandemic Preparedness, Surveillance, and Border Control Measures, by the Auditor General of Canada	Unresolved health surveillance issues	Pandemic plans were not regularly updated or tested GPHIN did not issue external early warnings or conduct comprehensive risk assessments of COVID-19 threat	Past recommendations on data-sharing agreements not implemented

Public health weaknesses were left unaddressed leading up to the COVID-19 pandemic. *Sources:* Bloodworth, Breton, and Gully 2021; Brewster 2021c.

Breton, and Gully 2021; Brewster 2021c). This indicates a systemic pattern of risk management that has not improved over time, even in the face of external criticism.

Staffing changes within PHAC have left the position of chief health surveillance officer unfilled since 2017 (Brewster 2021a), and restructuring in 2014 replaced the head of PHAC, a doctor, with a civil servant without a health background, and appointed several other generalist public servants to management roles (Robertson 2021c). Such changes allegedly left science "sidelined," compromising the ability to handle COVID-19 effectively (para. 64). PHAC staff said they struggled to move pertinent information about COVID-19 up the chain of command during January and February 2020 (Robertson 2021b). Recent federal reports (see table 11.1) indicate that public health deficiencies were left unaddressed leading up to COVID-19.

In sum, despite a comparatively good theoretical capability for pandemic response, Canada struggled to act during the early stages of COVID-19. Observed through a bureau-shaping lens, PHAC has shown a sustained preference for health promotion policy over emergency management. Internal interests left public health with deficiencies in gathering international information; in setting standards in terms of staffing, pandemic plans, and personal protective equipment (Office of Audit and Evaluation 2022); and in modifying behaviour in terms of coordination and data-sharing (Public Health Physicians of Canada 2022, 18).

EXTERNAL INTERESTS:
THE AMBIGUITY OF PRECAUTION

The precautionary principle emphasizes doing good by preventing harm, either through action or inaction (Government of Canada 2020b; Richter and Laster 2004, 10; Goldstein 2001, 1358; McArthur 2020; M.J. Smith, Komparic, and Thompson 2020, 110). In short, better safe than sorry (Huang 2020, 75; Sandin 2004). In practice it has limitations. Reasonableness plays a role in its application, but this concept is not precise (Resnik 2004, 281). What is "reasonable" may be informed by science but is subject to framing and interpretation and can change over time. Sandin (1999, 899) argues that the ineffective applications of precaution can be overcome if a potential threat is framed coherently and consistently. It may not be possible, however, to frame risks consistently or coherently when one is operating under conditions of uncertainty with stakeholders who have different and competing life experiences, values, incentives, and world views.

The precautionary principle is best suited for situations where there is significant uncertainty or ambiguity about a risk, when the consequences are potentially catastrophic and/or irreversible, and when there are externalities that would accrue to the public and society at large. However, critics argue that the precautionary principle can be unclear, incoherent, or ineffective because of the selective way in which it addresses risks (Boyer-Kassem 2017, 2027; M. Peterson 2017, 2035; Sunstein 2005b, 2); as noted in chapter 10, it can neglect trade-offs. This is particularly important when considering interests. A narrow approach from government can create opportunities for some while offloading the costs on others (Sunstein 2002a, 32; H. Miller and Engemann 2019, 251; Flood, Thomas, and Wilson 2020, 892). This also suggests that there is a power dynamic at play: different groups compete to frame uncertainty or ambiguity in a way that benefits their interests.

Precaution continued to be used to describe government's approach to COVID-19 even as policy-makers became more sensitive to costs and the fact that there was no zero-risk option. Managing the risks of COVID-19 inevitably created risks elsewhere; government officials were ill equipped to address these trade-offs in any transparent manner. Access to decision makers became important as organized groups advocated for their sectors. To understand this better, we shift to James Wilson (1980) to explore the dynamics and characteristics of lobbying, power, and regulatory politics.

INTEREST AND PRECAUTION:
WILSON'S INTEREST GROUP THEORY

The idea of regulatory costs and benefits is central to interest group theory. To illustrate the theory, Hood, Rothstein, and Baldwin (2001) draw on James Wilson's seminal book *The Politics of Regulation* (1980). Wilson's two-dimensional matrix of interest group configurations illustrates the key dynamics (table 11.2).

Each quadrant corresponds to a specific type of regulatory politics. When both benefits and costs are diffuse, or widely distributed, the matrix predicts that majoritarian politics will be present: no single group stands to gain or lose significantly from regulation. The opposite situation, where both benefits and costs are highly concentrated on fewer actors, produces interest group politics. This situation arises when a regulation threatens to benefit one set of business interests at the expense of other business interests: some groups win while others lose. Client politics occur in the presence of regulatory capture, which happens when regulatory decision making aligns with the preferences of large industry groups. Costs are diffuse, so no group perceives itself as losing. Entrepreneurial politics exist when a widely dispersed and loosely organized group, usually the public, benefits from regulation that involves a significant cost for a much smaller set of interests, such as a specific industry sector.

The Wilson typology, and by extension the risk regulation regime framework's interest group hypothesis (IGH), is ultimately about locating the sources of power in a regulatory regime. When power is

Table 11.2 | Interest group theory

		Distribution of benefits of risk regulation	
		Diffuse	Concentrated
Distribution of costs of risk regulation	Diffuse	Majoritarian politics	Client politics
	Concentrated	Entrepreneurial politics	Interest group politics

The concentration of the costs and benefits of risk regulation.
Sources: Adapted from J.Q. Wilson 1980; Hood, Rothstein, and Baldwin 2001.

concentrated among a few small groups, the regulatory regime exhibits client politics and regulatory capture. When power is diffuse, regulations are contested by multiple groups.

Governments made various regulatory decisions, ostensibly motivated by the scientific details of the risk of COVID-19. While some of these decisions were devastating for certain organizations, they were neutral or profitable for others.

PANDEMIC PRECAUTION AND INTERESTS

In the early stages of the COVID-19 pandemic there was concern about overreaction. Precaution was interpreted as maintaining stability, not inciting panic or overregulating the response.

By March 2020 the public health response was broad, shutting down all services deemed to be non-essential and encouraging people to stay home as much as possible. Essential services and activities remained open in a modified format and with health restrictions in place. As these certain functions of society had to continue, there was a degree of risk that was considered tolerable. Provinces and territories use largely the same categories of "essential" services but develop their specific lists and have the authority to address the public health risk as they see fit. It was in the best interest of businesses in the private sector to "self-identify" as essential (PS 2020b, para. 3) or at least to establish that one's business could abide by health guidelines and that there was a public interest in continuing operations.

Ostensibly, the government's first reaction was majoritarian and precautionary. Society was perceived to be on the precipice of a health calamity; one critical report that received international attention used epidemiological models to forecast that up to 81 per cent of the population of the US and the UK could be infected if government did not enact and enforce strict health protocols (Ferguson et al. 2020, 6). Canada, as a comparable Western country, could expect similar outcomes. (By 2 April 2022, cases of COVID-19 had been documented in about 10 per cent of Canada's population, and 0.1 per cent of the population had died.)

The costs and benefits of the government's new standards and enforced behaviours were widely distributed, affecting most of the country. Nearly three million jobs were lost in April and May 2020, with unemployment increasing to 13 per cent, up from 7.8 per cent in March 2020 (CBC News 2020d).

Everyone had something to gain from health protection, but everyone also had something to lose. "We are all in this together" was Prime Minister Justin Trudeau's mantra in news conferences in March (Cable Public Affairs Channel 2020, 23:18; Wherry 2020, para. 9). As more information was made available, it became clear that the costs and benefits of the standards and behaviours were not, in fact, equally distributed.

As more was learned about the disease and the economic consequences of the shutdown, governments had to make decisions that seemed reasonable even if the decision-making tools they had at their disposal were limited and decisions seemed at times to be extreme, arbitrary and/or contradictory (Dryden 2021; Rusnell 2021; Cecco and Lindeman 2022; B. Peterson 2020). By June, case counts were dropping. There was pressure from the business community and some members of the public for governments to reopen where and when it could. Reopening plans adhered to minimum health standards, such as wearing masks and maintaining social distancing, but also reflected trade-offs because the risk of onward transmission was always present.

Private interests do not necessarily initiate government change; more often industry engages with issues that are government priorities (Halpin and Fraussen 2019). Private sector interests that had existing relationships with government and could allocate both financial and human resources to lobbying efforts benefited. An examination of the federal lobby registry before and after the beginning of the pandemic shows an overall increase in lobbying activity during the first year of COVID-19, especially in the amount of documented communication between lobbyists and the federal government. There was a 23.5 per cent increase in total registrations, and a 64.0 per cent increase in communication reports during this time (Registry of Lobbyists 2022b, 2022c).

At the provincial level, journalists from the *Toronto Star* wrote exposés on former political staff who lobbied the Ontario Progressive

Conservative (PC) government for preferential treatment. Peter Van Loan, a former federal politician and president of the PC Party of Ontario, lobbied for five clients (including a toy company, housing developer, and manufacturers) to continue doing business (Warnica and Bailey 2021). Amazon hired lobbyists from a firm co-owned by one of Premier Ford's political advisors after a warehouse was closed due to a COVID-19 outbreak. Former PC Party of Ontario staffer Nick Kouvalis lobbied on behalf of Cinespace Film Studies to have film-set-personnel restrictions changed so that the company could continue filming. Less than fifty days after film-personnel restrictions had been imposed, the government issued a new set of film and television rules that greatly increased the number of performers permitted (Warnica and Bailey 2021). Two former political staff for Premier Doug Ford lobbied the Ontario government to continue allowing big-box stores to sell non-essential items while small businesses were closed; the president and CEO of Walmart Canada had a personal meeting with the premier.

Lobbying government is not new. Most governments allow it, and lobbyists with political experience are often skilled at doing it effectively. Moreover, big organizations, particularly in the hospitality sector, did not always benefit from pandemic health directives and suffered considerably instead. Nevertheless, lack of transparency and the sense that elite groups have privileged access erode trust in democratic governance; some governments regulate it better than others (Holman and Luneburg 2012). The federal government has lobbying-disclosure laws in place, which can be helpful. Notwithstanding these Ontario examples, the provinces are generally less transparent, so it is difficult to appreciate the full extent of the practice. These anecdotes, however, suggest that access helped organizations obtain preferred business outcomes in terms of continuing to operate.

Airlines provide an example of client politics in which the government is captured by the industry (Reynolds 2022). Air travel was extremely limited; Canada barred foreign nationals from entering the country from March 2020, and many flights were cancelled. Interprovincial travel saw such a decline that airlines suspended service to certain destinations (Evans 2020a, 2020b). In 2020 and 2021 combined, forty-seven airlines "ceased operations," including four in Canada (Tozer-Pennington 2021; 2022, 9). Consolidation of the industry also occurred (Al Mallees 2022). With new standards and severely reduced passenger capacity, Air Canada lost $1.16 billion in the fourth quarter of 2020 (R. Jones 2021a) and recorded a net loss of $4.6 billion for the entire year (Air Canada 2021b, 7). The size of Air

Canada, however, allowed it to benefit significantly from government programs such as the CEWS, available to many businesses to continue paying their employees in 2020 (R. Jones 2021a).

Air Canada made considerable lobbying efforts. According to the Office of the Commissioner of Lobbying of Canada (OCL), the airline hired several consultants and, between August 2020 and August 2021, filed ninety-seven monthly communications from seven different registrants (OCL, n.d.a, n.d.b). The efforts paid off in April 2021 with the delivery of a financial support package of $5.9 billion from the federal government (Air Canada 2021a; R. Jones 2021a; Rastello 2021). In exchange, Air Canada agreed to refund customers whose flights were cancelled in 2020 because of the pandemic, restore flights on nearly all suspended regional routes, and cap compensation for company executives at $1 million per year, among other stipulations.

Most Western governments had already announced significant support packages for national airlines (Rappeport and Chokshi 2020; Fife and Willis 2021; Alderman 2020; Karp 2020; Hurst and Butler 2020); it was unlikely that the Canadian government would not offer support to Air Canada, as part of what is ostensibly an oligopoly providing an essential service. Low-interest loans in the relief package suggest that taxpayers helped with this bailout, though Air Canada will be repaying the loan (Pittis 2021; Lao 2021a).

While aspects of big-box retail can be considered client politics at times, it also exemplifies an interest group regime. As with Air Canada, big-box retailers had privileged access to decision makers and resources to apply pressure (Warnica and Bailey 2021). Government policy resulted in these retailers growing their businesses at the expense of their competition. Large floor space allowed big-box retail to enforce social distancing; that they sold a variety of goods, often in addition to essential items like groceries, allowed them to support one-stop, in-person shopping. Smaller stores generally could not meet the same government standards and, if non-essential, were limited to offering curbside pickup and delivery. Many big-box retailers, such as Walmart, Dollarama, Best Buy, Costco, and Home Depot, experienced considerable revenue and share-value growth in 2020 and 2021 (Yahoo Finance 2020e, 2020l, 2021a–d, 2022a). Grocery stores also saw growth. Loblaws, the leading grocery retailer in the country, had its annual food retail sales increase from $33.7 billion in 2019 to $37.5 billion in 2020 (Loblaw Companies Limited 2021, 14). Sobeys saw a comparable boost in sales (Empire Company Limited 2021, 2). (For further discussion of market performance see chapter 9.)

While these big-box retailers enjoyed increased revenue and share values, smaller retailers paid a price as public health orders in many jurisdictions put a halt to in-person, non-essential shopping. Small businesses are normally vulnerable during high-impact, low-frequency events. They do not have extra staff, cash, or adequate insurance; they are usually ineffective at lobbying, partly because they neither have developed relationships with policy-makers nor have an easy route to them (Halpin and Fraussen 2019). The situation was made more difficult because public health in many jurisdictions set policy through public health directives, a process to which few small businesses had regular access; economic departments represented the interests of small business. Finally, most small businesses and any one small business can fail with minimal impact to the community. So it was with COVID-19: small businesses, unless they were able to operate online, were generally vulnerable.

Over a quarter of businesses with fewer than one hundred employees reported revenues down by at least 30 per cent compared to 2019 (Tam, Sood, and Johnston 2021a, 3). As of February 2021, 70 per cent of small businesses owners had taken on an average of $170,000 in debt (CFIB 2021). Roughly 58,000 small businesses closed their doors in 2020, and, as of January 2021, about one in six small business owners – an additional 181,000 – were seriously contemplating shutting down as well (CBC News 2021e).

CEWS assisted SMEs that experienced hardship and were at risk of failing due to COVID-19 restrictions. The government paid $95 billion through the CEWS. To be sure, for many retail businesses the government programs were a lifeline; for other businesses, the pandemic became a profitable opportunity that was made more lucrative by the nature of the disease and government interventions.

The final segment of regulatory politics, entrepreneurial politics, is represented by tourism, sports, and the arts. Here, provincial, territorial, and federal restrictions assumed a precautionary stance. These sectors were effectively closed and lost significant business. The hotel industry, for example, was plagued by empty rooms as travel restrictions and border closures came into effect (Tam, Sood, and Johnston 2021b). Losses were particularly stark in Montreal, Toronto, and Vancouver, with revenue in 2020 dropping by 79 per cent compared to 2019, for a total of $2.3 billion lost (Victor 2021). Cruise ships docked in ports, their lines carrying 80 per cent fewer passengers than they had the year before. Carnival, the world's largest cruise company, saw a 99 per cent decline in revenue in the third quarter of 2020, compared to the same period in 2019 (Yeginsu and Chokshi 2021). Live theatre and the performing arts, which generally rely on an in-person, intimate environment, also could not function. The entertainment and recreation sector in Canada was the hardest-hit area of the economy, after the airline industry, losing more than half its value in GDP (K. Taylor 2021). Even professional sports teams – historically one of the most reliable long-term investments for billionaires – recorded a decrease in value following shortened seasons played in a "bubble" or without fans (Birnbaum 2021). It is notable that professional sports leagues were quick to act in the initial shutdown of non-essential services, voluntarily moving faster to cancel games than the government was to implement public health restrictions (Aschburner 2020; Zucker 2020).

In the case of tourism, many small businesses were affected, but large businesses, such as hotels and cruise lines, also suffered (see chapter 8). Though the cost of these closures was the burden of businesses, the externalities or collective benefits accrued to communities as a whole. Because sectors supporting travel and large public gatherings in theatres and stadiums were closed, the COVID-19 transmission and community spread was limited, a positive consequence for society at large.

The self-named Freedom Convoy in early 2022 can also be thought of as resulting from entrepreneurial politics. Vaccine mandates for truckers crossing the Canada-US border were perceived as a cost concentrated on truckers, while the benefits of limited COVID-19 transmission and community spread were dispersed (see chapter 6 for further discussion on vaccine protests). The protest action of the truckers was poorly organized, lacked coherency (Jackman 2022; Kitroeff and Austen 2022), and resulted in less substantial changes when compared to lobbying efforts by other organized interests like Air Canada.

CONCLUSION

The role of public health viewed through a bureau-shaping lens offers insight into pandemic response. It might seem needlessly unkind to describe public health officials as bureau-shapers after they have endured unprecedented challenges throughout the pandemic – and certainly, we do not promote unwarranted distrust or suspicion of public servants. Managing COVID-19 was a complex task with high uncertainty, and addressing it resulted in considerable workload pressures and mental strife for those working in public health. While PHAC should be given credit for what it has done well, judging it only by its performance during the event would be narrow.

Bureau-shaping invites us to examine private interests and collective bureaucratic strategies that may precede these crises. These interests and strategies may not align with the public good, weakening emergency readiness. Bureau-shaping does not explain all the outcomes seen in public health; for example, there is limited competition between bureaus. Nonetheless, the actions of public health do reflect several bureau-shaping strategies. Restructuring in 2014 removed public health experts from the management and operations of PHAC and replaced them with generalist civil servants. Though it appears as if these changes were forced by political leaders, political overseers disputed this assessment, arguing that the changes reflected the preferences of senior public servants (K. Grant 2014). The proliferation of external advisory bodies for PHAC also reflects the bureau-shaping strategy of redefining relationships with external stakeholders to cut down on operational workloads while influencing policy (PHAC 2011a).

PHAC was created partly as a result of SARS with the intent of improving emergency management. In fact, there are few political and bureaucratic incentives to work on emergency response in the absence of an emergency. Though PHAC's overall budget has not increased over time, more of its existing budget has been directed towards health promotion, an area with long-term goals, unclear bureaucratic accountability, and limited operational responsibility. In the four years preceding COVID-19, spending on health security, of which emergency management is a part, trended down. These trends reflect transforming work practices to contain overall health costs and focus on policy over operations.

PHAC's long-term incentives and tendencies appear to be in the direction of health promotion. During the emergency management of COVID-19, this led to operational shortcomings. Canada's information-gathering system that successfully identified previous disease outbreaks was neglected, which is consistent with bureau-shaping tendencies of being research intensive and being accomplished at establishing new global networks but falling short in ongoing maintenance.

In terms of standards, a lack of comprehensive planning and foresight was evident in gaps in the NESS that had been left unaddressed after audits. Inconsistencies in standards surrounding travel, borders, and masks were exacerbated by poor provincial and territorial coordination regarding both policy and messaging.

Behaviour modification was the weakest. By mid-March and into April 2020, every day was considered crucial. January and February 2020 could have been valuable but instead were lost as caution and stability took precedence. Extracting Canadians from China and questioning travellers who had visited high-risk areas overseas seem naive given what was to come. The problem was far more advanced by then, and measures should have focused on preparing to mitigate the effects of COVID-19 within Canada. The responsibility for this failure is unclear; public health operates in an opaque environment, making it difficult to hold people to account, and there is blame-shifting between scientists, policy-makers, decision makers, and orders of government (Martin 2022; Cameron-Blake et al. 2021; C. Hall 2021). In any event, PHAC was not ready. Several partnerships with public health academic institutions were implemented to help with emergency response, and more are planned (PHAC 2021m, 35, 81), but such partnerships were lacking prior to the pandemic.

Other strategies should be taken, among them strong incentives and enforcement prioritizing operations and emergency management, and coordination when it comes to training and budgets and working with the provinces. The 2014 reorganization that brought in more public managers was not necessarily a mistake; it allowed people with expertise in management to do that job, while those with public health training could focus their energy on public health issues. PHAC needs more emphasis on operations, however, and a stronger integration and understanding of the relationship between science, policy, and management. Alas, PHAC is not alone among government departments in managing this complex trifecta.

In terms of external interests, despite the frequent references to precaution by politicians and policy-makers, the term is not without controversy in the risk community; scholars note the variation in definitions and methods of accountability, enforcement, use of evidence, transparency, and risk tolerance. Generally, it is criticized for being expensive and ambiguous; it fails to consider trade-offs and is vulnerable to the power of lobbyists (Renn 2008b; J. Tait 2008).

After weeks of lockdowns, people became less tolerant of restrictions. Government was trying to find the appropriate balance between containment and allowing society and the economy to function. The search for this elusive holy grail would recur throughout the pandemic. Even as more information became available, different world views underpinned how the data were interpreted; in cultural theory terms, there were individualistic-market, egalitarian-community, and bureaucratic-expert–led interpretations, which are not completely reconcilable (Hood 1998; see chapter 2).

Politicians, usually following the advice of CMOs, were left with the difficult task of reconciling the health and economic sides of the balance sheet, with no precise way to determine or communicate trade-offs. Generally, it was easier to side with less ambiguous health directives in the name of keeping people safe from the virus, but there was always pressure to get things "back to normal."

The IGH has much to offer in our understanding of government reaction to the pandemic. The ambiguity of the precautionary principle lent itself to lobbying. Many large organizations had the capacity to lobby extensively and reaped the business rewards of initial government interventions and health directives, as in the case of big-box retail, or subsequent government relief, as in the case of airlines. Poorly organized interests, such as the trucker convoy and small businesses generally, were less successful in doing so. While it is true that the pandemic affected various sectors, it is also clear that organized, concentrated interests with access to decision makers were in a stronger position to shape outcomes to their advantage.

PART FIVE

Living with It

We conclude the book by summarizing key observations about the context and governance of COVID-19 in Canada. We end with lessons for addressing low-probability, high-consequence events, considering the challenges associated with complex, uncertain, and ambiguous risks.

Conclusion

We find no villain in the federal government's officials and advisors then and think that anyone (ourselves included) might have done as they did – but we hope not twice.

R. Neustadt and H. Fineberg (1983),
The Epidemic That Never Was

In 1976 the US government initiated a massive vaccination program against an anticipated swine flu outbreak that, in the end, never materialized. Public health was criticized for the cost of the operation, the misinterpretation of the science, and the fact that some people may have died as a result of the vaccination (Neustadt and Fineberg 1983). Despite the magnitude of the case, little has been written about it, and it is largely a forgotten case study in public management (Moore 1995). In contrast, throughout the COVID-19 pandemic, governments were criticized for not responding quickly enough to a threat that did materialize in a devastating manner.

There are no perfect responses to risk. By their nature, they are underpinned by uncertainty. Risk management is not about being error free. The risk literature emphasizes that there will always be mistakes, trade-offs, winners and losers, different perspectives and biases, ideological clashes, and institutional fumbling; there will always be after-the-fact, even revisionist accounts assigning the roles of heroes and villains, and, as we have done here, selected criticisms of governments' approaches.

The risk now includes moving on without a serious examination of what happened, why it happened, and what we should learn from it. Thus far, there has been little interest in a government-wide and multi-jurisdictional review (Bubela et al. 2023). COVID-19 was indeed unprecedented in our lifetimes, but it does not mean that it could not happen again or that we cannot draw important observations about how we respond to pandemics or indeed low-probability, high-consequence events.

The pandemic serves as a powerful illustration of the challenges of governing in Beck's risk society. The threat was pervasive, invisible, and deadly; it transcended borders and, to a degree, many social categories like age, race, sex, and income, even if some were clearly more vulnerable than others. It exposed the fragility of global supply chains and the ease with which national borders reassert themselves. It also revealed the steadily increasing ambiguity in knowledge claims: that lab-like conditions are not replicated in the real world where power, politics, perspective, context, and experience make a difference in how information is gathered, directives are set, and people receive and act on risk messages. Hood, Rothstein, and Baldwin's (2001) framework and the four types of risk as described by the International Risk Governance Council help us to unmask these subtleties more clearly.

After a slow start, risk governance was focused on containing, then slowing COVID-19, which reduced some risks and increased others. Confronted by uncertainty, and forecasting a potentially immediate catastrophic outcome, governments assumed a precautionary approach on a vast scale, albeit with selected concessions and loopholes. The virus killed many people, which, to a point, further justifies the precautionary stance. While governments' approaches saved lives, they were also expensive and underprepared and at times lacked precision, prioritization, and nuance. The trade-offs were significant and not always clear.

This concluding chapter has three parts. First, using the concepts of cybernetics in the Hood, Rothstein, and Baldwin (2001) framework, we review the content of the government control mechanism, focusing on the regime's capacity to gather information, set standards, and change behaviour. Government response was fundamentally bureaucratic, which excelled at enacting standards and directing human and financial resources to address a potentially catastrophic threat to society that could not be adequately addressed by markets, the not-for-profit sector, or existing routine government operations. At the same time, it struggled with gathering and sharing the right information; adaptive capacity; scaling the response for purpose; diverse views; cost overruns; explaining trade-offs; and focusing on specific vulnerabilities. Second, we examine the contextual pressures, reviewing the three hypotheses of the Hood, Rothstein, and Baldwin framework. While no one hypothesis gives a fully satisfying account of the contextual pressure on government during such a far-reaching case, the examination of all three provides powerful insights into a complex dynamic with which government had to contend. While the context we have examined pressured the government regime, we also consider the extent to which the government control mechanism shaped the context. While governments acted at various times according to market failures, public anxiety, media coverage, and/or well-coordinated interests, the interplay between context and content was iterative and interactive. Governments changed the legal context by invoking emergency legislation, adopted aggressive communication plans to shape public opinion, and, through dynamics with interest groups, enabled and at times constrained the influence of different groups. Finally, we provide some thoughts on what the case reveals about risk governance of low-probability, high-consequence risk events, looking in particular at issues of complexity, uncertainty, and ambiguity.

BUREAUCRATIC CONTROL: ADDRESSING THE TENSION BETWEEN EGALITARIANISM AND INDIVIDUALISM

Gathering reliable and predictive information was difficult, particularly at the outset. With death and transmission rates initially seeming high, governments were pressured into a proactive precautionary stance, focused first on containment, and then on slowing transmission. Following the WHO declaration of a pandemic and a much more aggressive stance by the US CDC, in March 2020 Canadian officials framed the risk as pervasive, invisible, and deadly. Precaution meant acting dramatically and decisively in the face of the threat that had up until then been described as low risk. Data from global networks and dramatic action abroad, coupled with the conventions of infectious-disease containment and existing bureaucratic and constitutional design, shaped the reaction on a much larger scale than anyone had experienced in living memory or could even have imagined weeks earlier. In mid-March, governments enacted states of emergency, closed borders, distinguished between essential and non-essential services, and shut down large parts of daily life. The response was driven largely out of concern for the limited capacity of the health system to address the potential consequences in the near term. Large economic support programs followed to ensure stability.

By early April 2020, governments had started publishing models and projections, with regular public updates. The modelling was subject to the limitations of addressing complex risks, including dependence on expert opinion and reliance on data that were incomplete, derived from other jurisdictions, and based on various assumptions. While most leaders were grateful for the models (Grenier 2020b), and the short-term projections generally included the correct number, the published estimates of case and death count were wide ranging. The models prompted action by many, but there were challenges in collecting data, navigating various jurisdictional processes, mining and refining data for meaning, sharing with interested parties, making accurate longer-term forecasts, and communicating their meaning to the public. At times, models (particularly longer-term ones) are set up to fail; experts hope people will change their behaviour in light of the projections and, in so doing, change the trajectory of the disease. Uncertainty requires adaptive capacity from public agencies and the public. Although policies were updated as more information was gathered and the threat became better understood, governments seemed a step behind a threat that grew exponentially, subsided, and returned in waves, sometimes more aggressively.

The setting of standards, in the form of policies and directives, happened at the top: democratic accountability was executive-led, supported by senior and expert officials; parliamentary and legislative scrutiny through regular sittings was altered and often reduced, although the degree varied by jurisdiction. Provinces and territories were at once autonomous and highly interdependent. Most followed similar standards, but there continued to be weak coordination between provinces, at times described as a "patchwork" of systems (J. Ling 2020). They were responsible for their own jurisdictions but were constantly compared to others and subject to media scrutiny. As time went on, "follow the science" became a rallying cry for many, but science does not tell one what to do (Leonhardt 2022; J. Ball 2021). A way forward requires an ethical standard, as perhaps exemplified by the prime minister's declaration "We are all in this together"; true, people had to follow similar standards, even if they seemed disproportionate to the risk, to contain the disease. Then people were asked to follow restrictive health directives to protect others, "their grandparents," and the vulnerable (Rosenblatt 2020; Couto 2020); it was necessarily a collective responsibility.

Despite government policy leveraging of powerful market forces, in the acquisition of vaccines for example, behaviour modification at the organizational level was underpinned by a bureaucratic paradigm that tried to reconcile egalitarian and individualist impulses. Ostensibly our approach to public health focuses on population health (PHAC 2012). Government risk messages regarding health and wellness, however, are often tailored to individuals, as the state tries to provide information so that people can act in their own interests

(B. Brown and Baker 2012). This practice, which underscores individual responsibilities and incentivizes individual actions, is in tension with concepts like the social determinants of health, which put greater emphasis on context, environment, and collective responsibility for people's health. This tension is indicative of a broader conflict within health agencies and indeed medical practice and education about the appropriate focal point for analysis: the individual, the collective, or the environment (Arah 2009).

There was insufficient precedent for the prime minister's clarion call for egalitarianism on such a scale. Comparisons to phenomena like climate change exemplify how difficult it is to motivate collective action for which the benefits do not always accrue to the payer. There were also tensions in structure: government response was hierarchical by nature and design. Egalitarian forms of governance are difficult to operationalize on a large scale; they fracture. Bureaucracies, however, can specialize, organize, and standardize across large areas. There is also a steady hand at the top: accountability and authority are top-down. Efforts to standardize interventions across different populations in the name of broad social goals were supported by the majority, but they often overlooked the unique characteristics of subgroups. Women and people with disabilities, as well as low-income, racialized, and young people, carried different and underappreciated weight in the response. Arguably, bureaucratic design has the potential to strike a balance between competing pressures, but governments were slow to acknowledge and address the imbalance adequately in their responses.

Once the threat became better understood, it moved towards an ambiguous risk, yet there remained few tools to communicate how trade-offs were determined among different health risks, including COVID-19 and non-COVID-19. As well, trade-offs had to be made between containing COVID and mitigating the economic consequences of these measures. By 2021, most people had continued to support government restrictions, but consensus started to fray. This tension was more pronounced as vaccines and diagnostics became readily available. The clash of world views and lived experiences that underpinned many tensions with respect to reopening plans, vaccines, and vaccine mandates required a slower, more thoughtful and flexible process in which to engage communities. Rarely did governments have adequate processes in place. Time was short and the system ill-prepared, often struggling to address immediate concerns and act with foresight or outside of its existing bureaucratic design.

CONTEXT SHAPING CONTENT AND
CONTENT SHAPING CONTEXT

Despite popular comparisons to the Black Death (Varlik 2021; Wade 2020), this was not our ancestors' pandemic. The event took place in a modern legal, technological, psychological, and institutional context. The framework focuses our attention on how this context shapes content. It is also true that content changes context. Government intervention changed laws, public opinion, and the organization of interests. In many cases, governments had to intervene to achieve public policy goals. We examine this dynamic process here.

Market Failure: Readiness, Uncertainty and
the Challenge of Being Proportionate

The private sector played a key role. As outlined in chapter 9, some sectors prospered, some suffered, and others were up and down. Many businesses were opportunistic. Overall, governments could not have achieved their goals of trying to reduce disease transmission and protect public safety without a modern and responsive market.

Government responses dictated by market-failure logic are expected to be proportionate to the threat. Between March 2020 and the end of March 2022, 37,722 Canadians are known to have died of COVID-19 (and co-morbidities), which is about one person per one thousand (1.00), with an excess mortality rate of 7.4 per cent (Statistics Canada 2022j). Canada compares favourably, regarding deaths per thousand, to countries like the US (3.00) and UK (2.88) but not as well to Australia (0.25), Japan (0.07), and Taiwan (0.04). This gives us a glimpse of the magnitude of the problem but obviously does not include the number of people who would have died had governments not intervened in the manner they did.

With respect to the market failure hypothesis (MFH), Hood, Rothstein, and Baldwin (2001) examine information and opt-out costs. There is a strong case for the MFH in government response to COVID-19. Only government had the authority, credibility, and capacity to gather credible information and enable out-opt strategies, provide publicly funded health care, and secure PPE and effective vaccines in a highly competitive global market. Certainly, the government was not ready: it was a slow start, and enforcement was not always adequate. Still, governments came out strongly and did what only they could do: the federal government closed national borders, enforced the Quarantine Act and the Emergencies Act, and legislated massive economic programs to support businesses and those unable to work. Provincial and territorial governments enacted states of emergency that gave them sweeping powers to close businesses and schools and restrict movements, all by way of trying to contain the spread of the disease.

The response was expensive. The government ran the largest deficit in history, a bill to be paid by future generations. In 2020, Canada's spending and deficits were higher than thirty-four comparable high-income countries. Canada had the highest deficit-to-GDP ratio, 19.9 per cent, and was the second-highest spender (Fuss, Clemens, and Palacios 2020). Canada's debt grew faster than the debt of other developed countries in the first year of the pandemic. Its debt-to-GDP ratio had increased by about 80 per cent by December 2020, the highest of any developed country. This was mostly attributed to government borrowing for the CERB and a 38 per cent decline in GDP in the second quarter of 2020 (M. Lu 2020). Some measures were more reassuring from a financial point of view. In June 2021, Canada ranked best among the G7 in net debt as a share of GDP, which is arguably a better measure of Canada's ability to meet its financial obligations (Clemens and Palacios 2021). Government borrowing is not necessarily a bad thing; Canada borrowed significantly during the Second World War. There was a baby boom following the war, however, which led to increased productivity. Today, Canada's aging population makes increased productivity less likely; the debt, therefore, will probably be more burdensome (Poloz 2022a).

Despite the strength of the response, there was no consensus among government officials about what would constitute an appropriate size for the economic programs, and institutional divisions became apparent. The federal finance minister at the time, Bill Morneau, noted afterwards that CERB payouts had been necessary but were too generous for the need and driven more by the view of the prime minister's office of the politics, by the popular perception of the event, and by the media cycle rather than by the economic analysis provided by the Department of Finance (Morneau 2023). Morneau also argued that some payouts, like those to seniors, were largely unnecessary because their income was relatively stable; he felt that the programs were enacted to give an emotional lift to seniors and to secure the support of a politically active group.

The federal government's ability to support the economically vulnerable through transfer payments was generally successful, though the overall economic context was precarious. Inequality in Canada increased in the first half of 2020. In October 2020 one in five Canadians said they were better off financially, but almost two in five said the opposite and were more likely to have "overwhelming" debt (*Globe and Mail* 2020b). Inequality decreased as unemployment was offset by policy initiatives (Kuncl, McWhirter, and Ueberfeldt 2021, 5). The Bank of Canada noted that many Canadians ultimately saved extra money, including those in lower income groups (Schembri 2021). Low interest rates kept capital available, but those with assets benefited more; they also contributed to a volatile housing and rental market and the highest inflation in a generation, which is often hardest on the less well-off.

Forty per cent of the workforce could work from home. For those who had to go to work, employment and occupational health and safety legislation resulted in many businesses putting protective equipment and practices in place. These directives were not always enforced; those who were younger, less well-off, immigrants, foreign temporary workers, and racialized were more likely to have to go to work and were more at risk. Younger people were at much lower risk of becoming seriously ill, but the pandemic took a disproportionate toll on racialized groups in particular. Sick-leave benefits were available to some people and not others, which both raised questions of fairness and created incentives for one to keep working when sick.

Legal instruments were invoked at times by governments to shape the context. While the Quarantine Act was enforced inconsistently by the federal government, the Emergencies Act was much more powerful. As the prime minister noted at the Public Order Emergency Commission, the Emergencies Act was a tool that was on the books and so the government used it to end protests (J. Tunney 2022; S. Taylor, Berthiaume, and Tran 2022). While Justice Rouleau concluded that the federal government was justified in invoking the Act, he also noted several failures in policing, intelligence, and indeed federalism in a crisis (Rouleau 2023). In some respects, the use of the Emergencies Act was innocuous compared to what happened provincially and territorially. Alberta, Saskatchewan, Ontario, and Quebec, for example, enacted and retracted emergency legislation on several occasions. Other jurisdictions, like Nova Scotia, Nunavut, and the Northwest Territories, kept states of emergency or declarations of a public health emergency in place for two years, uninterrupted.

Although policing was at times "light touch" and was defended as necessary for a fast response, emergency orders granted significant power without the safeguards to ensure that action was "lawful and democratically legitimate" (Goudge 2021, 154). In Ontario the Emergency Management and Civil Protection Act gave government the power to suspend or rewrite certain laws. In contrast to the Public

Order Emergency Commission and perhaps with the exception of Alberta (Government of Alberta 2023), there has been little systematic review and reflection at the provincial order of government of the use of state power to limit people's rights.

By the end of 2021, tensions had been mounting over the government response. While health care is considered a market failure, the government intervention in its own way created other failures. Uncertain risks require adaptive capacity, but the health-care system operates largely at capacity and is limited in its ability to expand quickly. So much focus on the pandemic limited the system's ability to provide health services; people waited for months, and in some cases years, for care without a sense of how these trade-offs were determined and without reasonable alternatives.

According to B. Peterson (2020, 70), the pandemic forced us to evaluate trade-offs that pitted life against "broader costs to human flourishing" and overall well-being. One analysis found that the cost of lockdowns in Canada outweighed the benefits by seventeen to one (Joffe 2020). A study made a year into the pandemic found that many COVID-19 studies had relied on assumptions that turned out to be false, which led to overestimating the benefits and underestimating the costs of lockdowns (D. Allen 2021). For example, on the topic of sight restoration – one of the most cancelled surgeries during COVID-19 – a study found that one person suffering from severe visual impairment for five years is the equivalent of about four hundred moderate cases of infectious disease lasting two weeks each, when measured by health-adjusted life-years (Boyd et al. 2020).

Some called for cost-benefit analyses (A. Hunter 2022; *National Post* 2022), but such an analysis on a large scale would be practically impossible and should be treated with skepticism. It would require a consistent and logical model to reflect individual, institutional, and community-based knowledge and preference structures. The rational, psychological, sociological, and anthropological forces that we examine throughout this book would make such an analysis highly contested. The absence of a forum, and the high speed with which it would have to be done, makes it even more challenging.

Neither a precautionary approach nor a bureaucratic design is known for efficiency; rather, they are noted for their oversight and caution. When survival is at stake, risk can no longer be described as the product of probability and expected monetary losses (C. Jaeger et al. 2001). Long-term risk assessments do not hold when there is danger of massive operational failure and instability in the short term. Still, the largely universal approach that government took with restrictions, coupled with the absence of tools and transparency about how trade-offs were set for such extended periods with limited debate, is one problematic legacy of the pandemic, and one for which there continues to be no resolution.

Opinion-Responsive: Dread, Diversity, and Media Amplification

One might ask, in light of the opinion-responsive hypothesis (ORH), did governments do what people wanted? In some respects, the answer is largely yes. Most people were anxious about COVID-19 in the first year of the pandemic in particular; government response may have been more robust than one justified by the MFH, but people were highly supportive of their provincial, territorial, and federal governments. While former finance minister Morneau may be critical of the prime minister's decision to increase CERB spending and allocate funds to seniors, giving people an emotional lift in the face of anxious times was helpful in securing public support, which was crucial to the pandemic response.

Support waxed and waned, however, after the first year; people were fed up with the pandemic and at times were questioning governments' ability to get it under control. Yet even as late as the Freedom Convoy in early 2022, people were largely supportive of government policies on vaccines and vaccine mandates and disagreed with the tactics of the protesters even if they had some sympathy for them.

In fact, there are several challenges in interpreting public opinion. People's views change over time and because of various demographic considerations and psychological phenomena. Polling results can also be dubious. Polls can be done quickly, cheaply, and easily but not necessarily reliably (Quigley, Bisset, and Mills 2017, 165). People are also not very good at deliberating over trade-offs. Research showed that the same people held different and incompatible views about lockdowns depending on whether public health communications described them positively, with reference to protecting health, or negatively, with reference to economic costs (Carrieri, De Paola, and Gioia 2021).

People's support for policy was driven by the fact they were anxious about pandemics, more so than they would be about other risk events (Quigley, Bisset, and Mills 2017). As risk psychologists would anticipate, the high dread and unknown factors generated considerable anxiety. The threat was also magnified by a variety of social amplifiers, particularly the mainstream press. The media's role was indispensable in communicating important information to the public, scrutinizing government, and bringing attention to vulnerable populations. Media coverage was also alarming and divisive, more so than that of academic publications – although it is worth noting that many academics also published in popular media and made dramatic forecasts that turned out to be inaccurate. While media coverage was a concern for political offices, as indicated by Morneau, at times people felt that coverage was selective and exaggerated, which is consistent with traditional lay interpretation of the media (Edelman 2021, 25). The alarming nature of media coverage can cause both concern and skepticism.

By the end of 2022, anxiety levels had diminished considerably; people were generally much less concerned about the disease and its spread. Vaccinations and diagnostic tests were widely available. Many people had come to accept the residual risk. The drop in anxiety, however, did not necessarily correlate with case count. By February 2023, Nova Scotia, for example, was experiencing 3,310 new PCR-confirmed cases and 27 COVID-19–caused deaths per month, much higher than in 2020 when anxiety levels were at their highest, yet the case count in 2023 was hardly reported by the media or noticed by the public (Nova Scotia Department of Health and Wellness 2023).

Containing the disease was not just an individual responsibility but also a community one; collective action and shared responsibility were required. Costs for an individual may be disproportionate to the risk but necessary to protect the community. As noted in the control-mechanism section earlier in this chapter, this brings about the strengths and weaknesses of existing governance when it comes to egalitarian goals and raises important ethical considerations about what we owe to each other (C. Simpson 2022) and whether these questions should be left to individuals, communities, or governments to answer.

The rules were applied equally to many, but they were not experienced equally; this raises the possibility of strained alliances and factions. Older people, for example, were more likely to be in favour of health restrictions but less in favour of continuing government income-support programs, which disproportionately helped younger people. The middle-aged were the most likely to oppose health restrictions, which disproportionately benefited the elderly. The difference should not be overstated; the variation between age groups was not more than ten percentage points (Maru Blue 2021), but it does suggest a difference in demographic groups, which can lead to broader social divisions in addressing these issues. It is also a reminder that policy decisions frequently result in allocating resources to some groups over others. While the elderly were at higher risk of illness and death, many young people carried a disproportionate weight in other ways, from business, school, and daycare closures to mental health issues, for example. Their political priorities – climate change, social justice, housing – received less political and media attention. The middle-aged lost income during peak earning years. The imbalance between generations is not strictly a function of the different voting power of each group. It is also deeply embedded in cultural values about what constitutes a "good death" and a health system that focuses considerable effort on managing sickness and keeping people alive but struggles to reconcile what we spend on end-of-life care with what we should spend at different times to ensure a good life. Our low investments in public health compared to clinical health underscore this point.

The public was rightly concerned over the mistreatment if not outright neglect of many in LTC during the early stages of the pandemic. Media images of LTC residents were powerful not only because of the devastating circumstances due to the pandemic but also because of the images of many people as they approached the end of life, images that are rare and unsettling particularly in our current media culture (El-Bialy et al. 2022).

Public concern does not necessarily translate into government action. When the pandemic started, LTC facilities experienced high death counts. The episode revealed important weaknesses in the system, some of which have been detailed in one or several of 150 reports of long-term care since the start of Medicare in Canada (Picard 2021). By 2021, three-quarters of Canadians believed that the system needed an overhaul. There is also skepticism about the private sector's role in running LTC (Angus Reid Institute 2021b). Changes have been slow, and jurisdictional issues persist. In January 2023 the federal government introduced new voluntary standards for facilities, but there is no force of law, and the issue remains under provincial and territorial jurisdiction. On the day the guidelines were released, Ontario minister of long-term care Paul Calandra said that he would look at the guidelines but had "no interest in watering down what Ontario already has in place" (CBC News 2023a). Given the growing demand for and high expectations of LTC, it seems unlikely that the private sector's role will be reduced, particularly given the disposable income of many seniors.

While the public was greatly concerned about the pandemic, it is true that government tried to shape public opinion. Government needed to keep the public attentive and concerned to have them continue to follow mandates and strict directives. Governments accomplished this through extensive and relentless communications, typified by daily press briefings by the prime minister, premiers, and CMOs. Although government is not trusted by everyone in Canada, it is trusted by most (Edelman 2022). Trust in government, public health, and CMOs in particular helped governments implement standards successfully. This predisposition was particularly useful when government changed policies, as it did with masks, at first stating that masks did not help, then suggesting people wear one if they wished, and then finally mandating them. The complexity of the challenge did not always lend itself to short, simple media sound bites.

Government bureaucracies had a hard time accommodating different and competing views. Governments underestimated the number and significance of the vaccine-hesitant. In some respects, the views of the vaccine-hesitant did not seem rational: people with high levels of vulnerability throughout the pandemic were at times least likely to get vaccinated. These groups required targeted efforts that made a difference in First Nations and low-income neighbourhoods, for example, but government was slow both to recognize broader contextual issues shaping their views and to act to address them. Anti-vaxxers were a small group, about 8 per cent of the population, and could not be persuaded.

At a certain point more communication was not going to help. Although most agreed with government mandates, governments' positions became more precarious towards the end of 2021 and into early 2022. There was growing fatigue with the pandemic, sympathy for those who had lost their jobs, and evidence that Western governments as well as governments in Western Canada were starting to roll back measures (Rabson 2022; Malone 2022a, 2022b). In the same way that governments could not act before others at the start, they could not prolong standards as others ended theirs. As the risk became more ambiguous over costs and consequences, it became more overtly politicized; people gravitated towards the like-minded. In March 2022 when restrictions were winding down, opinion over government policies was divided along political lines. Among Conservatives, 84 per cent said Prime Minister Trudeau had done a bad or very bad job, while 88 per cent of Liberals said he had done a good or very good job (Boisvert 2022a). This polarization makes conflict more likely and the moderate middle-ground more elusive.

Interests: Insiders, Outsiders, and the Role of the State

Despite Parliament meeting much less often, between 2 March 2020 and 2 March 2021 there were 64 per cent more lobbyist communication reports compared to the previous year. Hiring skilled and well-connected lobbyists helped, as the film industry in Ontario discovered. Others, like big-box retailers, benefited from health regulations that allowed them to increase their market share at the expense of smaller competitors.

Like the other hypotheses, an interest group lens helps us detect important nuances to government response. Sectors that represent critical infrastructure have different characteristics, and they are important in understanding lobbying dynamics. Some sectors, like power supply, are often monopolies, and others, like banks and airlines, are oligopolies. There are significant regulatory barriers to market entry; benefits tend to be concentrated, and costs are highly dispersed. These companies are larger and well financed and have developed lobbying capacity and routines. Due to the nature of the services they provide, they cannot easily go out of business without significant disruption, and therefore governments take a keen interest in their stability. Companies like Air Canada knew this and were prepared to wait for government support. Most airlines in Western countries received support packages from their national governments (Rappeport and Chokshi 2020; Fife and Willis 2021; Alderman 2020; Karp 2020; Hurst and Butler 2020).

There are also critical infrastructure sectors predominantly composed of SMEs; any one business can fail and the economy is hardly affected. Most of these companies had to rely on general government-support programs to employers, like CEWS. Barriers to entry and exit are much lower. Trucking fits into this category. There are tens of thousands of trucking companies across Canada (Statistics Canada 2022q). There are some large organizations, but the vast majority are small, independent contractors. Any one business could fail, and it would have minimal impact when compared to banks and airlines. Much of the tourism sector outlined in chapter 8 is the same.

The limits to the trucking sector's power and organization provide some perspective on the Freedom Convoy. The truckers were not very well organized, nor did they understand government or lobbying, but they did receive extensive media coverage; the episode was initially framed as underdogs bound to take their message to Ottawa (Williams and Paperny 2022; F. MacDonald 2022). It became a crisis within the health crisis for government, with economic, security, and political dimensions. Some protesters presented a physical threat to citizens and public officials (Grant 2022), but the majority did not. Once it was clear they were causing economic disruption at the Ambassador Bridge, a key trade corridor that is privately owned and with few viable alternative routes (Brend 2022), the protesters were removed. It was harder for government to remove people from Ottawa due to jurisdictional complexity, disorganization, and inexperience with such an event. Although economic consequences are not identified in the Emergencies Act as a reason for invoking it, this was one of the reasons the government used to justify its action (C. Tunney 2022b). Finance Minister Chrystia Freeland described a call from the US secretary of state and meetings with executives from banks and the impact these interactions had on her decision to support invoking the Act. It was a glimpse into how power influences government decision making. At the same time, government's inability to engage with the protesters in a meaningful way, and in fact mocking them as a "fringe minority ... holding unacceptable views" (Rouleau 2023, 173), contributed to the instability. Although the episode ranged in appearance from a circus to an inconvenience to a bone fide security threat, the fact that many public health restrictions were dropped or reduced by March 2022 suggests that the frustration (if not the actions) of the protesters was not entirely at odds with public opinion or the overall policy direction in which public health was headed.

Finally, there is the role of interests working inside public institutions. Despite the important role of public servants, trust in these institutions declined, as we noted in chapter 11 (Edelman 2021, 2022, 2023). At times, anti-government rhetoric from a relatively small group became feverish and raised security concerns for politicians and policy-makers. The Freedom Convoy provided a high-profile platform for some of these views (Panneton 2022; Graham-Harrison and Lindeman 2022). Notably, CMO Dr Theresa Tam was accorded increased security during the pandemic, as were eight cabinet ministers (E. Thompson 2022).

Anti-government rhetoric is not new, although recent suspicions over the role of the state have been on the rise over the last eight years, perhaps most associated with some who support former US president Donald Trump and those who led the 6 January 2021 protests at the US Capitol Building (Pitcavage 2022; Kleinfeld 2022). There are growing concerns about the motivations of public servants, which some argue are more concerned with influence or advocacy (Galea 2023; Truss 2024). The more extreme views include conspiracy theories about unelected officials controlling the state. In comparison, this type of extremism has not been as openly pronounced in Canada (Perry and Scrivens 2016), though there has been a rise in extremist views in recent years (Carr 2022; McLeod 2022). In a polarized environment these extreme views can make it more challenging to raise questions about government performance. In cases like vaccines and vaccine mandates, and decisions to close businesses and schools, there were too often "yes/no" and "with us or against us" mindsets, with insufficient room for more nuanced discussions, which is necessary in order to address risks more successfully.

There are of course legitimate questions to ask about the performance of public health, particularly given that PHAC was created partly in response to SARS with the expectation that it would be better prepared to address the challenges of a pandemic. Bureau-shaping helps us focus on incentives and performance within bureaucracies but does not go so far as to disregard the role of political oversight. It recognizes that political overseers set limits on bureaucratic behaviours, and public servants work within those limits. The seventeen-year period between SARS and COVID-19 goes beyond any one elected government and prompts questions about the dynamics in the public service towards pandemic response and emergency management. While emergency response secures funds easily during a crisis, there is inadequate attention paid to it in other times; rather, the institutional behaviours at PHAC tended towards less operationally focused health promotion with sometimes opaque performance metrics.

Emergency response requires ongoing preparation to be successful. Once the pandemic had materialized, public health largely set the terms of the response, but there was insufficient accounting for why the response was initially slow and ill equipped to address the threat. In contrast to a conspiracy, this dynamic is the result of a system that rewards politicians and unelected officials for dramatic action in the face of a crisis but underestimates the more mundane operations, consistent care, and sometimes difficult choices that are necessary to address the possibility of such events in quieter times and with no clear time horizon.

FINAL THOUGHTS

Pandemics have been an issue for millennia, many contributing to the downfall of great societies (Ehrenreich 2020; Wazer 2016). Audits and studies in Canada have warned about pandemics for decades, and many organizations were tasked with addressing these challenges but had uneven success in doing so. After years of studies and recent early warnings through SARS and H1N1, we were forewarned but not forearmed.

With COVID-19, as with other prolonged crises, people are exhausted, fed up, and uneasy about mistakes in the response. Most people are grateful to be moving on. The fact that people can continue to look forward even after calamity is a powerful comment about their resiliency. There is also very little political payoff for looking back. By living through it, people have changed their way of thinking about it and could not easily go back to an earlier, less informed perspective. They have also come to realize the difficult trade-offs required with these types of problems – the "wicked problems" (Churchman 1967) – and so they move their gaze to the next big thing (Downs 1967).

While there are concerns about pandemic revisionism (Murdoch and Caulfield 2023), studies with insights are emerging. A review of COVID-19 responses from twenty-eight countries, not including Canada, highlights the interdependence of health and other policy areas and emphasizes the importance of the broader social and economic context that must be considered. The authors emphasize a need to "[activate] comprehensive responses, which are responses that address health and well-being as intertwined with social and economic considerations" (Haldane et al. 2021, 978). In other words, crises do not respect bureaucratic lines of responsibility. The recommendations underscore the broad approach that governments and indeed society at large must take to understand and respond to a pandemic.

There is no guarantee that public agencies will learn the right lessons. Cultural theorists warn that organizations will only learn lessons that reinforce the organizational culture, not challenge it. Douglas (2001, 145) notes: "Certainty is only possible because doubt is blocked institutionally: most individual decisions about risk are taken under pressure from institutions." Health is a large policy domain with many entrenched interests. Insofar as public health is an expert-led bureaucratic enterprise, as is the auditing of it, post-mortems are likely to reinforce bureaucratic tendencies. This leaves public health and other public agencies at risk of repeating the mistakes of the past. A far-reaching post-mortem that goes beyond public health to examine risk governance is required.

Such an inquiry can help us think about future crises. Can anyone imagine what a large-scale cyber failure would look like, or how we could respond? How a tsunami on the west coast of Canada could overwhelm Vancouver? Experts have studied these questions for decades. If these events were to take place, should we really be surprised? And yet, would we be ready? While it is common to refer to the "climate crisis," action on climate change is slow, with much longer time frames than the pandemic had, which renders accountability even more opaque. Experts predicted a 9/11 event years before 9/11; the US government's inability to mobilize resources and prepare for such an event was famously called a failure of imagination (National Commission on Terrorist Attacks 2004).

At the time of our writing this book, it is hard to use the word *crisis* without thinking about the pandemic. In some respects, governments showed us throughout the pandemic that they can act with speed, force, and conviction. How then should we apply this power?

When we consider the three types of risk from the International Risk Governance Council's framework that we addressed in this book – complex, uncertain, and ambiguous – important issues emerge from COVID-19 that require urgent and sustained attention from government. With respect to complex risks, some politicians were persuaded by COVID-19 of the importance of a reliable scientific community (Borins 2020); this commitment to science needs to continue. Scientists, however, do not get a free pass. They need to continue to earn the trust of the citizenry. Trust depends on being open, knowledgeable, and concerned. Generally, scientists score well in these areas, but important fault lines came to light. First, openness in addressing complex risks is not merely a question of making data available for re-examination by others. It requires a capacity to communicate science and its limitations effectively to policy-makers and lay people. Policy-makers in turn need to be more transparent about how they use science to inform policy. Second, with regard to knowledge, the pandemic demonstrated that experts and lay people have access to a plethora of local to international data in real time, but developing useful knowledge requires accessing the right data at the right time and interpreting it appropriately. This was constrained not simply by the complexity of disease transmission but also by limitations in governance. At times, there were failures. China did not share information. South Africa shared information about new variants and was isolated by other countries for it. The US was slow to react, and its elected leaders politicized the interpretation of the science and government response. The usefulness of the UN was undermined by these dynamics. Social-media echo chambers amplified conspiracy theories with inadequate responses. Canada's federal, provincial, and territorial governance impeded information sharing and collective learning. It struggled to identify more efficient and reliable ways to share information across jurisdictions. Finally, with respect to concern, most would agree that scientists and policy leaders were concerned about disease transmission. Over time, however, the challenges became so far reaching that some people doubted whether leaders shared their concerns, which went beyond COVID-19 to other health, social, economic, and ideological issues. More expertise from more disciplines including the social sciences can help to frame issues more broadly and thereby make us more sensitive to them earlier. How we frame the issue and how we gather relevant data also raise insights into how to address ambiguous risks, which we will discuss in more detail.

With respect to uncertain risks, governments need to develop adaptive capacity, guard against consequential and cascading failures, and identify trade-offs and weaknesses in responses, including their own. Bureaucracies are premised on a command-and-control dynamic, but increasingly public servants need tools and skills that allow them to anticipate, address, and communicate risks that are global in reach and highly personalized in impact and over which they have limited control. They have to have a greater appreciation for the context that shapes government response, by seizing opportunities and reducing vulnerabilities within it.

Governments also need to have a better understanding of our willingness and capacity to tolerate uncertain risk. Various psychological and economic dimensions of the threat made it clear that there was neither one view of risk nor one measure of risk tolerance. We need to be sensitive to the psychological phenomena that cause over- and under-reaction to risk events, and to work to reduce their impact. We also need to acknowledge that people have different views and vulnerabilities, and our collective response must be aware of them and manage different groups with some sensitivity about diverse views and expectations. This is a challenge for bureaucratic agencies.

Precaution over precision and prioritization can be necessary when there are such high levels of uncertainty and the consequences are potentially catastrophic or irreversible, but precautionary approaches are nervous by nature and resource intensive and need to be used sparingly, with clear rationales and in a time-limited manner. Inevitably, they direct resources and attention away from other important policy areas. In an effort to have a stable response in one policy area, we create instability in other areas. Sometimes those trade-offs are experienced immediately, but they can also be deferred unwittingly to a future date and generation.

Uncertain risks can lend themselves to dire forecasts. Despite anxieties about social media and protesters, we need to allow people to be skeptical and questioning. Increasing polarization leads to a type of "with us or against us" reasoning; we need more tolerance for reasoned debate in the grey areas. Democratic institutions should be scrutinized constructively during crises as well as in anticipation of them; elected officials need to hold these institutions and those who lead them to account, not to acquiesce in the name of unusual circumstances. Practically and figuratively, we cannot simply close borders; we have to be clear eyed about the risks to which we expose ourselves and prepare to adapt and cooperate with like-minded jurisdictions in light of global threats and with a greater sense of global justice (Borins 2020). We cannot rally around the concept of solidarity at home and then leave poor countries behind; it exposes the hypocrisy and fragility of the claim.

In the same way that uncertain risk can lead to fear, anxiety, and over- and under-reaction, ambiguous risk can lead to anything from neglect to antagonism to stalemate; how it is addressed can depend on how power is distributed in society. If there were another similar pandemic, when the proportion of elderly people were even greater, the cost of a precautionary stance would be greater. If the burden continues to fall disproportionately on vulnerable members of society, then we have to accept the injustice, inadequacy, and instability inherent in our collective response.

Like the virus itself, poverty and social injustice are pervasive yet invisible to many of us. The pandemic brought inequalities and suffering into sharp focus, from the poor to the neglected elderly to marginalized racial groups. These inequalities predated the pandemic and continue today. To provide greater stability during a crisis, we need to furnish more than funding for public bureaucracies as well as an expanded organizational design. Those responsible for policy require a greater appreciation of the ambiguity in risks; they need to commit to a governance process that tries harder to understand ambiguities and address them in a fair and inclusive manner. This requires greater effort in clarifying and reconciling the epistemological challenges at the heart of risk governance, distinguishing between uncertainty and ambiguity for instance, instilling compassion in government response, and affording dignity to those who are subject to it.

Emergency response deceives us with its name. It is not something we do in a moment. Diseases can kill and debilitate; how we anticipate and respond is up to us. A crisis is a product of governance and social and economic context. The solutions require ongoing collaborative, ethical, and democratic processes, an informed public, and different types of organizational design, from markets to NGOs to networks, to ready ourselves for these challenges. Containment and control as a strategy sits comfortably within a rationalist bureaucratic paradigm, but it is slow, expensive, selective in its focus, and dangerous in its own way; it must be applied carefully and with scrutiny.

Indeed, the pandemic emphasizes the increasingly ambiguous nature of Beck's risk society. While there was often broad agreement among Canadians about pandemic policy, as more information became available the episode revealed public agencies that struggled with interpreting diverse contexts, establishing standards, and engaging in debate and with dissension. Despite their best efforts, governments had blind spots in their response that took them too long to acknowledge and address in a polycentric society that is increasingly ill suited to bureaucratic control. The pandemic did not cause these problems in governance; it merely revealed them.

Methods

This book is an analytical compilation of data we collected and observations we made about Canada's response to the COVID-19 pandemic from its beginning in January 2020 until the end of March 2022. The objective of our work has been to describe the control mechanisms that the federal, provincial, and territorial governments enacted to contain the pandemic, using a cybernetic definition of control, which includes information gathering, standard setting, and behaviour modification. We applied Hood, Rothstein, and Baldwin's (2001) risk regulation regimes framework, which emphasizes social and economic context for studying regulatory responses, including markets, law and insurance, media, polling data, and the role of organized interests. Although most of our research focused on the first two years of the pandemic (1 January 2020 to 31 March 2022), our research necessarily extended to several years before COVID-19.

We conducted secondary research and applied a mixed-methods approach to our data collection and analysis. For our quantitative research and analysis we consulted numerous reports and data sets from Statistics Canada and other government resources, including federal, provincial, and territorial economic and COVID-19 data. We also consulted sources such as Yahoo Finance to collect and track changes in the share values and the revenues of Canadian and global companies throughout the pandemic. In our qualitative research we reviewed a combination of academic literature, including risk governance literature and studies on previous pandemics, and media sources, particularly CBC News, the New York Times, the Globe and Mail, and the Economist. Data on the COVID-19 pandemic have been updated over time, including case numbers and fatality information.

The majority of data used in this work was collected by the end of September 2022; reports published after September 2022 may have slightly different data from the data in this book owing to updates and reporting adjustments.

COVID-19 DATA COLLECTION

We collected research about the COVID-19 pandemic in real time between March 2020 and September 2022 and focused our analysis on the period between January 2020 and 31 March 2022.[1] We looked to reputable sources during our research and analysis, including official government and NGO publications, statistics, audits, high-quality broadsheet media, and academic literature. Key sources included Statistics Canada; Our World in Data; the Public Health Agency of Canada; academic literature such as peer-reviewed journal articles; federal, provincial, and territorial government websites, press releases, and publications, including those of public health agencies and legislative assemblies; along with websites, press releases, and publications produced by the World Health Organization and various NGOs. We also referred to media publications from the *Globe and Mail*, the *New York Times,* and CBC *News*. Due to the changing nature of the virus and governments' responses, we checked sources frequently and updated our research regularly. We have also included the most up-to-date information unless our analysis refers to knowledge from a specific time, which we have specified within chapters.

We used media, government, and NGO sources to describe key events throughout the pandemic, including governments' policy decisions. We conducted some statistical analysis to discuss broad trends and context at different times, including calculating percentage change over time and per capita, using Microsoft Excel. *Coronavirus,* COVID-*19, testing, contact tracing, enforcement, behaviour,* PPE, *public health,* ICU, *standards, legislation,* and *healthcare* were among the key terms we used while conducting research. While we relied primarily on Canadian data, some international data were used, including data from the US and the UK.

Overall, tracking and compiling data on COVID-19 in real time was challenging. Throughout the first two years of the pandemic, provinces' and territories' reporting on COVID-19 changed from daily updates to weekly and monthly ones. Governments also refined their statistical reporting methods over time, which required us to be specific about and make connections between datasets.

MEDIA ANALYSIS

In our media analysis (chapter 10) we focused on three Canadian publications or media sources: *Toronto Star*, *National Post*, and CBC *News*. We selected 1 July 2019 to 30 June 2020 – the last six months of 2019 and the first six months of 2020 – as the central date range for our analysis. This time frame allowed us to examine how COVID-19 affected media coverage. Specifically, we compared media coverage of issues leading up to and following the 2019 federal election to the onset of the pandemic. We subsequently expanded our scope to March 2022 to align with the book's focus on the first two years of COVID-19.

We accumulated articles using the database NexisUni, focusing on the front section of the news. We used a qualitative approach to identify our media search terms, which included tracking terms commonly used by the media in our selected date ranges and unstructured discussions among the research team. Polling data on Canadians' priorities going into the 2019 federal election, such as pharmacare and climate change, also helped us identify media search terms.

When determining the ratio of COVID-19 coverage from a health perspective versus an economic perspective, we used the two search terms *COVID-19 and health* and *COVID-19 and economy*. Subsequently we narrowed our search using specific health- and economy-related terms to determine the extent of media coverage of other issues, such as mental health and unemployment.

To understand whether political bias played a role in which topics were covered by different media outlets, we compared the use of key terms in the *National Post*'s and the *Toronto Star*'s coverage of COVID-19. Overall, coverage of the health, social, and COVID-19–specific terms varied little between the two newspapers. While mentions of most terms were largely the same, there were some exceptions. The *National Post* referred to the Freedom Convoy about 1.7 times more often than the *Toronto Star* did. The *National Post* also referred to economic terms, such as *unemployment* and *debt*, more often than the *Toronto Star* did.

In accordance with the opinion-responsive hypothesis, polling data were also part of our research and analysis. We focused on examining how people's attitudes towards different topics aligned with what happened and how they changed over time. Leger (in partnership with the Association for Canadian Studies and Canadian Press), Edelman, Ipsos, and Maru Blue were the key sources we consulted while examining public opinion polling.

BUREAU-SHAPING

We examined and applied the bureau-shaping model in chapter 11. To start, we examined academic literature on public choice theory, primarily focused on Dunleavy's bureau-shaping argument. Looking at budgets, we used data from the Canadian Institute for Health Information to discern how public health budgets compared to overall health expenditures. We also relied on corporate management reporting from the Public Health Agency of Canada. We looked at evaluation reports and internal audits but mostly used information from departmental results reports. We examined available departmental results reports, starting in 2006–07 and ending in 2021–22, to examine trends in spending leading up to and throughout the COVID-19 pandemic. In these reports we looked at the spending for core responsibilities related to emergency management and health promotion. To create the figures in the chapter, we used the data of "actual spending (authorities used)" (as opposed to "planned spending" or "total authorities available for use"). We also noted any reasons given in the reports for drastic changes in spending in certain years. This sometimes related to pandemic spending (e.g., H1N1); at other times it pertained to certain programs beginning or ending that had a significant effect on budgets.

Next, we accessed publicly available reports from the chief public health officer since 2008 to see the extent to which infectious disease, pandemic preparedness, and emergency response were addressed. We did this by searching the documents for key terms, such as *pandemic*, *epidemic*, and *emergency*, and by examining any hits more closely. We examined audits after health crises since the early 2000s published by Health Canada, the Auditor General of Canada, and PHAC to determine which problems within the organization had been raised repeatedly. We also looked at federal reports about the COVID-19 response published in 2021. In addition to Government of Canada websites, we relied on media reporting for information about the National Emergency Strategic Stockpile and the Global Public Health Intelligence Network. For PHAC's role in the early stages of the pandemic, we looked for reporting from sources such as the *Globe and Mail* and CBC News published between December 2019 and early March 2020.

THE LOBBY REGISTRY

Registration in the context of federal lobbying is defined as the legal requirement, when one or more employees who represent clients and communicate with public office holders, to report these activities as per subsection 5 (1) of the Lobbying Act (Government of Canada 2008). Registrants are defined as the individuals or lobbyists identified in registrations who conduct these activities or who are accountable for the activities of other junior lobbyists (Registry of Lobbyists 2022a).

Monthly communication reports are defined as mandatory reports that detail "each oral and arranged communication with a designated public office holder" and include the name of the most senior registrant and other registrants who conducted direct communication, as required (Registry of Lobbyists 2022a, sec. 2). These reports document individual communications and identify the general subject matter of communications (e.g., housing) but do not provide specific details of the communication.

Measurement of the quantity of lobbyist registrations and monthly communication reports was conducted using the Registry of Lobbyists' dashboard. This dashboard has an internal database search function to refine results by specific dates and, for registrations, specific submission types (e.g., new registrations). Fifteen total searches were conducted using the "recent registrations" and "recent monthly communication reports" dashboard tools to find total results posted in specific time periods. The time periods for the searches were 1 March 2019 to 1 March 2020; 2 March 2020 to 2 March 2021; and 14 March 2020 to 22 September 2020 (a period of COVID-19–related parliamentary closure; Parliament of Canada, n.d.). Registration searches were filtered to identify the three subcategories of registrations within the reported totals: new registrations, updated registrations, and reactivations. Quantitative totals were produced directly from the website.

Years of Life Lost to COVID-19 Compared to World Wars

Table A.2

	Average age of death during event	Life expectancy for a person who has survived to the average age of death for the event	Estimated Canadian lives lost during event	Estimated total years lost
COVID-19 (March 2020– 2 April 2022)	84	89	37,722	188,610
First World War (1914–18)	25	63*	61,000	2,318, 000
Second World War (1939–45)	26*	68*	45,400	1,906, 800

*American data used instead of Canadian data.

The total years of lives lost refers specifically to military lives lost and not total civilian lives lost. The fatality totals used include Canadian lives lost and do not include total lives lost on both sides of the conflict (e.g., Germans). Canadian data are primarily used; however, the average life expectancy at the age of death is from American data.

Average age of death for soldiers in the Second World War is from American data. Average years of life lost is calculated using the average life expectancy at age of death, and not life expectancy from birth (Statistics Canada 2021).

Years of Life Lost to COVID-19
Compared to Road Fatalities

Table A.3

	Average age of death during event	Life expectancy for a person who has survived to the average age of death for the event	Estimated total lives lost during time frame	Estimated total years of life lost
COVID-19 (2020)	84	89	16,151	80,755 years lost
COVID-19 (March 2020– 2 April 2022)	84	89	37,722	188,610 years lost
Vehicle-related fatalities (2019)	50	81	1,762	60,387 years lost
Vehicle-related fatalities (2018 and 2019)	50	81	3,701	128,562 years lost
Vehicle-related fatalities (2009–19)	50	81	21,689	642,810 years lost*

*Average years of life lost between 2018 and 2019 used to estimate total years of life lost.

The total years lost were calculated using the average age of death for each listed age group for road fatalities multiplied by the number of deaths for that specific age group, except for the age group over the age of sixty-five, where the age of seventy-seven is used as the average age of death because it is a halfway point between the age of sixty-five and the average age of life-expectancy at time of death (eighty-nine years old) (Transport Canada 2021). The years lost in Canada were calculated using average life expectancy at each age interval (Statistics Canada 2021l). For the estimated total of lives lost between 2009 and 2019, the average years of life lost between 2018 and 2019 is used to estimate the total years of life lost (noted with *).

We used Transport Canada data to determine an average age of death for road fatalities. Over the past ten years, vehicle-related deaths have occurred more often among people between thirty-five and sixty-four years old, but the margin is small between people aged thirty-five to sixty-four, and zero to thirty-four.

These data include fatalities and not serious injuries, and approximately 50 per cent of deaths occur among drivers (Transport Canada 2021). It should be noted that before the pandemic, 2019 had the the greatest number of recorded vehicle-related fatalities. Data from 2018 were also used to compare estimated average years of life lost between COVID-19 and road fatalities, rather than the 2019 data.

There is a noted discrepancy in the data. The reported total deaths for 2018 were listed in 2018 data from Transport Canada as 1,922. This was updated to 1,939 total fatalities in 2019, so the total 1,939 number is used for total deaths in 2018.

Consumer Purchases at Retail (× 1,000) by Category (2019–21)

Purchases of cannabis products, sporting and leisure products, and hardware tools at retail increased the most in 2020 compared to 2019. Vehicle-related sales, clothing, jewellery, and luggage had significant increases between 2020 and 2021.

Table A.4

North American Product Classification System (NAPCS) Canada 2017 version	Total 2019 (C$)	Total 2020 (C$)	Total 2021 (C$)	Change 2019–20 (%)	Change 2020–21 (%)
Total commodities, retail trade commissions, and miscellaneous services	616,544,409	608,330,375	680,101,033	–1.33	11.80
Food, at retail	109,135,750	120,785,089	122,141,744	10.67	1.12
Soft drinks and alcoholic beverages, at retail	36,146,805	38,977,254	40,203,374	7.83	3.15
Cannabis products, at retail	1,189,951	2,613,217	3,834,766	119.61	46.75
Clothing, at retail	31,105,010	23,561,500	27,729,947	–24.25	17.69
Footwear, at retail	7,467,167	5,859,334	6,690,428	–21.53	14.18
Jewellery and watches, luggage and briefcases, at retail	5,047,880	3,856,117	4,844,159	–23.61	25.62
Home furniture, furnishings, housewares, appliances and electronics, at retail	52,506,123	56,052,824	59,538,725	6.75	6.22
Sporting and leisure products (except publications, audio and video recordings, and game software), at retail	10,763,378	12,773,741	14,620,623	18.68	14.46
Publications, at retail	3,054,472	2,410,919	2,143,967	–21.07	–11.07
Audio and video recordings, and game software, at retail	1,236,449	921,987	805,835	–25.43	–12.60
Motor vehicles, at retail	128,452,848	114,326,178	136,081,950	–11.00	19.03

Table A.4 continued

North American Product Classification System (NAPCS) Canada 2017 version	Total 2019 (C$)	Total 2020 (C$)	Total 2021 (C$)	Change 2019–20 (%)	Change 2020–21 (%)
Recreational vehicles, at retail	8,952,625	10,166,337	11,765,752	13.56	15.73
Motor vehicle parts, accessories and supplies, at retail	23,083,628	22,850,970	26,826,316	–1.01	17.40
Automotive and household fuels, at retail	53,179,877	40,535,410	54,453,737	–23.78	34.34
Home health products, at retail	39,071,914	40,243,054	43,461,291	3.00	8.00
Infant care, personal and beauty products, at retail	14,152,553	14,291,710	14,938,190	0.98	4.52
Hardware, tools, and renovation and lawn and garden products, at retail	43,432,524	49,169,339	56,722,305	13.21	15.36
Miscellaneous products, at retail	28,726,022	29,754,803	31,382,572	3.58	5.47
Total retail trade commissions and miscellaneous services	19,839,432	19,180,592	21,915,350	–3.32	14.26

Light-shaded cells represent categories where purchases at retail increased between 2019 and 2020; dark-shaded cells represent categories where purchases at retail decreased. *Source:* Statistics Canada 2021n.

Notes

INTRODUCTION

1 Data on the COVID-19 pandemic have been updated over time, including cases and fatality information. The majority of the data was collected by the end of September 2022; some data points may be updated in subsequent reporting. See further comments in the introduction and appendix 1 for more information about methods.

2 Unless otherwise noted, all dollar amounts refer to Canadian dollars.

3 Formal testing refers to polymerase chain reaction (PCR) and antigen testing. It does not capture those who tested positive on a home test and did not report the case or have a PCR test to confirm the case.

4 Organ transplants are a different issue. For example, smokers are generally not listed for heart transplantation until they have stopped smoking for six months (Canadian Cardiac Transplant Network 2011, 5).

CHAPTER ONE

1 Inanimate objects capable of transmitting viruses or infections between individuals are referred to as "fomites" (Goldman 2020). Examples include doorknobs, railings, and clothing.

2 Provisional figures at the national, provincial, and territorial levels were not available for December 2021 and onwards at the time of writing. The true numbers of deaths attributed to certain causes may be underrepresented due to lengthy investigations to determine cause of death and related reporting delays.

3 Social and structural determinants of health refer to the economic and social conditions that influence differences in health status (e.g., race, gender, income).

CHAPTER TWO

1 Provisional figures at the national, provincial, and territorial levels were not available for December 2021 and onwards at the time of writing. True numbers of deaths attributed to certain causes may be under-represented due to lengthy investigations to determine cause of death and related reporting delays.
2 Herd immunity occurs when the majority of people in a community develop immunity, or protection, against a contagious virus or disease.
3 Hood's (1998) book won the 1998 Mackenzie Book Prize for the best book in political science.
4 University of Toronto Joint Centre for Bioethics' Pandemic Influenza Working Group (2005, 6–7).

CHAPTER THREE

1 Government of Manitoba, n.d.; Government of New Brunswick, n.d.; Office of the Premier of New Brunswick 2020a; Government of Quebec, n.d.; Government of Newfoundland and Labrador, n.d.; Provincial Laboratory Services 2020; Government of Northwest Territories 2022; Government of Prince Edward Island 2022.

CHAPTER FOUR

1 New Brunswick was the first province to hold an election in September 2020 (Garnett et al. 2021).
2 The provincial election in Newfoundland and Labrador was held in March 2021.

CHAPTER FIVE

1 While the data are still limited and preliminary, rates for cardiovascular disease increased in Canada between 2018 and 2022. Crude rates for cardiac care across Canada increased from 2.3 (2013–16) to 2.4 (2018–21) (CIHI 2017, 2022a).

2 The *World Happiness Report* is published by the Sustainable Development Solutions Network, powered by the Gallup World Poll data. The *World Happiness Report* reflects a worldwide demand for more attention to happiness and well-being as criteria for government policy. It reviews the state of happiness in the world today and shows how the science of happiness explains personal and national variations in happiness.

3 Economic impacts of poor mental health and mental illness include employer costs (e.g., absenteeism, presenteeism, employee turnover), private and public disability insurance costs, costs of public income support and social programs, lost tax revenue due to unemployment and underemployment, and costs incurred by caregivers (MHCC 2017). Care for dementia accounts for most of the spending for mental-health-care services. Total public and private non-dementia-related direct costs for mental-health care and supports in 2015 were estimated at $23.8 billion (MHCC 2017).

4 Crisis Services Canada is a network of existing distress, crisis, and suicide prevention services across the country.

5 Alcohol-induced deaths relate to diseases and conditions from the over-consumption of alcohol, and not unintentional deaths such as vehicle-related accidents.

6 Remaining travellers are categorized as "other travellers," including transportation crews.

7 The WE Charity scandal was a Canadian political scandal in 2020 involving a contract from the federal government to the WE Charity to administer the $912 million Canada Student Service Grant program. Financial and personal connections between the WE Charity and Prime Minister Trudeau, Finance Minister Bill Morneau, and their families were revealed and spurred controversy when neither Trudeau nor Morneau recused himself from the decision to award the contract to WE (J. Murphy 2020).

CHAPTER EIGHT

1 "Subjective well-being refers to how people experience and evaluate their lives and specific domains and activities in their lives" (National Research Council 2013, 15).

2 "Natural capital includes land, beaches, coastal and marine areas, national parks, rivers, etc." (UNWTO 2018, 19).

3 Monthly communication reports are defined as mandatory reports that detail each oral and arranged communication with a designated public

office holder and include the name of the most senior registrant and other registrants who conducted direct communication, as required (Registry of Lobbyists 2022a).

4 The financial year ended on 31 August 2019.

5 Close to 50 per cent of the 110,000 businesses that closed across Canadian industries in March and April 2020 had reopened by August 2020. Therefore, businesses that reopened by December 2020 were typically not included in the total number of business closures (Lafrance-Cooke 2021, 6).

CHAPTER NINE

1 Supply chain issues, including material and worker shortages and disruptions in transportation, continued throughout 2020, 2021, and into 2022. Experts predict that supply chain problems could persist for several years (Farrer 2021).

2 House prices continued to increase throughout 2021, setting a record in December 2021 when they were up by 26.6 per cent from the previous year (Younglai 2022).

3 Pharmaceuticals, mental health services, and non-medically-necessary LTC services are among those that are not publicly funded. Since the 1960s, some physicians in Canada have worked in privately owned and operated practices through fee-for-service payment arrangements with provincial governments. They have considerable autonomy over how, where, when, and what they practise, making physicians, in a sense, private agents working in a largely public system (McKay et al. 2022).

4 This amount is based on official reports and most likely under-represents the real total.

5 These data are derived from the AWCBC's National Work/Injury Disease Statistics Program, which includes data for twenty major industrial groups (2021b, 1–2).

6 Enforcement authorities in Alberta, Saskatchewan, and the territories cannot issue fines for Quarantine Act offences.

CHAPTER TEN

1 *Senior residences, assisted living, seniors' homes, nursing homes*, and *retirement homes* are other related terms included in the search on LTC.

2 The terms *gay* and *queer* were also included in the media search.

3 *Guaranteed basic income* is a related term included in the search.

CHAPTER ELEVEN

1 In some situations public health does have a decision-making role, for example, by licensing food producers and distributors (a provincial and territorial responsibility) or setting standards and regulations related to food safety, a responsibility of Health Canada.

2 These public health expenditures are made for disease-prevention and health-promotion activities, community mental health and addictions services, and occupational health services to promote and enhance health and safety in the workplace (CIHI 2020c). Financial support of activities related to food and water safety are not included in health budgets.

3 PHAC's responsibilities for health security include such activities as inspecting Canadian laboratories, acquiring antiviral drugs for the NESS, and responding to notifications regarding ill travellers. Border security and related costs also fall under the mandate of the CBSA, with PHAC providing guidance in some areas.

4 The US and the UK were ranked first and second, respectively.

5 This action was taken even though the federal pandemic plan used during H1N1 was predicated on an assumption that the next pandemic would most likely emerge from Asia (Sharon 2009).

APPENDIX ONE

1 In many cases 2 April 2022 is used because it is the closest reporting date to 31 March 2022.

References

Abdullah, M.M.H., C.P.F. Marinangeli, P.J.H. Jones, and J.G. Carlberg. 2017. "Canadian Potential Healthcare and Societal Cost Savings from Consumption of Pulses: A Cost-of-Illness Analysis." *Nutrients* 9 (7): 793–815. http://dx.doi.org/10.3390/nu9070793.

Abraham, J., and S. Plowman. 2021. "Dalhousie Considers Suspension, Students Apologize after Police Ticket 22 for 'Large Social Gathering.'" CTV News, 26 April 2021. https://atlantic.ctvnews.ca/dalhousie-considers-suspension-students-apologize-after-police-ticket-22-for-large-social-gathering-1.5400848.

Adam, D. 2020. "Special Report: The Simulations Driving the World's Response to COVID-19." *Nature*, 3 April 2020. https://doi.org/10.1038/d41586-020-01003-6.

Adams, J. 1995. *Risk*. London: UCL Press.

Adecco. 2020. "COVID-19 and the Effect on the Manufacturing Sector." https://www.adecco.ca/en-ca/blog/covid-19-and-the-effect-on-the-manufacturing-sector.

Adriano, L. 2020. "Canadian Home Insurance Companies Saved over $1 Billion in 2020 – Study." *Insurance Business Canada*, 2 December 2020. https://www.insurancebusinessmag.com/ca/news/breaking-news/canadian-home-insurance-companies-saved-over-1-billion-in-2020--study-240827.aspx.

Ahsan, S. 2021. "Isn't It Time We Had Data on the Health of BIPOC in Canada?" *Healthing*, 6 December 2021. https://www.healthing.ca/wellness/isnt-it-time-we-knew-how-bipoc-communities-interact-with-the-healthcare-system.

Aiello, R. 2020. "The Challenge of Our Lifetime: Federal Deficit to Hit $343 Billion This Year." CTV News, 8 July 2020. https://www.ctvnews.ca/politics/the-challenge-of-our-lifetime-federal-deficit-to-hit-343-billion-this-year-1.5015467.

– 2021. "Vaccine Mandate Coming to House of Commons, MPs Rule." CTV News, 19 October 2021. https://www.ctvnews.ca/politics/vaccine-mandate-coming-to-house-of-commons-mps-rule-1.5629447.

Aiello, R., and J. Forani. 2020. "'V-Day': First COVID-19 Vaccines Administered in Canada." CTV News, 14 December 2020. https://www.ctvnews.ca/health/coronavirus/v-day-first-covid-19-vaccines-administered-in-canada-1.5230184.

Air Canada. 2020. "Air Canada Discontinues Service on 30 Domestic Regional Routes and Closes Eight Stations in Canada." 30 June 2020. https://aircanada.mediaroom.com/2020-06-30-Air-Canada-Discontinues-Service-on-30-Domestic-Regional-Routes-and-Closes-Eight-Stations-in-Canada.

– 2021a. "Air Canada and Government of Canada Conclude Agreements on Liquidity Program." 12 April 2020. https://aircanada.mediaroom.com/2021-04-12-Air-Canada-and-Government-of-Canada-Conclude-Agreements-on-Liquidity-Program.

– 2021b. Air Canada Reports 2020 Annual Results. https://www.aircanada.com/content/dam/aircanada/portal/documents/PDF/en/quarterly-result/2020/2020_q4_release.pdf.

Alberta Court of Appeal. 2020. "Notice – COVID-19 – Electronic Hearing Procedural Information Notice." 8 April 2020. https://www.albertacourts.ca/ca/publications/announcements/notice---electronic-hearings.

Alderman, L. 2020. "Air France-KLM Gets €10 Billion Bailout as Coronavirus Hits Travel." New York Times, 25 April 2020. https://www.nytimes.com/2020/04/25/business/air-france-klm-bailout.html.

Aldrich, D.P. 2013. "A Normal Accident or a Sea-change? Nuclear Host Communities Respond to the 3/11 Disaster." Japanese Journal of Political Science 14 (2): 261–76. https://doi.org/10.1017/S1468109913000066.

Alhakami, A.S., and P. Slovic. 1994. "A Psychological Study of the Inverse Relationship between Perceived Risk and Perceived Benefit." Risk Analysis 14 (6): 1085–96.

Alini, E. 2021. "'The Universe Has Really Expanded.' How 3 Small Businesses Pivoted in the Pandemic." Global News, 17 March 2021. https://globalnews.ca/news/7664743/canadian-small-business-pivot-covid-19-pandemic.

Allen, D.W. 2021. "Covid Lockdown Cost/Benefits: A Critical Assessment of the Literature." https://www.sfu.ca/~allen/LockdownReport.pdf.

Allen, K. 2020. "Ontario Received 100,000 Contaminated, Unusable Swabs for COVID-19 Tests." Toronto Star, 10 April 2020. https://www.thestar.com/news/canada/2020/04/10/ontario-received-100000-contaminated-unusable-swabs-for-covid-19-tests.html.

Allin, S., T. Fitzpatrick, G. Marchildon, and A. Quesnel-Vallée. 2022. "The Federal Government and Canada's COVID-19 Responses: From 'We're Ready, We're Prepared' to 'Fires are Burning.'" *Health Economics, Policy and Law* 17 (1): 76–94. https://doi.org/10.1017/S1744133121000220.

Allin, S., G. Marchildon, and S. Merkur, 2021. *Health Systems in Transition: Canada.* 3rd edition. Toronto: University of Toronto Press. https://doi.org/10.3138/9781487537517.

Al Mallees, N. 2022. "WestJet Airlines to Acquire Sunwing." CBC News, 2 March 2022. https://www.cbc.ca/news/business/westjet-sunwing-acquisition-1.6370021.

Alper, A. 2020. "Trump Says U.S. in 'Great Shape' with Plan for Coronavirus." Reuters, 22 January 2020. https://www.reuters.com/article/us-davos-meeting-trump-coronavirus-idUSKBN1ZL13C.

Altman, M.J. 2020. "Q&A with Dr Peter Hotez: Behind the Scenes of COVID-19 Vaccine Research." United Nations Foundation, 15 May 2020. https://unfoundation.org/blog/post/qa-with-dr-peter-hotez-behind-the-scenes-of-covid-19-vaccine-research.

Alves, J.P., C. Eusébio, M.J. Carneiro, L. Teixeira, and S. Mesquita. 2023. "Living in an Untouchable World: Barriers to Recreation and Tourism for Portuguese Blind People during the COVID-19 Pandemic." *Journal of Outdoor Recreation and Tourism* 42: 100637. https://doi.org/10.1016/j.jort.2023.100637.

Amin, F., and M. Bond. 2020. "Nurses, PSWs Leaving Health Care Industry amid COVID-19 Pandemic." CityNews Toronto, 22 September 2020. https://toronto.citynews.ca/2020/09/22/nurses-psws-leaving-health-care-industry-amid-covid-19-pandemic.

Anderson, B. 2021. "2.4 Million Are Vaccine 'Maybes,' Another 2.4 Million Say 'No.' More than 5 Million Doubt the Second Shot is Essential." Abacus Data, 21 July 2021. https://abacusdata.ca/second-shot-faster-together-vaccine.

Anderson, M., H. Angus, R. Steele, and D. Cole. 2020. "Temporary Pause on Transitioning Hospital Patients to Long-Term Care and Retirement Homes." Government of Ontario, 15 April 2020. https://www.oha.com/Bulletins/DMs%20memo%20hospital%20transfers%20v3%20(2020-04-15).pdf.

Anderssen, E. 2022. "Two Weeks in the Life of Ottawans Trapped by the Convoy's Chaos." *Globe and Mail*, 13 February 2022. https://www.theglobeandmail.com/canada/article-two-weeks-in-the-life-of-ottawans-trapped-by-the-convoys-chaos.

Angus Reid Institute. 2020a. "Philanthropy, Pandemic & Political Scandal: COVID-19 Curtails Donor Giving; WE Affair Weakens Trust in Charities." https://angusreid.org/covid-we-charity-giving.

– 2020b. "Social Values in Canada: Consensus on Assisted Dying and LGBTQ2 Rights, Division over Abortion Rights, Diversity." http://angus reid.org/social-values-canada.

– 2020c. "So Long, Office Space? Two-Thirds of Canadians Who Work from Home Expect It to Continue after Pandemic." https://angusreid.org/ coronavirus-work-from-home.

– 2021a. "Long-Term Care in Canada: For Those with Family in LTC Facilities during COVID-19 Pandemic, Size Mattered." 25 May 2021. https://angusreid.org/long-term-care-covid.

– 2021b. "Long-Term Care in Canada: Three-Quarters Say Significant Change Is Needed; Only One-in-Five Believe It Will Happen." 26 July 2021. https://angusreid.org/canada-long-term-care-policy.

– 2021c. "Unvaccinated? Meet the Unsympathetic: Most Inoculated Canadians Indifferent to Whether the Non-Jabbed Get Sick." 17 August 2021. https://angusreid.org/unvaccinated-covid-sympathy.

– 2022. "Blockade Backlash: Three-in-Four Canadians Tell Convoy Protesters, 'Go Home Now.'" 14 February 2021. https://angusreid.org/ trudeau-convoy-trucker-protest-vaccine-mandates-covid-19.

Annable, K. 2020. "Surprise Inspections Reveal 'Filthy' Floors, Uncleaned Rooms, Stool-Stained Blankets at Winnipeg Nursing Homes." CBC News, 8 June 2020. https://www.cbc.ca/news/canada/manitoba/pch-covid-winnipeg-1.5596568.

Arah, O.A. 2009. "On the Relationship between Individual and Population Health." *Medicine, Health Care and Philosophy* 12 (3): 235–44. https:// doi.org/10.1007%2Fs11019-008-9173-8.

Armstrong, P., and J. Mazerolle. 2021. "Playstations Scarce, Automakers Stalled amid Semiconductor Shortage Brought On by Pandemic." CBC News, 25 February 2021. https://www.cbc.ca/news/business/semiconductor-shortage-1.5925709.

Arthur, B. 2021. "Dr. David Williams Leaves a Clear, Tragic Legacy as He Rides Off into the Fog." *Toronto Star*, 25 June 2021. https://www.thestar.com/ opinion/star-columnists/2021/06/25/the-wrong-man-for-the-pandemic-dr-david-williams-leaves-a-clear-tragic-legacy-as-he-rides-off-into-the-fog.html.

Arya, A. 2020. "Palliative Care Has Been Lacking for Decades in Long-Term Care." *Policy Options*, 16 July 2020. https://policyoptions.irpp.org/ magazines/july-2020/palliative-care-has-been-lacking-for-decades-in-long-term-care.

Aschburner, S. 2020. "Coronavirus Pandemic Causes NBA to Suspend Season after Player Tests Positive." National Basketball Association, 12 March 2020. https://www.nba.com/news/coronavirus-pandemic-causes-nba-suspend-season.

Asquith, A. 2020. "Edmonton Taxi Drivers Shocked by Insurance Charges during Pandemic." CBC News, 1 May 2020. https://www.cbc.ca/news/canada/edmonton/edmonton-taxi-drivers-shocked-by-insurance-charges-during-pandemic-1.5552528.

Assailly, J.P. 2009. *The Psychology of Risk*. Hauppauge, NY: Nova Science Publishers.

Assembly of First Nations COVID-19 Data Working Group. 2021. *Lost in the Numbers: Learning about First Nations Health Data from the COVID-19 Pandemic*. https://www.afn.ca/wp-content/uploads/2021/12/3.-21-08-23-COVID-Data-Position-Paper-Executive-Summary.pdf.

Associated Press. 2020. "China Didn't Warn Public of Likely Pandemic for 6 Key Days." 15 April 2020. https://apnews.com/article/virus-outbreak health-ap-top-news-international-news-china-clamps-down-68a9e1b-91de4ffc166acd6012d82c2f9.

Association of Canadian Community Colleges. 2012. *Canadian Educational Standards for Personal Care Providers: Environmental Scan*. https://cacce.ca/wp-content/uploads/2021/11/Canadian-Standards-Environmental-Scan.pdf.

Aston, J., O. Vipond, K. Virgin, and O. Youssouf. 2020. "Retail E-commerce and COVID-19: How Online Shopping Opened Doors While Many Were Closing." StatCan COVID-19: Data to Insights for a Better Canada, catalogue no. 45280001. https://www150.statcan.gc.ca/n1/en/pub/45-28-0001/2020001/article/00064-eng.pdf?st=j2GRWtSi.

Atkins, E., and M. Habibinia. 2022. "How Labour Shortages at Canada's Busiest Airports Are Slowing the Aviation Industry's Resurgence." *Globe and Mail*, 9 May 2022. https://www.theglobeandmail.com/business/article-flight-delays-labour-shortage-travel-problems.

Attorney General of British Columbia. 2020. "Province Suspends Legal Time Limitations Due to COVID-19." Government of British Columbia, 8 April 2020. https://news.gov.bc.ca/releases/2020AG0028-000578.

Aucoin, P. 1990. "Administrative Reform in Public Management: Paradigms, Principles, Paradoxes and Pendulums." *Governance* 3 (2): 115–37. https://doi.org/10.1111/j.1468-0491.1990.tb00111.x.

– 1997. "The Design of Public Organizations for the 21st Century: Why Bureaucracy Will Survive in Public Management." *Canadian Public Administration* 40 (2): 167–386. https://onlinelibrary.wiley.com/toc/17547121/1997/40/2.

Auerswald, P.E., L.M. Branscomb, T.M. La Porte, and E.O. Michel-Kerjan. 2006. *Seeds of Disaster, Roots of Response: How Private Action Can Reduce Public Vulnerability*. Cambridge: Cambridge University Press.

Austen, I., and V. Isai. 2022. "Canadian Trucker Convoy Descends on

Ottawa to Protest Vaccine Mandates." *New York Times,* 10 February 2022. https://www.nytimes.com/2022/01/29/world/americas/canada-trucker-protest.html.

Austen-Smith, D., and J.R. Wright. 1994. "Counteractive Lobbying." *American Journal of Political Science* 38 (1): 25–44. https://doi.org/10.2307/2111334.

Australian Bureau of Statistics. 2019. "National, State and Territory Population." Government of Australia, December 2019. https://www.abs.gov.au/statistics/people/population/national-state-and-territory-population/dec-2019.

Aven, T., and O. Renn. 2018. "Improving Government Policy on Risk: Eight Key Principles." *Reliability Engineering and System Safety* 176 (August): 230–41. https://doi.org/10.1016/j.ress.2018.04.018.

Aviram, A. 2005. "Network Responses to Network Threats: The Evolution into Private Cybersecurity Associations." In *The Law and Economics of Cybersecurity*, edited by M.F. Grady and F. Parisi, 143–92. New York: Cambridge University Press.

Aviram, A., and A. Tor. 2004. "Information Sharing in Critical Infrastructure Industries: Understanding the Behavioral and Economic Impediments." George Mason Law & Economics Research Paper, 03–30; FSU College of Law, Public Law Research Paper no. 103. https://dx.doi.org/10.2139/ssrn.427540.

Avraham, E. 2020. "Nation Branding and Marketing Strategies for Combatting Tourism Crises and Stereotypes toward Destinations." *Journal of Business Research* 116 (August): 711–20. https://doi.org/10.1016/j.jbusres.2018.02.036.

AWCBC (Association of Workers' Compensation Boards of Canada). 2021a. *2017–2019 National Work Injury, Disease and Fatality Statistics.* https://awcbc.org/wp-content/uploads/2021/04/National-Work-Injury-Disease-and-Fatality-Statistics-2017-2019.pdf.

– 2021b. *Fact Sheet: National Work Injury Statistics Program.* https://awcbc.org/wp-content/uploads/2021/09/AWCBC_FactSheet_NWISP_2021-09c_PRINT.pdf.

– 2022. *Canadian Workers' Compensation System – 2020 Year at a Glance.* https://awcbc.org/en/statistics/canadian-workers-compensation-system-year-at-a-glance.

Ayre, P. 2001. "Child Protection and the Media: Lessons from the Last Three Decades." *British Journal of Social Work* 31 (6): 887–901. https://doi.org/10.1093/bjsw/31.6.887.

Ayres, S. 2020. "Pandemic in the Fields: The Harsh Realities Temporary Foreign Workers Face in Canada." CTV News, 26 September 2020.

https://www.ctvnews.ca/w5/pandemic-in-the-fields-the-harsh-realities-temporary-foreign-workers-face-in-canada-1.5120806.

Bailey, I. 2022. "Public Health Agency's Data-Gathering Program during Pandemic Lockdown Leads to Ethics Probe." *Globe and Mail*, 11 January 2022. https://www.theglobeandmail.com/politics/article-commons-ethics-committee-to-probe-data-gathering-program.

Bain, J. 2021. "Visitor Stats Reveal How Canada's Parks and Historic Sites Fared in 2020." *National Parks Traveller*, 13 March 2021. https://www.nationalparkstraveler.org/2021/03/visitor-stats-reveal-how-canadas-parks-and-historic-sites-fared-2020.

Bains, C. 2020. "How One Montreal Long-Term Care Home Has Kept COVID-19 at Bay." *Globe and Mail*, 2 August 2020. https://www.theglobeandmail.com/canada/article-how-one-montreal-long-term-care-home-has-kept-covid-19-at-bay.

Ball, J. 2011. "September 11's Indirect Toll: Road Deaths Linked to Fearful Flyers." *Guardian*, 5 September 2011. https://www.theguardian.com/world/2011/sep/05/september-11-road-deaths.

Ball, P. 2020. "The Lightning-Fast Quest for COVID Vaccines – and What It Means for Other Diseases." *Nature*, 18 December 2020. https://www.nature.com/articles/d41586-020-03626-1.

– 2021. "What the COVID-19 Pandemic Reveals about Science, Policy and Society." *Interface Focus* 11 (6): 1–10. http://doi.org/10.1098/rsfs.2021.0022.

Banerjee, A. 2007. "An Overview of Long-Term Care in Canada and Selected Provinces and Territories." Women and Health Care Reform Group. https://www.researchgate.net/profile/Albert_Banerjee/publication/284652528_Long-term_care_in_Canada_An_overview/links/5b7ddda492851c1e122919a3/Long-term-care-in-Canada-An-overview.pdf.

Banerjee, S. 2021. "Families Reach $5.5 Million Settlement in Lawsuit against Quebec Long-Term Care Home." *Canadian Underwriter*, 1 April 2021. https://www.canadianunderwriter.ca/insurance/families-reach-5-5-million-settlement-in-lawsuit-against-quebec-long-term-care-home-1004205966.

– 2022a. "Canada's Public Health Leaders Navigate Choppy Waters as Pandemic Drags On." *National Post*, 15 January 2022. https://nationalpost.com/news/canada/canadas-public-health-leaders-navigate-choppy-waters-as-pandemic-drags-on.

– 2022b. "Officials Report Nearly 3 Million Quebecers Were Hit by Omicron Wave." *Yahoo News*, 23 February. https://ca.news.yahoo.com/quebec-reports-17-more-covid-163727162.html.

Bank of Canada. 2021. "Toward 2021: Consultations with Canadians." https://www.bankofcanada.ca/core-functions/monetary-policy/monetary-policy-framework-renewal/toward-2021-outreach/lets-talk-inflation/consultations-with-canadians.

– n.d.a. "COVID-19: Actions to Support the Economy and Financial System." Accessed 17 March 2022. https://www.bankofcanada.ca/markets/market-operations-liquidity-provision/covid-19-actions-support-economy-financial-system.

– n.d.b. "Interest Rates Charged for New and Existing Household Lending by Chartered Banks." Accessed 25 January 2022. https://www.bankofcanada.ca/rates/banking-and-financial-statistics/interest-rates-for-new-and-existing-lending-by-chartered-banks.

– n.d.c. "Policy Interest Rate." Accessed 25 January 2022. https://www.bankofcanada.ca/core-functions/monetary-policy/key-interest-rate.

Barbalet, J. 2009. "A Characterization of Trust, and Its Consequences." *Theory and Society* 38 (4): 367–82.

Barrett, F. 2018. "Interest Growth Differentials and Debt Limits in Advanced Economies." International Monetary Fund, working paper no. 18/82. https://www.imf.org/en/Publications/WP/Issues/2018/04/11/Interest-Growth-Differentials-and-Debt-Limits-in-Advanced-Economies-45794.

Barrie, D. 2016. "Comment: It's Time for a Hard Look at Health-Care System." *Times Colonist*, 19 September 2016. https://www.timescolonist.com/opinion/comment-its-time-for-a-hard-look-at-health-care-system-4641093.

Bascaramurty, D., N. Bhatt, and U. Rana. 2021. "In India and Canada's International Student Recruiting Machine, Opportunity Turns into Grief and Exploitation." *Globe and Mail*, 6 November 2021. https://www.theglobeandmail.com/canada/article-india-canada-international-student-recruitment.

Bator, F.M. 1958. "The Anatomy of Market Failure." *Quarterly Journal of Economics* 72 (3): 351–79.

Batt, S. 2017. *Health Advocacy Inc.: How Pharmaceutical Funding Changed the Breast Cancer Movement*. Vancouver: UBC Press.

Baum, K.B., C. Tait, and T. Grant. 2020. "How Cargill Became the Site of Canada's Largest Single Outbreak of COVID-19." *Globe and Mail*, 3 May 2020. https://www.theglobeandmail.com/business/article-how-cargill-became-the-site-of-canadas-largest-single-outbreak-of.

Baum, T. 2019. "Hospitality Employment 2033: A Backcasting Perspective." *International Journal of Hospitality Management* 76, part B (January): 45–52. https://doi.org/10.1016/j.ijhm.2018.06.027.

Baumann, A., M. Crea-Arsenio, M. Lavoie-Tremblay, A. Meershoek, P. Norman, and R. Deber. 2022. "Exemplars in Long-Term Care during COVID-19: The Importance of Leadership." Special Issue, *Healthcare Policy* 17: 27–39. https://www.longwoods.com/content/26856/health-care-policy/exemplars-in-long-term-care-during-covid-19-the-importance-of-leadership.

Baumgartner, F.R., and B. Jones. 1993. *Agendas and Instability in American Politics*. Chicago: University of Chicago Press.

Baystreet Staff. 2021. "Canada's Big Banks to Make COVID-19 Vaccines Mandatory." *Baystreet*, 23 August 2021. https://www.baystreet.ca/articles/economiccommentary/69689/Canadas-Big-Banks-To-Make-COVID-19-Vaccines-Mandatory.

BBC. 2015. "Tunisia Attack on Sousse Beach 'Kills 39.'" 27 June 2015. https://www.bbc.com/news/world-africa-33287978.

– 2021. "Covid: New WHO Group May Be Last Chance to Find Virus Origins." 13 October 2021. https://www.bbc.com/news/health-58905945.

BC Centre for Disease Control. 2020a. "Phases of COVID-19 Testing in B.C." http://www.bccdc.ca/health-professionals/clinical-resources/covid-19-care/covid-19-testing.

– 2020b. "The Story of B.C.'s Leading-Edge COVID-19 Test Development." http://www.bccdc.ca/about/news-stories/stories/2020/the-story-of-b-c-s-leading-edge-covid-19-test-development.

Beaunoyer, E., S. Dupéré, and M.J. Guitton. 2020. "COVID-19 and Digital Inequalities: Reciprocal Impacts and Mitigation Strategies." *Computers in Human Behaviour* 111 (October). https://doi.org/10.1016/j.chb.2020.106424.

Beck, U. 1992. *Risk Society: Towards a New Modernity*. London: Sage Publications.

Béland, L.P., A. Brodeur, D. Mikola, and T. Wright. 2020. "The Short-Term Economic Consequences of COVID-19: Occupation Tasks and Mental Health in Canada." Global Labour Organization Discussion Paper Series 542. https://ideas.repec.org/p/zbw/glodps/542.html.

Belvedere, M. 2020. "Trump Says He Trusts China's Xi on Coronavirus and the US Has It 'Totally under Control.'" CNBC, 22 January 2020. https://www.cnbc.com/2020/01/22/trump-on-coronavirus-from-china-we-have-it-totally-under-control.html.

Bendaoud, M. 2020. "Understanding Public Policy Agenda Setting Using the 4 P's Model: Power, Perception, Potency and Proximity." National Collaborating Centre for Healthy Public Policy. http://www.ncchpp.ca/docs/2020-ProcessPP-AgendaSetting.pdf.

Benjamin, G. 2020. "Airline Passengers Voice Frustrations after WestJet Cuts Services, Refunds with Vouchers." *Global News*, 15 October 2020. https://globalnews.ca/news/7399874/westjet-cuts-services.

Bentham, J. 1824. *The Book of Fallacies: From Unfinished Papers of Jeremy Bentham*. Edited by P. Bingham. London: J. and H.L. Hunt.

Bernier, L., L. Juillet, and C. Deschamps. 2022. "Why Create Government Corporations? An Examination of the Determinants of Corporatization in the Canadian Public Sector." *Public Administration* 100 (2): 216–31. https://doi.org/10.1111/padm.12791.

Berry, D.A., S. Berry, P. Hale, L. Isakov, A.W. Lo, K.W. Siah, and C.H. Wong. 2020. "A Cost/Benefit Analysis of Clinical Trial Designs for COVID-19 Vaccine Candidates." *PLOS One* 15 (12): e0244418. https://doi.org/10.1371/journal.pone.0244418.

Berta, W., A. Laporte, D. Zarnett, V. Valdmanis, and G. Anderson. 2006. "A Pan-Canadian Perspective on Institutional Long-Term Care." *Health Policy* 79 (2–3): 175–94. https://doi.org/10.1016/j.healthpol.2005.12.006.

Berthiaume, L. 2020a. "Civic Duty or Infringing Freedom? Surveying Canadians' Attitudes about Masks." CTV News, 22 September 2020. https://www.ctvnews.ca/health/coronavirus/civic-duty-or-infringing-freedom-surveying-canadians-attitudes-about-masks-1.5114694.

– 2020b. "Lack of Canadian Vaccine Production Means Others Will Get Inoculations First: PM." *National Observer*, 25 November 2020. https://www.nationalobserver.com/2020/11/24/news/-canadian-vaccine-production-inoculations-PM-Trudeau-COVID-19.

Bertin, P., K. Nera, and S. Delouvée. 2020. "Conspiracy Beliefs, Rejection of Vaccination, and Support for Hydroxychloroquine: A Conceptual Replication-Extension in the COVID-19 Pandemic Context." *Frontiers in Psychology* 11 (September 2020): 565128. https://doi.org/10.3389/fpsyg.2020.565128.

Betsch, T., and D. Pohl. 2002. "The Availability Heuristic: A Critical Examination." In *Etc. –Frequency Processing and Cognition*, edited by P. Sedlmeier and T. Betsch, 109–19. Oxford: Oxford University Press.

Bholla, C. 2020. "Teachers at Scarborough School Refusing to Work after COVID-19 Outbreak." *Toronto Star*, 2 November 2020. https://www.thestar.com/news/gta/2020/11/02/ontario-reports-71-new-cases-of-covid-19-in-public-schools-including-41-more-students-in-latest-report.html.

Bianchi, R.V., and M.L. Stephenson. 2018. "Tourism, Border Politics, and the Fault Lines of Mobility." In *Borderless Worlds for Whom? Ethics, Moralities, and Morbidities*, edited by A. Paasi, E.K. Prokkola, J. Saarinen, and K. Zimmerbauer, 121–38. London: Routledge.

Birch, S. 2019. "Demand-Based Models and Market Failure in Health Care: Projecting Shortages and Surpluses in Doctors and Nurses." *Health Economics, Policy and Law* 14 (2): 291–4. doi.org/10.1017/S1744133118000336.

Birkland, T.A. 1998. "Focusing Events, Mobilization, and Agenda Setting." *Journal of Public Policy* 18 (1): 53–74. https://doi.org/10.1017/S0143814X98000038.

Birnbaum, J. 2021. "Major Sports Leagues Lost Jaw-Dropping Amount of Money in 2020." *Forbes*, 6 March 2021. https://www.forbes.com/sites/justinbirnbaum/2021/03/06/major-sports-leagues-lost-jaw-dropping-amount-of-money-in-2020/?sh=2a4b15a969c2.

Bizzabo. 2020. "2021 Marketing Statistics, Trends, and Data for the Events Industry." 15 December 2020. https://www.bizzabo.com/blog/event-marketing-statistics#top-event-statistics.

Black, J., and the To3 Management Team. 2004. *Assessment of the Toronto3 Alliance's Tourism Recovery Efforts.* https://civicaction.ca/app/uploads/2021/03/To3Assessment.pdf.

Blackwell, T. 2021. "COVID-19 Fight Has Relied Too Much on Uncertain Math Modelling, Some Scientists Say." *National Post*, 1 March 2021. https://nationalpost.com/news/canada/covid-19-fight-has-relied-too-much-on-uncertain-math-modelling-some-scientists-say.

Blais, A., and S. Dion. 1990. "Are Bureaucrats Budget Maximizers? The Niskanen Model & Its Critics." *Polity* 22 (4): 655–74. https://doi.org/10.2307/3234823.

Blalock, G., V. Kadiyali, and D.H. Simon. 2009. "Driving Fatalities after 9/11: A Hidden Cost of Terrorism." *Applied Economics* 41 (14): 1717–29. https://doi.org/10.1080/00036840601069757.

Bloodworth, M., M. Breton, and P. Gully. 2021. *Signals: The Global Public Health Intelligence Network (GPHIN) Independent Review Panel Final Report.* Public Health Agency of Canada. https://www.canada.ca/en/public-health/corporate/mandate/about-agency/external-advisory-bodies/list/independent-review-global-public-health-intelligence-network/final-report.html.

Bloomberg. 2023. "China's True COVID Death Toll Estimated To Be in Hundreds of Thousands." *Time*, 16 January 2023. https://time.com/6247534/china-covid-death-toll-underreporting.

BNN Bloomberg. 2021. "Home Prices Up 16% in June for Largest 12-Month Gain on Record." 20 July 2021. https://www.bnnbloomberg.ca/home-prices-up-16-in-june-for-largest-12-month-gain-on-record-1.1630973.

Bogart, N. 2020. "Anti-mask Rallies Held across Canada despite Increased

Support for Mandatory Masks." CTV News, 20 July 2020.
https://www.ctvnews.ca/health/coronavirus/anti-mask-rallies-held-across-canada-despite-increased-support-for-mandatory-masks-1.5031078.

– 2022. "Nearly $12 Million in CERB Payments Sent to Applicants with Foreign Addresses." CTV News, 10 February 2022. https://www.ctvnews.ca/health/coronavirus/nearly-12-million-in-cerb-payments-sent-to-applicants-with-foreign-addresses-1.5776607.

Boin, A., P.'t. Hart, E. Stern, and B. Sundelius. 2016. *The Politics of Crisis Management: Public Leadership under Pressure.* Cambridge: Cambridge University Press.

Boisvert, N. 2022a. "Canadians Sharply and Evenly Divided over Trudeau's Pandemic Performance, Poll Suggests." CBC News, 15 March 2022. https://www.cbc.ca/news/politics/angus-reid-pandemic-poll-politics-1.6384927.

– 2022b. "GoFundMe Ends Payments to Convoy Protest, Citing Reports of Violence and Harassment." CBC News, 5 February 2022. https://www.cbc.ca/news/politics/gofundme-stops-payments-1.6340526.

Bokat-Lindell, S. 2020. "Is the Coronavirus Killing the World Health Organization?" *New York Times,* 7 July 2020. https://www.nytimes.com/2020/07/07/opinion/coronavirus-world-health-organization.html.

– 2021. "Overdoses Have Skyrocketed during the Pandemic. How Do We Stop Them?" *New York Times,* 2 December 2021. https://www.nytimes.com/2021/12/02/opinion/drug-overdose-prevention.html.

Borins, S. 2020. "Interviews: Episode 12 – Sandford Borins." Observatory of Public Sector Innovation: Government after Shock Interview Series. https://gov-after-shock.oecd-opsi.org/interviews.

Born, K., V. Yiu, and T. Sullivan. 2014. "Provinces Divided over Mandatory Vaccination for School Children." *Healthy Debate,* 22 May 2014. https://healthydebate.ca/2014/05/topic/health-promotion-disease-prevention/mandatory-school-entry-vaccinations.

Bou-Karroum, L., J. Khabsa, M. Jabbour, N. Hilal, Z. Haidar, P. Abi Khalil, R.A. Khalek, J. Assaf, G. Honein-AbouHaidar, C.A. Samra et al. 2021. "Public Health Effects of Travel-Related Policies on the COVID-19 Pandemic: A Mixed-Methods Systematic Review." *Journal of Infection* 83 (4): 413–23. https://doi.org/10.1016/j.jinf.2021.07.017.

Bowden, O. 2020. "Divorces Have Increased during the Coronavirus Pandemic and Lawyers Are Expecting More." Global News, 19 July 2020. https://globalnews.ca/news/7188797/divorce-couples-coronavirus.

Boyd, M.J., D.A.R. Scott, D.M. Squirrell, and G.A. Wilson. 2020. "Proof-of-Concept Calculations to Determine the Health-Adjusted Life-Year

Trade-Off between Intravitreal Anti-VEGF Injections and Transmission of COVID-19." *Clinical & Experimental Ophthalmology* 48 (9): 1276–85. https://doi.org/10.1111/ceo.13855.

Boyer-Kassem, T. 2017. "Is the Precautionary Principle Really Incoherent?" *Risk Analysis* 37 (11): 2026–34. https://doi.org/10.1111/risa.12774.

Boyle, M. 2020. "COVID-19 and work." McInnes Cooper. PowerPoint presentation, 25 March 2020. https://cdn.dal.ca/content/dam/dalhousie/pdf/dept/maceachen-institute/March%2026,%202020%200828%20hrs%20COVID-19%20and%20the%20Workplace.pdf.

Boynton, S. 2021. "Majority of Canadians Support Mandatory Vaccines, Say COVID-19 a Top Election Issue: Poll." Global News, 19 August 2021. https://globalnews.ca/news/8124103/canada-election-mandatory-vaccines-covid-poll.

Brans, M., and S. Rossbach. 1997. "The Autopoiesis of Administrative Systems: Niklas Luhmann on Public Administration and Public Policy." *Public Administration* 75 (3): 417–39. https://doi.org/10.1111/1467-9299.00068.

Brend, Y. 2020. "Distillers Scrambled to Make Hand Sanitizer for Free. Then the Federal Government Moved On." CBC News, 8 December 2020. https://www.cbc.ca/news/business/distillers-hand-sanitizer-pandemic-1.5813509.

– 2022. "Why Economists Say It's a Bad Idea to Rely on a Privately Owned Bridge for 25% Of Canada's Trade with U.S." CBC News, 1 March 2022. https://www.cbc.ca/radio/costofliving/ambassador-bridge-protests-trade-us-canada-border-cargo-trucks-convoy-1.6355981.

Brenot, J., S. Bonnefous, and C. Marris. 1998. "Testing the Cultural Theory of Risk in France." *Risk Analysis* 18 (6): 729–39.

Brewster, M. 2020. "Military Mission to COVID-Hit Long Term Care Homes Cost Taxpayers about $53 Million." CBC News, 16 November 2020. https://www.cbc.ca/news/politics/covid-pandemic-coronavirus-canadian-armed-forces-1.5804063.

– 2021a. "Canada's Pandemic Warning System Was Understaffed and Unready When COVID Hit, Review Finds." CBC News, 12 July 2021. https://www.cbc.ca/news/politics/global-pandemic-early-warning-1.6098988.

– 2021b. "Military Medical Intelligence Warnings Gathered Dust as Public Health Struggled to Define COVID-19." CBC News, 13 January 2021. https://www.cbc.ca/news/politics/covid-military-medical-intelligence-1.5866627.

– 2021c. "Public Health Agency Was Unprepared for the Pandemic and 'Underestimated' the Danger, Auditor General Says." CBC News, 25 March 2021. https://www.cbc.ca/news/politics/auditor-general-pandemic-covid-phac-1.5963895.

Bricker, D. 2019. "Healthcare (35%), Cost of Living (27%), Climate Change (25%) Top Voter Issues as Campaign Season Kicks Off." Ipsos, 20 September 2019. https://www.ipsos.com/en-ca/news-polls/ Healthcare-Cost-of-Living-Climate-Change-Top-Voter-Issues.

– 2020. "Majority (60%) See Racism as Serious Problem in Canada Today, up 13 Points since Last Year." Ipsos, 24 July 2020. https://www.ipsos. com/en-ca/majority-60-see-racism-serious-problem-canada-today-13-points-last-year.

Bridgman, A., E. Merkley, P.J. Loewen, T. Owen, D. Ruths, L. Teichmann, and O. Zhilin. 2020. "The Causes and Consequences of COVID-19 Misperceptions: Understanding the Role of News and Social Media." *Harvard Kennedy School Misinformation Review* 1 (3): 1–18. https://doi. org/10.37016/mr-2020-028.

Briggs, P. 2020. "Canada's News Media Tries to Regain Trust during COVID-19 Outbreak." *Insider Intelligence*, 25 March 2020. https://www. emarketer.com/content/canada-news-media-tries-to-regain-trust-during-covid-19-outbreak.

Brioux, B. 2020. "News Ratings in Canada Take Big Leap during COVID-10 Coverage." *Brioux.tv* (blog), 20 March 2020. https://brioux.tv/ blog/2020/03/20/news-ratings-in-canada-take-big-leap-during-covid-19-coverage.

Britneff, B. 2020a. "Food Banks' Demand Surges amid COVID-19. Now They Worry about Long-Term Pressures." Global News, 15 April 2020. https://globalnews.ca/news/6816023/food-bank-demand-covid-19-long-term-worry.

– 2020b. "'People Are Livid': Advocates Call on Feds to Make Airlines Give Refunds amid COVID-19." Global News, 22 May 2020. https://global news.ca/news/6968756/coronavirus-airlines-refunds-canada.

Brooks, J.T., and J.C. Butler. 2021. "Effectiveness of Mask Wearing to Control Community Spread of SARS-COV-2." *Journal of the American Medical Association* 325 (10): 998–9. https://doi.org/10.1001/jama. 2021.1505.

Broster, A. 2021. "Coronavirus Hasn't Lead [*sic*] to the Baby Boom That Was Anticipated, According to a New Study." *Forbes*, 3 February 2021. https://www.forbes.com/sites/alicebroster/2021/02/03/coronavirus-hasnt-lead-to-the-baby-boom-that-was-anticipated-according-to-a-new-study.

Brown, B.J., and S. Baker. 2012. *Responsible Citizens: Individuals, Health, and Policy under Neoliberalism*. London: Anthem Press.

Brown, C., E. Seville, and J. Vargo. 2016. "Efficacy of Insurance for Organisational Disaster Recovery: Case Study of the 2010 and 2011

Canterbury Earthquakes." *Disasters* 41 (2): 388–408. https://doi. org/10.1111/disa.12201.

Brown, K.A., N.M. Stall, T. Vanniyasingam, S.A. Buchan, N. Daneman, M.P. Hillmer, J. Hopkins et al. 2021. "Early Impact of Ontario's COVID-19 Vaccine Rollout on Long-Term Care Home Residents and Health Care Workers." *Science Briefs of the Ontario COVID-19 Science Advisory Table* 2 (13). https://doi.org/10.47326/ocsat.2021.02.13.1.0.

Browne, C. 2021. "Hundreds of Anti-lockdown, Anti-mask Protesters Take to the Streets Again in Downtown Barrie." *Toronto Star*, 21 May 2021. https://www.thestar.com/news/canada/hundreds-of-anti-lockdown-anti-mask-protesters-take-to-the-streets-again-in-downtown-barrie/article_b8cfae99-8770-5b67-8d05-03214cb1888e.html.

Brownell, C. 2018. "Canada's First World War Sacrifice by the Numbers." *Maclean's*, 4 October 2018. https://www.macleans.ca/news/canada/canadas-first-world-war-sacrifice-by-the-numbers.

Bubela, T., C.M. Flood, K. McGrail, S.E. Straus, and S. Mishra. 2023. "How Canada's Decentralised Covid-19 Response Affected Public Health Data and Decision Making." *BMJ* 382: e075665. https://doi.org/10.1136/bmj-2023-075665.

Buchanan, J., and G. Tullock. 1999. *The Calculus of Consent: Logical Foundations of Constitutional Democracy*. 3rd ed. Indianapolis, IN: Liberty Fund.

Bui, Q., J. Katz, A. Parlapiano, and M. Sanger-Katz. 2020. "What 5 Coronavirus Models Say the Next Month Will Look Like." *New York Times*, 22 April 2020. https://www.nytimes.com/interactive/2020/04/22/upshot/coronavirus-models.html.

Bulmer, L., and J. Penny. 2022. "Title Protection for Unregulated Care Providers in Canada." Canadian Association of Continuing Care Educators. https://cacce.ca/wp-content/uploads/2022/09/Title-Protection-Report-PDF-Final-Sept-2022-3.pdf.

Burch, A.D.S., and A. Schoenfeld Walker. 2021. "Why Many Black Americans Changed Their Minds about Covid Shots." *New York Times*, 16 October 2021. https://www.nytimes.com/2021/10/13/us/black-americans-vaccine-tuskegee.html.

Burke, A. 2020. "Grounded Travellers Call on Government to Force Airlines to Issue Refunds for Cancelled Flights." *CBC News*, 22 May 2020. https://www.cbc.ca/news/politics/canadian-airlines-refunds-consumer-complaints-1.5580042.

Burns, C. 2012. "Implicit and Explicit Risk Perception." Paper presented at the European Academy of Occupational Health Psychology. Zurich, Switzerland.

Bush, G.W. 2002. *Proposal to Create the Department of Homeland Security.* https://www.dhs.gov/sites/default/files/publications/book_0.pdf.

Business Research & Economic Advisors. 2021. *The Economic Contribution of the International Cruise Industry in 2019.* https:// clia-nwc.com/wp-content/uploads/2021/04/CLIA-2019-Canada-EIS-Report-Final.pdf.

Butcher, J. 2020. "Constructing Mass Tourism." *International Journal of Cultural Studies* 23 (6): 898–915. https://doi.org/10.1177%2F136787 7920911923.

Cable Public Affairs Channel. 2020. "PM Trudeau Announces U.S. Border Closure, Economic Package in Response to COVID-19 – March 18, 2020." Filmed 18 March 2020 in Ottawa. Video, 30:44. https://www. youtube.com/watch?v=NrNDt2JVEdE.

CAF (Canadian Armed Forces). 2020a. "Observation sur les centres d'hébergement de soins longues durées de Montréal." https://cdn-contenu. quebec.ca/cdn-contenu/sante/documents/Problemes_de_sante/covid-19/ Rapport_FAC/Observation_FAC_CHSLD.pdf?1590587216.

– 2020b. "OP Laser – JTFC Observations in Long-Term Care Facilities in Ontario." http://s3.documentcloud.org/documents/6928480/OP-LASER-JTFC-Observations-in-LTCF-in-On.pdf.

Cagle, T. 2021. "Until Now, What's the Quickest a Vaccine Has Ever Been Developed?" *Nautilus*, 21 July 2021. https://coronavirus.nautil.us/ until-now-whats-the-quickest-a-vaccine-has-ever-been-developed.

Calkins, M., and C. Cassella. 2007. "Exploring the Cost and Value of Private versus Shared Bedrooms in Nursing Homes." *The Gerontologist* 47 (2): 169–83. https://doi.org/10.1093/geront/47.2.169.

Cameron-Blake, E., C. Breton, P. Sim, H. Tatlow, T. Hale, A. Wood, J. Smith, J. Sawatsky, Z. Parsons, and K. Tyson. 2021. "Variation in the Canadian Provincial and Territorial Responses to COVID-19." BSG Working Paper Series. https://www.bsg.ox.ac.uk/sites/default/files/2021-03/BSG-WP-2021-039.pdf.

Campbell, A. 2004. *SARS and Public Health in Ontario: First Interim Report.* The SARS Commission (4). http://www.archives.gov.on.ca/en/e_records/sars/report/v4.html.

Campbell, K. 2021a. "Pandemic Shows EI System in Need of Significant Retooling, Committee Finds." CBC News, 17 June 2021. https://www. cbc.ca/news/canada/prince-edward-island/ pei-employment-insurance-pandemic-reform-gig-economy-1.6069900.

– 2021b. "P.E.I. Hospitality Industry Struggling to Find Staff as Tourism Booms." CBC News, 16 August 2021. https://www.cbc.ca/news/canada/ prince-edward-island/pei-workers-shortage-murphy-wages-1.6140548.

Canada Helps. 2021. *The Giving Report 2021*. https://www.canadahelps. org/media/The-Giving-Report-2021_EN.pdf.

Canada Revenue Agency. 2022. "Table 2: Approved Canada Emergency Wage Subsidy (CEWS) Claims by Period and Industry, Canada." Government of Canada, 22 May 2022. https://www.canada.ca/content/ dam/cra-arc/serv-info/tax/business/topics/cews/statistics/ cews_p1-p21_tbl2_ac_en.pdf.

Canadian Anti-Fraud Centre. 2022. "Recent Scams and Fraud." Modified 9 February 2022. https://www.antifraudcentre-centreantifraude.ca/index-eng.htm.

Canadian Cardiac Transplant Network. 2011. "Cardiac Transplantation: Eligibility and Listing Criteria in Canada 2012." https://ccs.ca/app/ uploads/2020/12/CCTN_Cardiac_Transplantation_Eligibility_and_ Listing_Criteria_in_Canada_2012.pdf.

Canadian Centre for Cyber Security. 2020. *National Cyber Threat Assessment 2020*. https://cyber.gc.ca/sites/default/files/publications/ncta-2020-e-web.pdf.

Canadian Federation of Nurses Unions. 2022. "Canada's Nursing Shortage at a Glance: A Media Reference Guide." https://nursesunions.ca/wp-content/uploads/2022/07/nurses_shortage_media_ref_guide_comp.pdf.

Canadian Fraud News. 2020. "CAFC's List of Top Frauds in 2019." https:// www.canadianfraudnews.com/cafcs-list-of-top-frauds-in-2019.

Canadian Healthcare Technology. 2020. "Ontario Invests $1 Billion in COVID Testing, Tracing." 7 October 2020. https://www.canhealth. com/2020/10/07/ontario-invests-1-billion-in-covid-testing-tracing.

Canadian Health Coalition. 2018. *Policy Brief: Ensuring Quality Care for All Seniors*. http://www.healthcoalition.ca/wp-content/uploads/2018/11/ Seniors-care-policy-paper-.pdf.

Canadian Hub for Applied and Social Research. 2021. "COVID-19 Regulations." https://news.usask.ca/documents/chasr_ttpoc_june-omnibus-full_data.pdf.

Canadian Medical Association. 2020. *Clearing the Backlog: The Cost to Return Wait Times to Pre-Pandemic Levels*. https://www.cma.ca/sites/ default/files/pdf/Media-Releases/Deloitte-Clearing-the-Backlog.pdf.

Canadian Mental Health Association. n.d. *Summary of Findings – Mental Health Impacts of COVID-19: Wave 2*. Accessed 3 February 2022. https:// cmha.ca/wp-content/uploads/2020/12/CMHA-UBC-wave-2-Summary-of-Findings-FINAL-EN.pdf.

Canadian Real Estate Association. n.d. "Try the MLS HPI Tool – MLS Home Price Index." Accessed 16 February 2022. https://www.crea.ca/ housing-market-stats/mls-home-price-index/hpi-tool.

Cardoso, T. 2022. "Data Leak Reveals Canadians, Americans Donated Millions to Fund Trucker Convoy Protests." *Globe and Mail,* 15 February 2022. https://www.theglobeandmail.com/canada/article-data-leak-reveals-canadians-americans-donated-millions-to-fund-convoy.

Cardoso T., and P. Brethour. 2021. "Bankrupt Firms Tapped Federal Wage Subsidy despite Long Odds of Survival." *Globe and Mail,* 13 May 2021. https://www.theglobeandmail.com/business/article-bankrupt-firms-tapped-federal-wage-subsidy-despite-long-odds-of.

CARP (Canadian Institute of Retired Persons). 2021. "CARP Priority – Home Care." 5 July 2021. https://www.carp.ca/2021/07/05/c-a-r-p-priority-home-care.

Carr, J. 2022. *The Rise of Ideologically Motivated Violent Extremism in Canada: Report of the Standing Committee on Public Safety and National Security.* House of Commons. https://publications.gc.ca/collections/collection_2022/parl/xc76-1/XC76-1-1-441-6-eng.pdf.

Carrieri, V., M. De Paola, and F. Gioia. 2021. "The Health-Economy Trade-Off during the Covid-19 Pandemic: Communication Matters." *PLOS ONE* 16 (9): e0256103. https://doi.org/10.1371/journal.pone.0256103.

Carrigg, D. 2021. "COVID-19 Patients Taking Up a Third of All Intensive Care Unit Beds in BC." *Vancouver Sun,* 22 September 2021. https://vancouversun.com/news/local-news/covid-19-patients-taking-up-a-third-of-all-intensive-care-unit-beds-in-b-c.

Carvin, S., and N. Tishler. 2020. "Made in Canada: The Evolution of Canadian Counter-Terrorism Policy in the Post-9/11 World." *Canadian Public Administration* 63 (1): 53–70. http://dx.doi.org/10.1111/capa.12359.

Casler, J.G. 2014. "Revisiting NASA as a High Reliability Organization." *Public Organization Review* 14 (2): 229–44. http://dx.doi.org/10.1007/s11115-012-0216-5.

Cassia, F., P. Castellani, C. Rossato, and C. Baccarani. 2020. "Finding a Way towards High-Quality, Accessible Tourism: The Role of Digital Ecosystems." *TQM Journal* 33 (1): 205–21. https://doi.org/10.1108/TQM-03-2020-0062.

Caton, K., and C.A. Santos. 2008. "Closing the Hermeneutic Circle? Photographic Encounters with the Other." *Annals of Tourism Research* 35 (1) 7–26. https://doi.org/10.1016/j.annals.2007.03.014.

CBC News. 2020a. "Alberta Moves to Provincewide COVID-19 Testing Available to All – Symptoms or Not." 29 May 2020. https://www.cbc.ca/news/canada/edmonton/alberta-moves-to-provincewide-covid-19-testing-available-to-all-symptoms-or-not-1.5590332.

– 2020b. "B.C. Families Demand Changes to Rules So They Can See Loved Ones in Long-Term Care More Often." 30 September 2020. https://www. cbc.ca/news/canada/british-columbia/ltc-rally-september-29-1.5744153.

– 2020c. "Calgary Police Chief Says the Time to Debate COVID-19 Laws Is Not 'On the Rink.'" 21 December 2020. https://www.cbc.ca/news/ canada/calgary/calgary-police-covid-enforcement-update-1.5850409.

– 2020d. "Canada Lost Nearly 2 Million Jobs in April amid COVID-19 Crisis: Statistics Canada." 8 May 2020. https://www.cbc.ca/news/ business/canada-jobs-april-1.5561001.

– 2020e. "Ontario Taking Over 5 Long-Term Care Homes Following 'Gut-Wrenching' Military Report." 27 May 2020. https://www.cbc.ca/news/ canada/toronto/covid-19-coronavirus-ontario-update-may-27-emergency-order-1.5586256.

– 2020f. "Ontario to Provide COVID-19 Liability Protection to Businesses, Workers and Some Organizations." 20 October 2020. https://www.cbc. ca/news/canada/toronto/covid-19-liability-protection-legislation-ontario-1.5769801.

– 2020g. "Shelters Struggle to Keep Up with Skyrocketing Demand for Pet Adoptions during COVID-19." 4 June 2020. https://www.cbc.ca/news/ canada/british-columbia/high-demand-for-pets-1.5637516.

– 2020h. "Timeline of COVID-19 Cases across Canada." 13 March 2020. https://www.cbc.ca/news/health/canada-coronavirus-timeline-1.5482310.

– 2020i. "Toronto Breaks Down Geographic Spread of COVID-19, Showing Local Hot Spots in Detail for First Time." 28 May 2020. https://www. cbc.ca/news/canada/toronto/toronto-postal-code-covid19-1.5586860.

– 2020j. "Your Rights at Work under COVID-19 – 8 Questions for an Expert in Employment Law." 7 June 2020. https://www.cbc.ca/news/ canada/hamilton/cbc-asks-labour-law-covid-1.5600567.

– 2021a. "Alberta Doubles Fines, Brings in New Enforcement Protocol for COVID-19 Rule-Breakers." 5 May 2021. https://www.cbc.ca/news/ canada/edmonton/alberta-doubles-fines-brings-in-new-enforcement-protocol-for-covid-19-rule-breakers-1.6015710.

– 2021b. "All N.W.T. Gov't Employees Will Have to Show Proof of Vaccination by Nov. 30." 18 October 2021. https://www.cbc.ca/news/ canada/north/nwt-gov-t-vaccine-mandate-1.6215509.

– 2021c. "Average Cost for COVID-19 ICU Patients Estimated at More than $50,000: Report." 9 September 2021. https://www.cbc.ca/news/ health/cihi-covid19-canada-hospital-cost-1.6168531.

– 2021d. "Canada Doubles Dollar Contribution to COVAX Alliance – But Still Isn't Sharing Doses." 2 June 2021. https://www.cbc.ca/news/politics/ covax-summit-canada-contribution-1.6050212.

– 2021e. "Crime Down in First 8 Months of Pandemic, but Mental Health Calls Rise, Says StatsCan." 27 January 2021. https://www.cbc.ca/news/politics/crime-down-during-pandemic-canada-1.5890059.

– 2021f. "Essential Workers Should Be Prioritized for AstraZeneca Vaccine, Experts Suggest." 2 March 2021. https://www.cbc.ca/news/astrazeneca-essential-vaccine-1.5933006.

– 2021g. "Ford Won't Impose COVID-19 Vaccine Mandate for Ontario Health-Care Workers." 3 November 2021. https://www.cbc.ca/news/canada/toronto/ford-no-vaccine-mandate-for-healthcare-workers-1.6235828.

– 2021h. "N.S. Says All Health-Care Workers, School Staff Must Be Fully Vaccinated by Nov. 30." 29 September 2021. https://www.cbc.ca/news/canada/nova-scotia/vaccine-mandate-health-care-workers-teachers-1.6193798.

– 2021i. "Ontario Announces Mandatory Vaccine Plans for Health, Education Workers; 3rd Doses for Some." 18 August 2021. https://www.cbc.ca/news/canada/toronto/ontario-covid-vaccines-requirement-health-care-education-1.6143378.

– 2021j. "Ontario to Replace Dr. David Williams as Chief Medical Officer of Health." 30 May 2021. https://www.cbc.ca/news/canada/toronto/ontario-top-doctor-pandemic-retirement-1.6046068.

– 2021k. "Opioid Overdoses in Indigenous Communities Increased Sharply during Pandemic: Reports." 6 December 2021. https://www.cbc.ca/news/canada/hamilton/first-nations-opioids-pandemic-1.6274614/.

– 2021l. "Violent Deaths of Women in Canada Increased in 2020, Study Finds." 18 March 2021. https://www.cbc.ca/news/canada/femicide-canada-1.5953953.

– 2022a. "Canadians Fined at Least $15M for Breaking COVID Quarantine Rules for 1st 8 Months of Year: Data." 27 December 2022. https://cbc.ca/news/politics/covid-quarantine-fines-2022-1.6698395.

– 2022b. "Day 6: Animal Shelters Are Being Overwhelmed with Surrendered Pandemic Pets." 23 July 2022. https://www.cbc.ca/listen/live-radio/1-14/clip/15926819.

– 2022c. "End of Coutts' Protest Relieves Some Supply Chain Pressures, but Retailers Wary of Future Blockades." 18 February 2022. https://www.cbc.ca/news/canada/calgary/coutts-protest-business-relief-1.6355448.

– 2022d. "Multiple Border Crossings Blocked amid Canada-Wide Protests against COVID-19 Rules." 13 February 2022. https://www.cbc.ca/news/canada/pandemic-mandate-protests-feb12-2022-1.6349468.

– 2022e. "Trudeau Concerned Blockades Could Return in Ottawa, Says Convoy Stopped en Route." 21 February 2022. https://www.cbc.ca/news/canada/manitoba/trudeau-convoy-blockades-return-1.6359605.

– 2023a. "'I Have No Interest in Watering Down What Ontario Already Has in Place': Paul Calandra on LTC Standards." Video, 8:54. https://www.cbc.ca/player/play/2167639107727.

– 2023b. "Insolvency Filings in Canada Nearing Pre-pandemic Levels, Bankruptcy Office Says." 6 January 2023. https://www.cbc.ca/news/canada/british-columbia/canada-insolvency-filings-rising-1.6705343.

CBSA (Canada Border Services Agency). 2020. "Changes to Travel Restrictions for Immediate Family Members of Canadian Citizens and Permanent Residents." Government of Canada, modified 8 June 2020. https://www.canada.ca/en/border-services-agency/news/2020/06/changes-to-travel-restrictions-for-immediate-family-members-of-canadian-citizens-and-permanent-residents.html.

CCLA (Canadian Civil Liberties Association) and Policing the Pandemic Mapping Project. 2021a. *By the Numbers: The Second Wave of COVID-19 Law Enforcement in Canada*. https://ccla.org/wp-content/uploads/2021/06/2021-05-12-The-second-wave-by-the-numbers.pdf.

– 2021b. *COVID-19 and Law Enforcement in Canada: The Second Wave.* https://ccla.org/wp-content/uploads/2021/06/2021-05-13-COVID-19-and-Law-Enforcement-The-second-wave.pdf.

CCOHS (Canadian Centre for Occupational Health and Safety). 2019. "OH&S Legislation in Canada – Basic Responsibilities." Updated 8 April 2019. https://www.ccohs.ca/oshanswers/legisl/responsi.html.

– 2021. "National Day of Mourning." Modified 20 April 2021. https://www.ccohs.ca/events/mourning.

CDC (Centers for Disease Control and Prevention). 2020a. "Overdose Deaths Accelerating during COVID-19." 18 December 2020. https://www.cdc.gov/media/releases/2020/p1218-overdose-deaths-covid-19.html.

– 2020b. "Public Health Responses to COVID-19 Outbreaks on Cruise Ships – Worldwide, February–March 2020." *Morbidity and Mortality Weekly Report* 69 (12): 347–52. http://dx.doi.org/10.15585/mmwr.mm6912e3.

– 2021. "Cost-Effectiveness Analysis." 20 October 2021. https://www.cdc.gov/policy/polaris/economics/cost-effectiveness/index.html.

– 2022a. "National Pandemic Strategy." https://www.cdc.gov/flu/pandemic-resources/national-strategy/index.html.

– 2022b. "Omicron Variant: What You Need to Know." Updated 2 February 2022. https://www.cdc.gov/coronavirus/2019-ncov/variants/omicron-variant.html.

Cecco, L. 2022. "Ottawa Protests: Conspiracy Theories and Accusations of Betrayal as Police End Blockade." *Guardian*, 20 February 2022. https://www.theguardian.com/world/2022/feb/20/ottawa-protests-capital-police-clear-blockade.

Cecco, L., and T. Lindeman. 2022. "'Carnival of Chaos': Ottawa Police Face Growing Flak for Failure to End Protests." *Guardian*, 16 February 2022. https://www.theguardian.com/world/2022/feb/16/ottawa-protests-police-face-pressure-over-response.

CFIB (Canadian Federation of Independent Businesses). 2020. "More than One Quarter of Small Firms Report Workers Refusing to Return to Work; Preference for CERB Top Reason Given." https://www.cfib-fcei.ca/en/media/news-releases/more-one-quarter-small-firms-report-workers-refusing-return-work-preference.

– 2021. "Canada's Small Businesses Now Collectively Owe $135 Billion as a Result of the Pandemic." https://www.cfib-fcei.ca/en/media/news-releases/canadas-small-businesses-now-collectively-owe-over-135-billion-result-pandemic.

CFOJA (Canadian Femicide Observatory for Justice and Accountability). 2020. *#Callitfemicide: Understanding Sex/Gender-Related Killings of Women and Girls in Canada*. https://femicideincanada.ca/callit femicide2020.pdf.

Chamberlain, S.A., W. Duggleby, J. Fast, P.B. Teaster, and C.A. Estabrooks. 2019. "Incapacitated and Alone: Prevalence of Unbefriended Residents in Alberta Long-Term Care Homes." *Sociology of Health and Illness* 9 (4): 1–7. https://doi.org/10.1177%2F2158244019885127.

Chamberlain, S.A., A. Gruneir, M. Hoben, J.E. Squires, G.G. Cummings, and C.A. Estabrooks. 2017. "Influence of Organizational Context on Nursing Home Staff Burnout: A Cross-Sectional Survey of Care Aides in Western Canada." *International Journal of Nursing Studies* 71: 60–9. https://doi.org/10.1016/j.ijnurstu.2017.02.024.

Chamberlain, S.A., M. Hoben, J.E. Squires, G.G. Cummings, P. Norton, and C.A. Estabrooks. 2019. "Who Is (Still) Looking After Mom and Dad? Few Improvements in Care Aides' Quality-of-Work Life." *Canadian Journal on Aging* 38 (1): 35–50. https://doi.org/10.1017/S0714980818000338.

Chappell, N.L. 2011. "Population Aging and the Evolving Care Needs of Older Canadians: An Overview of the Policy Challenges." Institute for Research on Public Policy. https://irpp.org/wp-content/uploads/assets/research/faces-of-aging/population-aging-and-the-evolving-care-needs-of-older-canadians/IRPP-Study-no21.pdf.

Charities Aid Foundation. 2021. "COVID-19: The Effect on Global Civil Society." https://www.cafonline.org/about-us/international/coronavirus-effect-on-charities-globally.

Charity Village. 2021. "Human Resources Impact of COVID-19 on Canadian Charities and Non-profits." 30 April 2021. https://charity

village.com/ report-reveals-significant-negative-impact-on-volunteerism-due-to-covid-19.

Charlebois, S., and J. Music. 2021. "New Report Suggests 42.3% of Canadians Have Gained Extra Weight Unintentionally during Pandemic." Agri-Food Analytics Lab, 27 April 2021. https://cdn.dal.ca/content/dam/dalhousie/pdf/sites/agri-food/COVID%20Well%20Being%20(April%20 18%202021)%20EN.pdf.

Cheng, Y., N. Ma, C. Witt, S. Rapp, P.S. Wild, M.O. Andrea, U. Poschl, and H. Su. 2021. "Face Masks Effectively Limit the Probability of SARS-COV-2 Transmission." *Science* 372 (6549): 1439–43. https://doi.org/10.1126/science.abg6296.

Chirico, F., J.A. Teixeira da Silva, and N. Magnavita. 2020. "'Questionable' Peer Review in the Publishing Pandemic during the Time of COVID-19: Implications for Policy Makers and Stakeholders." *Croatian Medical Journal* 61 (3): 300–1. https://doi.org/10.3325/cmj.2020.61.300.

Chiu, P., S. Duncan, and N. Whyte. 2020. "Charting a Research Agenda for the Advancement of Nursing Organizations' Influence on Health Systems and Policy." *Canadian Journal of Nursing Research* 52 (3): 185–93. https://doi.org/10.1177/0844562120928794.

Christakis, N. 2020. *Apollo's Arrow: The Profound and Enduring Impact of Coronavirus on the Way We Live.* 1st ed. New York, Boston, London: Little, Brown Spark.

Christensen, B. 2005. "The Problematics of a Social Constructivist Approach to Science." *Comparative Literature and Culture* 7 (3). http://dx.doi.org/10.7771/1481-4374.1267.

Christou, P.A. 2022. "Tourism during the Late Modern Period (1750–1945)." In *The History and Evolution of Tourism*, 56–75. Oxford: CAB International.

Chung, E. 2020. "Mandatory Mask Laws Are Spreading in Canada." CBC News, 17 June 2020. https://www.cbc.ca/news/health/mandatory-masks-1.5615728.

Chung, H., K. Fung, L.E. Ferreira-Legere, B. Chen, L. Ishiguro, G. Kalappa, P. Gozdyra et al. 2020. *COVID-19 Laboratory Testing in Ontario: Patterns of Testing and Characteristics of Individuals Tested, as of April 30, 2020.* Toronto: ICES. https://www.ices.on.ca/Publications/Atlases-and-Reports/2020/COVID-19-Laboratory-Testing-in-Ontario.

Churchman, C.W. 1967. "Guest Editorial: Wicked Problems." *Management Science* 14 (4): B141–2. https://www.jstor.org/stable/i344811.

CIHI (Canadian Institute for Health Information). 2016. *Care in Canadian ICUs.* Ottawa. https://secure.cihi.ca/free_products/ICU_Report_EN.pdf.

– 2017. *Cardiac Care Quality Indicators Report.* https://www.cihi.ca/sites/default/files/document/cardiac-care-quality-indicators-report-en-web.pdf.
– 2020a. "1 in 9 New Long-Term Care Residents Potentially Could Have Been Cared for at Home." Modified 6 August 2020. https://www.cihi.ca/en/1-in-9-new-long-term-care-residents-potentially-could-have-been-cared-for-at-home.
– 2020b. "Long-Term Care Homes in Canada: How Many and Who Owns Them?" 24 September 2020. https://www.cihi.ca/en/long-term-care-homes-in-canada-how-many-and-who-owns-them.
– 2020c. "National Health Expenditure Trends, 2020." https://www.cihi.ca/en/national-health-expenditure-trends#data-tables.
– 2020d. *Pandemic Experience in the Long-Term Care Sector: How Does Canada Compare with Other Countries?* https://www.cihi.ca/sites/default/files/document/covid-19-rapid-response-long-term-care-snapshot-en.pdf.
– 2021a. "The Impact of COVID-19 on Long-Term Care in Canada: Focus on the First 6 Months." https://www.cihi.ca/en/long-term-care-and-covid-19-the-first-6-months.
– 2021b. "National Health Expenditure Trends." https://www.cihi.ca/en/national-health-expenditure-trends#Key-Findings.
– 2021c. "Over Half a Million Fewer Surgeries Have Been Performed in Canada since the Start of the Pandemic." https://www.cihi.ca/en/over-half-a-million-fewer-surgeries-have-been-performed-in-canada-since-the-start-of-the-pandemic.
– 2022a. "COVID-19 Intervention Timeline in Canada." Updated 13 January 2022. https://www.cihi.ca/en/covid-19-intervention-timeline-in-canada.
– 2022b. "National Health Expenditure Trends, 2022 – Snapshot." 3 November 2022. https://www.cihi.ca/en/national-health-expenditure-trends-2022-snapshot.
– 2023. "Hospital Stays in Canada." 23 February 2023. https://www.cihi.ca/en/hospital-stays-in-canada.
Cinelli, M., W. Quattrociocchi, A. Galeazzi, C.M. Valensise, E. Brugnoli, A.L. Schmidt, P. Zola, F. Zollo, and A. Scala. 2020. "The COVID-19 Social Media Infodemic." *Scientific Reports* 10 (1): 1–10. https://doi.org/10.1038/s41598-020-73510-5.
CityNews Toronto. 2021. "Ontario Hospitals Ramp Down Elective Surgeries as COVID-19 Cases Surge." 9 April 2021. https://toronto.citynews.ca/2021/04/09/ontario-hospitals-directed-to-ramp-down-elective-surgeries-non-emergent-activities.
City of Toronto. n.d. "Property Tax, Water & Solid Waste Relief Programs." Accessed 24 January 2022. https://www.toronto.ca/

services-payments/property-taxes-utilities/property-tax/property-tax-rebates-and-relief-programs/property-tax-and-utility-relief-program.

Clarke, C. 2023. "ArriveCan Contracting Wasn't That Bad. It Was Worse." *Globe and Mail*, 23 January 2023. https://www.theglobeandmail.com/politics/article-arrivecan-contracting-wasnt-that-bad-it-was-worse.

Clarke, M.C., and R.L. Payne. 1997. "The Nature and Structure of Workers' Trust in Management." *Journal of Organisational Behaviour* 18 (3): 205–24.

Clemens, J., and M. Palacios. 2021. "Caution Required When Comparing Canada's Debt to That of Other Countries." Fraser Institute, 1 June 2021. https://www.fraserinstitute.org/studies/caution-required-when-comparing-canadas-debt-to-that-of-other-countries.

Clement, D. 2020. "Is Business Interruption Insurance a Lost Cause?" Auckland District Law Society, 2 October 2020. https://adls.org.nz/Story?Action=View&Story_id=219.

Clemmensen, C., M.B. Petersen, and T.I.A. Sørensen. 2020. "Will the COVID-19 Pandemic Worsen the Obesity Epidemic?" *Nature Reviews Endocrinology* 16 (September): 469–70. https://doi.org/10.1038/s41574-020-0387-z.

Cléroux, P. n.d. "Canada's Manufacturing Sector: Trends, Challenges and the Way Forward." Business Development Bank of Canada. Accessed 31 January 2022. https://www.bdc.ca/en/articles-tools/blog/canada-manufacturing-sector-trends-challenges-way-forward.

Closing the Gap Healthcare Group Inc. 2019. "Long-Term Care Homes vs. Retirement Homes vs. Home Care in Ontario." Modified 8 February 2019. https://www.closingthegap.ca/long-term-care-homes-vs-retirement-homes-vs-home-care-in-ontario.

Cobb, R.W., and C.D. Elder. 1983. *Participation in American Politics: The Dynamics of Agenda-Building.* Baltimore, MD: Johns Hopkins University Press.

Cochrane, D., and K. Harris. 2020. "Canada Building Its Own PPE Network in China." CBC News, 16 April 2020. https://www.cbc.ca/news/politics/canada-building-own-ppe-supply-chain-in-china-1.5530259.

Cochrane, J.H., and J. Hartley. 2022. "The Most Important Source of Canada's Inflation: The Government Borrowed More than $700-Billion." *Globe and Mail*, 14 November 2022. https://www.theglobeandmail.com/business/commentary/article-inflation-canadian-government-borrowing-billions.

Cohen, M., T. Subramaniam, and C. Hickey. 2020. "The Lost Month." CNN, 18 April 2020. https://www.cnn.com/interactive/2020/04/politics/trump-covid-response-annotation.

Cohen, P. 2021. "Recession with a Difference: Women Face Special Burden." *New York Times*, 8 March 2021. https://www.nytimes. com/2020/11/17/business/economy/women-jobs-economy-recession.html.

Cohen, P., and T. Hsu. 2020. "Pandemic Could Scar a Generation of Working Mothers." *New York Times*, 3 June 2020. https://www.nytimes. com/2020/06/03/business/economy/coronavirus-working-women.html.

Colaço, J., C. Duvinage, and C. Mahony. 2020. *State of the Canadian Commercial Property & Casualty Insurance Market: Pressures Facing the Canadian Commercial Insurance Market in 2020.* https://businessinsur ancehelp.ca/wp-content/uploads/2020/11/State-of-the-Canadian-Commercial-Property-Casualty-Insurance-Market-Full-Report.pdf.

Coletto, D. 2021. "Pandemic Pets: Did Canada See a Pandemic Pet Boom?" *Abacus Data*, 10 June 2021. https://abacusdata.ca/pets-pandemic-canada.

Colleges & Institutes Canada. 2023. "A National Standard Means the Care Economy Is a Bit Easier to Navigate (SDGs 3 & 8)." 23 March 2023. https://www.collegesinstitutes.ca/national-standard-means-the-care-economy-is-a-bit-easier-to-navigate-sdgs-3-8.

Colley, R.C., T. Bushnik, and K. Langlois. 2020. "Exercise and Screen Time during the COVID-19 Pandemic." *Health Reports* 31 (6), catalogue no. 82-003-X: 3–11. https://www.doi.org/10.25318/82-003-x2020006 00001-eng.

Comfort, L. 2002. Rethinking Security: Organizational Fragility in Extreme Events. *Public Administration Review* 62 (1): 98–107.

Compton, N., and H. Sampson. 2020. "Is It Safer to Fly or Drive during the Pandemic? 5 Health Experts Weigh In." *Washington Post*, 5 October 2020. https://www.washingtonpost.com/travel/tips/drive-fly-safe-covid.

Connolly, A. 2021. "Nearly Half of Canadians Gather outside of Household over Holidays: Ipsos." Global News, 12 January 2021. https:// globalnews.ca/news/7568826/coronavirus-christmas-gathering-rules.

Contandriopoulos, D. 2011. "On the Nature and Strategies of Organized Interests in Health Care Policy Making." *Administration & Society* 43 (1): 45–65. https://doi.org/10.1177/0095399710390641.

Contandriopoulos, D., A. Brousselle, C. Larouche, M. Breton, M. Rivard, M.D. Beaulieu, J. Haggerty, G. Champagne, and M. Perroux. 2018. "Healthcare Reforms, Inertia Polarization and Group Influence." *Health Policy* 122 (9): 1018–27. https://doi.org/10.1016/j.healthpol. 2018.07.007.

Convery, S. 2021. "'You Can Make Money out of Us': The Disabled People Demanding More Accessible Travel and Tourism." *Guardian*, 26 December 2021. https://www.theguardian.com/australia-news/2021/

dec/27/you-can-make-money-out-of-us-the-disabled-people-demanding-more-accessible-travel-and-tourism.

Cope, S. 2000. "Assessing Rational-Choice Models of Budgeting – From Budget-Maximising to Bureau-Shaping: A Case Study of British Local Government." *Journal of Public Budgeting, Accounting & Financial Management* 12 (4): 598–624. http://doi.org/10.1108/JPBAFM-12-04-2000-B004.

Costa, C.S. 2011. "Tourism Policy Instruments: An Empirical Analysis of Portuguese Local Governments." In *EGPA Annual Conference 2011.* Bucharest, Romania: European Group for Public Administration. http://hdl.handle.net/10198/21474.

Council of Canadian Academies. 2023. *Fault Lines Expert Panel on the Socioeconomic Impacts of Science and Health Misinformation.* https://www.cca-reports.ca/wp-content/uploads/2023/01/Report-Fault-Lines-digital-1.pdf.

Couto, M. 2020. "Cases Going Down, but Experts Urge against Visiting Grandparents during Pandemic." CTV News, 28 May 2020. https://www.ctvnews.ca/health/coronavirus/cases-going-down-but-experts-urge-against-visiting-grandparents-during-pandemic-1.4958289.

COVID-19 Canada Open Data Working Group. 2021. "Dataset: Comprehensive Data on Canada's COVID-19 Epidemic." https://opencovid.ca/work/dataset.

COVID-19 National Preparedness Collaborators. 2022. "Pandemic Preparedness and COVID-19: An Exploratory Analysis of Infection and Fatality Rates, and Contextual Factors Associated with Preparedness in 177 Countries, from Jan 1, 2020, to Sept 30, 2021." *Lancet* 399 (10334): 1489–1512. https://doi.org/10.1016/S0140-6736(22)00172-6.

Cowley, S., and A. Haimerl. 2020. "These Businesses Thrived as Others Struggled to Survive." *New York Times,* 24 December 2020. https://www.nytimes.com/2020/12/24/business/small-business-coronvirus.html.

Cox, W., and J. Keller. 2021. "Western Canada: The Struggle to Maintain COVID-19 Contact Tracing." *Globe and Mail,* 2 February 2021. https://www.theglobeandmail.com/canada/british-columbia/article-western-canada-the-struggle-to-maintain-covid-19-contact-tracing.

CPHA (Canadian Public Health Association). 2018. *Racism and Public Health – Position Statement.* https://www.cpha.ca/sites/default/files/uploads/policy/positionstatements/racism-positionstatement-e.pdf.

– 2021. *Review of Canada's Initial Response to the COVID-19 Pandemic.* https://www.cpha.ca/review-canadas-initial-response-covid-19-pandemic.

– n.d. "Making the Economic Case for Investing in Public Health and the SDH." https://www.cpha.ca/making-economic-case-investing-public-health-and-sdh.

Craven, M., A. Sabow, L. Van der Veken, and M. Wilson. 2020. "Not the Last Pandemic: Investing Now to Reimagine Public-Health Systems." McKinsey & Company, 21 May 2020. https://www.mckinsey.com/indus tries/public-and-social-sector/our-insights/not-the-last-pandemic-investing-now-to-reimagine-public-health-systems.

Crawford, B. 2022. "Convoy Class Action Claim Increased to $306M as Downtown Restaurateurs Join Lawsuit." *Ottawa Citizen*, 18 February 2022.https://ottawacitizen.com/news/local-news/convoy-class-action-claim-increased-to-306m-as-downtown-restaurateurs-join-lawsuit.

Crawley, M. 2021a. "Ontario Largely Ignored Long-Term Care as COVID-19 Crisis Began, Internal Documents Reveal." CBC News, 28 April 2021. https://www.cbc.ca/news/canada/toronto/covid-19-ontario-long-term-care-coronavirus-1.6004572.

– 2021b. "Ontario Orders Hospitals to Halt Non-emergency Surgeries as COVID-19 Patients Fill ICUs." CBC News, 9 April 2021. https://www. cbc.ca/news/canada/toronto/covid-19-ontario-hospitals-elective-surgery-icu-patients-1.5980755.

– 2021c. "What's Behind Ontario's Abrupt Shift toward Vaccinating Everyone in COVID-19 Hotspots." CBC News, 10 April 2021. https:// www.cbc.ca/news/canada/toronto/ontario-covid-19-vaccine-hotspots-postal-code-1.5979774.

Crea-Arsenio, M., A. Baumann, and V. Smith. 2022. "Inspection Reports: The Canary in the Coal Mine." Special issue, *Healthcare Policy* 17: 122–32. https://www.longwoods.com/content/26850/healthcare-policy/inspection-reports-the-canary-in-the-coal-mine.

Crenshaw, K. 1995. *Critical Race Theory: The Key Writings that Formed the Movement*. New York: New Press.

Crowley, M. 2020. "Some Experts Worry as a Germ-Phobic Trump Confronts a Growing Epidemic." *New York Times*, 10 February 2020. https://www.nytimes.com/2020/02/10/us/politics/trump-coronavirus-epidemic.html.

C-SPAN. 2020a. "President Trump News Conference in India." Filmed 25 February 2020. Video, 46:33. https://www.c-span.org/video/?469669-1/president-trump-holds-news-conference-delhi-india.

– 2020b. "President Trump with Coronavirus Task Force Briefing." Filmed 26 February 2020. Video, 1:02:42. https://www.c-span.org/video/? 469747-1/president-trump-announces-vice-president-pence-charge-coronavirus-response.

CTV News Calgary Staff. 2021. "Proof of Vaccination Program Announced in Alberta as State of Public Health Emergency Declared." CTV News, 16 September 2020. https://calgary.ctvnews.ca/proof-of-vaccination-program-announced-in-alberta-as-state-of-public-health-emergency-declared-1.5586827.

CTV News Edmonton Staff. 2021. "Alberta Health Services Makes COVID-19 Vaccine Mandatory for All Staff." CTV News, 1 September 2021. https://edmonton.ctvnews.ca/alberta-health-services-makes-covid-19-vaccine-mandatory-for-all-staff-1.5568524.

Curry, B. 2023a. "CERB Audit of High-Risk Cases Find 65 Per Cent Went to Ineligible Recipients." *Globe and Mail*, 3 March 2023. https://www.theglobeandmail.com/politics/article-cerb-ineligible-recipients-cra-audit.

– 2023b. "Review of Billions of COVID-19 Wage Benefits Not Worth the Effort, CRA Head Says." *Globe and Mail*, 27 January 2023. https://www.theglobeandmail.com/politics/article-covid-wage-benefits-cra.

Cutler, D.M., and L.H. Summers. 2020. "The COVID-19 Pandemic and the $16 Trillion Virus." *Journal of the American Medical Association* 324 (15): 1495–6. https://doi.org/10.1001/jama.2020.19759.

Czeisler, M.E., R.I. Lane, E. Petrosky, J.F. Wiley, A. Christensen, R. Njai, M.D. Weaver et al. 2020. "Mental Health, Substance Use, and Suicidal Ideation during the COVID-19 Pandemic – United States, June 24–30, 2020." *Morbidity and Mortality Weekly Report* 69 (32): 1049–57. http://dx.doi.org/10.15585/mmwr.mm6932a1.

Dacombe, R. 2021. "Conspiracy Theories: Why Are They Thriving in the Pandemic?" *The Conversation*, 29 January 2021. https://theconversation.com/conspiracy-theories-why-are-they-thriving-in-the-pandemic-153657.

Dadashzadeh, N., T. Larimian, U. Levifve, and R. Marsetič. 2022. "Travel Behaviour of Vulnerable Social Groups: Pre, During, and Post COVID-19 Pandemic." *International Journal of Environmental Research and Public Health* 19 (16): 10065. https://doi.org/10.3390/ijerph191610065.

Dake, K. 1991. "Orienting Dispositions in the Perception of Risk: An Analysis of Contemporary Worldviews and Cultural Biases." *Journal of Cross-Cultural Psychology* 22 (1): 61–82.

Dalhousie University. 2021. "Quarantine Plan for Dalhousie International Students." 7 January 2021. https://www.dal.ca/covid-19-information-and-updates/updates/2021/01/07/quarantine_plan_for_dalhousie_international_students.html.

Daly, T. 2015. "Dancing the Two-Step in Ontario's Long-Term Care Sector: Deterrence Regulation = Consolidation." *Studies in Political Economy* 95 (1): 29–58. https://doi.org/10.1080/19187033.2015.11674945.

Daly, T., J. Struthers, B. Muller, D. Taylor, M. Goldmann, M. Doupe, and F. Jacobsen. 2016. "Prescriptive or Interpretive Regulation at the Frontlines of Care Work in the 'Three Worlds' of Canada, Germany and Norway."

Labour: Journal of Canadian Labour Studies 77:37–71. https://doi.
org/10.1353/llt.2016.0029.

Dangerfield, K. 2021. "Canada's 'Slow' Rollout of Coronavirus Vaccine
'Embarrassing': Experts." Global News, 5 January 2021. https://global
news.ca/news/7553419/coronavirus-vaccine-canada-distribution-slow.

Darcy, S., B. McKercher, and S. Schweinsberg. 2020. "From Tourism and
Disability to Accessible Tourism: A Perspective Article." *Tourism Review*
75 (1): 140–4. https://doi.org/10.1108/TR-07-2019-0323.

Daugbjerg, C., and P. Fawcett. 2017. "Metagovernance, Network Structure,
and Legitimacy: Developing a Heuristic for Comparative Governance
Analysis." *Administration & Society* 49 (9): 1223–45. https://doi.org/
10.1177/0095399715581031.

Dawson, T. 2020. "As the COVID-19 Pandemic Hit, Provinces Declared
States of Emergency. Now Many Are Up for Renewal." *National Post*, 15
April 2020. https://nationalpost.com/news/provincial-states-of-
emergencies-were-issued-a-month-ago-most-are-coming-up-for-renewal.

– 2021. "More than $636M in CERB Benefits Paid to 300,000 Teens Aged
15 to 17, Documents Show." *National Post*, 28 January 2021. https://
nationalpost.com/news/politics/more-than-636m-in-cerb-benefits-was-paid-
to-300000-teens-between-ages-of-15-and-17-documents.

DC (Destination Canada). 2019. "2019 Tourism Fact Sheet." https://www.
destinationcanada.com/sites/default/files/archive/1241-2019%20
Tourism%20Fact%20Sheet/coretourismfacts_Nov20_EN.pdf.

– 2020a. *Weekly COVID-19 Resident Sentiment, 11 May 2020.*
https://www.destinationcanada.com/sites/default/files/archive/1029-
Canadian%20Resident%20Sentiment%20-%20May%2011%2C%20
2020/Resident%20Sentiment%20Tracking_May%2011_EN.pdf.

– 2020b. *Weekly COVID-19 Resident Sentiment, 1 September 2020.*
https://www.destinationcanada.com/sites/default/files/archive/1160-
Canadian%20Resident%20Sentiment%20-%20September%20
1%2C%202020/Resident%20Sentiment%20Tracking_September%201_
EN.pdf.

– 2021a. *Revisiting Tourism: Canada's Visitor Economy One Year into the
Global Pandemic – March 2021,* https://www.destinationcanada.com/
sites/default/files/archive/1342-Revisiting%20Tourism%20Report%20
-%20March%208%2C%202021/Revisiting%20Tourism%20
Report-%20Mar%208%2C%202021.pdf.

– 2021b. *Weekly COVID-19 Resident Sentiment, 5 January 2021.*
https://www.destinationcanada.com/sites/default/files/archive/1281-
Canadian%20Resident%20Sentiment%20-%20January%205%2C%20
2021/Resident%20Sentiment%20Tracking_January%205_EN.pdf.

– 2021c. *Weekly COVID-19 Resident Sentiment, 4 May 2021.* https://www. destinationcanada.com/sites/default/files/archive/1378-Canadian%20 Resident%20Sentiment%20-%20May%204%2C%202021/ Resident%20Sentiment%20Tracking%20May%204_EN_FOR%20 PUBLICATION.pdf.

– 2021d. *Weekly COVID-19 Resident Sentiment, 7 September 2021.* https://www.destinationcanada.com/sites/default/files/archive/1467- Canadian%20Resident%20Sentiment%20-%20September%20 7%2C%202021/Resident%20Sentiment%20Tracking_September%207_ EN.pdf.

– 2022a. *Weekly COVID-19 Resident Sentiment, 11 January 2022.* https://www.destinationcanada.com/sites/default/files/archive/1541- Canadian%20Resident%20Sentiment%20-%20January%2011%2C%20 2022/Resident%20Sentiment%20Tracking_January%2011%202022_ EN.pdf.

– 2022b. *Weekly COVID-19 Resident Sentiment, 22 March 2022.* https://www.destinationcanada.com/sites/default/files/archive/1585-Cana dian%20Resident%20Sentiment%20-%20March%2022%2C%202022/ Resident%20Sentiment%20Tracking_March%2022%202022_EN.pdf.

– n.d.a. "Canada Tourism Fact Sheet 2020." Accessed 3 August 2021. https://www.destinationcanada.com/sites/default/files/archive/1410-2020 %20Tourism%20Fact%20Sheet/Destination%20Canada%20Tourism% 20Fact%20Sheet%202020_EN.pdf.

– n.d.b. "Who We Are." Accessed 3 August 2021. https://www.destination canada.com/en/about-us#whoweare.

De Bruijne, M., and M. Van Eeten. 2007. "Systems That Should Have Failed: Critical Infrastructure Protection in an Institutionally Fragmented Environment." *Journal of Contingencies and Crisis Management* 15 (1): 18–29. http://dx.doi.org/10.1111/j.1468-5973.2007.00501.x.

de Lange, D., and R. Dodds. 2017. "Increasing Sustainable Tourism through Social Entrepreneurship." *International Journal of Contemporary Hospitality Management* 29 (7): 1977–2002. https://doi.org/10.1108/ IJCHM-02-2016-0096.

Del Vicario, M., A. Bessi, F. Zollo, and F. Petroni. 2016. "The Spreading of Misinformation Online." *Proceedings of the National Academy of Sciences* 113 (3): 554–9. https://doi.org/10.1073/pnas.1517441113.

Deng, Z., R. Morissette, and D. Messacar. 2020. "Running the Economy Remotely: Potential for Working from Home during and after COVID-19." StatCan COVID-19: Data to Insights for a Better Canada, catalogue no. 45280001. https://www150.statcan.gc.ca/n1/en/pub/45-28- 0001/2020001/article/00026-eng.pdf?st=6A3uJ8Pu.

Department of Health. 2020. "Nunavut Extends Public Health Emergency." Government of Nunavut, 10 December 2020. https://gov.nu.ca/health/news/nunavut-extends-public-health-emergency-6.

Department of Health and Social Care. 2021. *JCVI Statement on COVID-19 Vaccination of Children and Young People Aged 12 to 17 Years: 15 July 2021*. Public Health England, 19 July 2021. https://www.gov.uk/government/publications/covid-19-vaccination-of-children-and-young-people-aged-12-to-17-years-jcvi-statement/jvci-statement-on-covid-19-vaccination-of-children-and-young-people-aged-12-to-17-years-15-july-2021.

Department of Justice Canada. 2020. "Government of Canada Further Facilitates Enforcement of the Federal Quarantine Act." Government of Canada, modified 14 April 2020. https://www.canada.ca/en/department-justice/news/2020/04/government-of-canada-further-facilitates-enforcement-of-the-federal-quarantine-act.html.

Derfel, A. 2020a. "Government Report Finds Fault with Operators of Herron Seniors' Residence." *Montreal Gazette*, 24 September 2020. https://montrealgazette.com/news/local-news/government-report-finds-fault-with-operators-of-herron-seniors-residence.

– 2020b. "Public Health, Police Find Bodies, Feces at Dorval Seniors' Residence: Sources." *Montreal Gazette*, 11 April 2020. https://montrealgazette.com/news/local-news/public-health-police-find-bodies-feces-at-dorval-seniors-residence-sources.

Deschamps, T. 2021. "Companies Entice Vaccinated Canadians with Freebies, Discounts." CTV News, 9 May 2021. https://www.ctvnews.ca/health/coronavirus/companies-entice-vaccinated-canadians-with-freebies-discounts-1.5420299.

Deshman, A. 2020. "Stay Off the Grass: COVID-19 and Law Enforcement in Canada." Canadian Civil Liberties Association, 23 June 2020. https://ccla.org/criminal-justice/police-powers-accountability/stay-off-the-grass-covid-19-and-law-enforcement-in-canada.

Desson, Z., E. Weller, P. McMeekin, and M. Ammi. 2020. "An Analysis of the Policy Responses to the COVID-19 Pandemic in France, Belgium, and Canada." *Health Policy and Technology* 9 (4): 430–46. https://doi.org/10.1016/j.hlpt.2020.09.002.

Dickson, C. 2021. "B.C. Orders Mandatory COVID-19 Vaccination for Workers in Assisted Living and Long-Term Care." CBC News, 12 August 2021. https://www.cbc.ca/news/canada/british-columbia/bc-mandatory-vaccination-workers-1.6138703.

Dickson, J., M. Walsh, and J. Hunter. 2022. "Ottawa Police to Implement Hard-Line Approach toward Pandemic-Restriction Protesters." *Globe and Mail,* 5 February 2022. https://www.theglobeandmail.com/politics/article-ottawa-police-say-more-officers-will-be-deployed-downtown-as-thousands.

Dietsch, P., and J. Best. 2021. "The Bank of Canada Must Seize the Pandemic Moment and Do More for Canadians." *The Conversation,* 4 May 2021. https://theconversation.com/the-bank-of-canada-must-seize-the-pandemic-moment-and-do-more-for-canadians-159034.

Dietz, L., P.F. Horve, D.A. Coil, M. Fretz, J.A. Eisen, and K. Van Den Wymelenberg. 2020. "2019 Novel Coronavirus (COVID-19) Pandemic: Built Environment Considerations to Reduce Transmission." *mSystems* 5 (2): e00245-20. https://doi.org/10.1128/msystems.00245-20.

Djuric, M., and L. Osman. 2021. "Canada Has Thrown Away More than One Million COVID-19 Vaccine Doses: Survey." *Globe and Mail,* 19 November 2021. https://www.theglobeandmail.com/canada/article-canada-has-thrown-away-more-than-one-million-covid-19-vaccine-doses.

Dolny, T., A. Iqbal, and K.R. Rosenstein. 2020. *Business Interruption Insurance and COVID-19: A Discussion of Future Implications.* Miller Thomson, 29 September 2020. https://www.millerthomson.com/en/publications/communiques-and-updates/financial-services-restructuring-communique/september-29-2020-fsi/business-interruption-insurance-and-covid-19-a-discussion-of-future-implications.

Douglas, M. 1982. *Essays in the Sociology of Perception.* London: Routledge & Kegan Paul.

– 1992. *Risk and Blame: Essays in Cultural Theory.* London: Routledge.

– 2001. "Dealing with Uncertainty." *Ethical Perspectives* 8 (3): 145–55. http://doi.org/ 10.2143/EP.8.3.583185.

Douglas, M., and A.B. Wildavsky. 1982. *Risk and Culture: An Essay on the Selection of Technical and Environmental Dangers.* Berkeley: University of California Press.

Downs, A. 1967. *Inside Bureaucracy.* Boston: Little, Brown.

Drahokoupil, J., and T. Müller. 2021. *Job Retention Schemes in Europe: A Lifeline during the Covid-19 Pandemic.* European Trade Union Institute, July 2021. Brussels: ETUI aisbl. https://www.etui.org/sites/default/files/2021-09/Job%20retention%20schemes%20in%20Europe%20-%20A%20lifeline%20during%20the%20Covid-19%20pandemic_2021_0.pdf.

Dryden, J. 2021. "Alberta's Updated COVID-19 Modelling Projects Close to 2,000 Daily Cases in 4th Wave 'High Scenario.'" CBC News, 3 September 2021. https://www.cbc.ca/news/canada/calgary/alberta-jason-kenney-deena-hinshaw-covid-modelling-1.6164280.

Dryden, J., and S. Rieger. 2020. "Inside the Slaughterhouse." CBC News, 6 May 2020. https://newsinteractives.cbc.ca/longform/cargill-covid19-outbreak.

Dunham, J. 2020. "Majority of Canadians Support Closing Non-essential Businesses during Second Wave: Nanos Survey." CTV News, 10 October 2020. https://www.ctvnews.ca/health/coronavirus/majority-of-canadians-support-closing-non-essential-businesses-during-second-wave-nanos-survey-1.5141296.

Dunleavy, P. 1986. "Explaining the Privatisation Boom: Public Choice versus Radical Approaches." *Public Administration* 64 (1): 13–34. https://doi.org/10.1111/j.1467-9299.1986.tb00601.x.

– 1991. *Democracy, Bureaucracy and Public Choice: Economic Explanations in Political Science.* New York: Prentice Hall.

Dunn, C. 2020. "Anger, Grief and Exhaustion: A City Is Left Raw after George Floyd's Death." CBC News, 4 June 2020. https://www.cbc.ca/news/world/minneapolis-after-george-floyd-death-1.5597735.

Dunsire, A. 1995. "Administrative Theory in the 1980s: A Viewpoint." *Public Administration* 73 (1): 17–40. https://doi.org/10.1111/j.1467-9299.1995.tb00815.x.

Duong, D. 2021. "Canada's Health System Is at a Breaking Point, Say Medical Leaders." *CMAJ* 193 (42): e1638. https://doi.org/10.1503/cmaj.1095965.

Earle, T.C. 2007. *Trust in Cooperative Risk Management: Uncertainty and Scepticism in the Public Mind.* London: Earthscan.

Eaton, M. 2021. *Investing in Community-Based Mental Health Services for Long-Term Pandemic Recovery.* Canadian Mental Health Association. https://cmha.ca/wp-content/uploads/2021/04/CMHA-Submission-to-LetsTalkBudget-March2021.pdf.

Economist. 2021a. "Assessing the Theory That Covid-19 Leaked from a Chinese Lab." 29 May 2021. https://www.economist.com/international/2021/05/29/assessing-the-theory-that-covid-19-leaked-from-a-chinese-lab.

– 2021b. "Did Covid-19 Leak from a Chinese Lab?" 18 June 2021. https://www.economist.com/films/2021/06/18/did-covid-19-leak-from-a-chinese-lab.

– 2021c. "Vaccine Nationalism Means That Poor Countries Will Be Left Behind." 28 January 2021. https://www.economist.com/graphic-detail/2021/01/28/vaccine-nationalism-means-that-poor-countries-will-be-left-behind.

– 2022. "Trudeau Invokes Emergency Powers to Shut Down Canada's Protests." 19 February 2022. https://www.economist.com/the-americas/

justin-trudeau-invokes-emergency-powers-to-shut-down-canadas-freedom-convoy/21807705.

Edelman. 2021. *2021 Canadian Edelman Trust Barometer.* https://www.edelman.ca/sites/g/files/aatuss376/files/trust-barometer/2021%20Canadian%20Edelman%20Trust%20Barometer_0.pdf.

– 2022. *2022 Canadian Edelman Trust Barometer.* https://www.edelman.ca/sites/g/files/aatuss376/files/trust-barometer/2022%20Canadian%20Edelman%20Trust%20Barometer.pdf.

– 2023. *2023 Edelman Trust Barometer: Canada Report.* https://www.edelman.ca/sites/g/files/aatuss376/files/2023-03/2023%20Edelman%20Trust%20Barometer%20EN.pdf.

Egan, M. 2007. "Anticipating Future Vulnerability: Defining Characteristics of Increasingly Critical Infrastructure-Like Systems." *Journal of Contingencies and Crisis Management* 15 (1): 4–17. http://dx.doi.org/10.1111/j.1468-5973.2007.00500.x.

Eggleton, A., and K.K. Ogilvie. 2010. *Canada's Response to the 2009 H1N1 Influenza Pandemic.* Ottawa, ON: The Standing Senate Committee on Social Affairs, Science and Technology. https://publications.gc.ca/collections/collection_2011/sen/yc17-0/YC17-0-403-15-eng.pdf.

Ehrenreich, B. 2020. "How Do You Know When Society Is about to Fall Apart?" *New York Times Magazine,* 4 November 2020. https://www.nytimes.com/2020/11/04/magazine/societal-collapse.html.

Einstein, A.J., L.J. Shaw, C. Hirschfeld, M.C. Williams, T.C. Villines, N. Better, J.V. Vitola et al. 2021. "International Impact of COVID-19 on the Diagnosis of Heart Disease." *Journal of the American College of Cardiology* 77 (2): 173–85. https://doi.org/10.1016/j.jacc.2020.10.054.

Eiser, J.R., and M.P. White. 2005. "A Psychological Approach to Understanding How Trust Is Built and Lost in the Context of Risk." CARR Conference "Taking Stock of Trust," London School of Economics. https://www.kent.ac.uk/scarr/events/Eiser%20+%20White%20Isepaper.pdf.

El-Bialy, R., L. Funk, G. Thompson, M. Smith, P. St John, K. Roger, J. Penner, and H. Luo. 2022. "Imperfect Solutions to the Neoliberal Problem of Public Aging: A Critical Discourse Analysis of Public Narratives of Long-Term Residential Care." *Canadian Journal on Aging* 41 (1): 121–34. https://doi.org/10.1017/S0714980821000325.

Elections Canada. 2019. "The 43rd Federal Election by the Numbers." https://www.elections.ca/content.aspx?section=med&document=oct2219&dir=pre&lang=e.

– 2021. "The 44th Federal Election by the Numbers." https://elections.ca/content.aspx?section=med&dir=pre&document=sep2921&lang=e.

Eligh, B. 2020. "COVID-19 Exposes Gaps in Canadian Home-Care System: U of T Researcher." *U of T News*, 7 May 2020. https://www.utoronto.ca/news/covid-19-exposes-gaps-canadian-home-care-system-u-t-researcher.

El Jaouhari, M., R. Edjoc, L. Waddell, P. Houston, N. Atchessi, M. Striha, and S. Bonti-Ankomah. 2021. "Impact of School Closures and Re-openings on COVID-19 Transmission." *Canada Communicable Disease Report* 47 (12): 515–23. https://doi.org/10.14745/ccdr.v47i11 2a02.

Emanuel, E.J. 2020. *Which Country Has the World's Best Health Care?* New York: PublicAffairs.

Emanuel, E.J., G. Persad, R. Upshur, B. Thome, M. Parker, A. Glickman, C. Zhang, C. Boyle, M. Smith, and J.P. Phillips. 2020. "Fair Allocation of Scarce Medical Resources in the Time of COVID-19." *New England Journal of Medicine* 382 (21): 2049–55. https://www.nejm.org/doi/10.1056/NEJMsb2005114.

Emeto, T.I., F.O. Alele, and O.S. Ilesanmi. 2021. "Evaluation of the Effect of Border Closure on COVID-19 Incidence Rates across Nine African Countries: An Interrupted Times Series Study." *Transactions of the Royal Society of Tropical Medicine and Hygiene* 115 (10): 1174–83. https://doi.org/10.1093/trstmh/trab033.

Empire Company Limited. 2021. *2021 Annual Report.* https://www.empireco.ca/en/investor-centre/financial-reports/annual-reports.

English, J., and T. Murphy. 2020. "Support for Atlantic Bubble Remains Strong even as Some Question Its Constitutionality." CBC News, 16 September 2020. https://www.cbc.ca/news/canada/nova-scotia/atlantic-bubble-covid-19-pandemic-borders-1.5718807.

Estabrooks, C.A., J.E. Squires, H.L. Carleton, G.G. Cummings, and P.G. Norton. 2015. "Who Is Looking After Mom and Dad? Unregulated Workers in Canadian Long-Term Care Homes." *Canadian Journal on Aging* 34 (1): 47–59. https://doi.org/10.1017/S0714980814000506.

Estabrooks, C.A., S. Straus, C.M. Flood, J. Keefe, P. Armstrong, G. Donner, V. Boscart, F. Ducharme, J. Silvius, and M. Wolfson. 2020. "Restoring Trust: COVID-19 and the Future of Long-Term Care." Royal Society of Canada. https://rsc-src.ca/sites/default/files/LTC%20PB%20%2B%20ES_EN_0.pdf.

Eurostat. 2021. "Life Expectancy Decreased in 2020 across the EU." https://ec.europa.eu/eurostat/web/products-eurostat-news/-/edn-20210407-1.

– 2022. "Mortality and Life Expectancy Statistics." https://ec.europa.eu/eurostat/statistics-explained/index.php?title=Mortality_and_life_expectancy_statistics.

Evans, P. 2020a. "Air Canada Cancels 30 Domestic Routes, Closes 8 Stations at Regional Airports." CBC News, 1 July 2020. https://www.cbc.ca/news/business/air-canada-service-cuts-1.5632874.

– 2020b. "WestJet Shuts Down Most of Its Operations in Atlantic Canada." CBC News, 14 October 2020. https://www.cbc.ca/news/business/westjet-cuts-1.5761526.

– 2022. "Canada's Inflation Rate Jumps to New 31-Year High of 6.7%." CBC News, 20 April 2022. https://www.cbc.ca/news/business/canada-inflation-1.6424388.

Expert Panel on SARS and Infectious Disease Control (Walker). 2003. *Initial Report*. Toronto: Ontario Ministry of Health and Long-Term Care.

Fafard, P., B. McNena, A. Suszek, and S.J. Hoffman. 2018. "Contested Roles of Canada's Chief Medical Officers of Health." *Canadian Journal of Public Health* 109 (August): 585–9. https://doi.org/10.17269/s41997-018-0080-3.

Falvo, N. 2020. "The Long-Term Impact of the COVID-19 Recession on Homelessness in Canada: What to Expect, What to Track, What to Do." Nick Falvo Consulting, December 2020. https://nickfalvo.ca/wp-content/uploads/2020/11/Falvo-Final-report-for-ESDC-FINAL-28nov2020.pdf.

Fang, L. 2021. "Drugmakers Promise Investors They'll Soon Hike COVID-19 Vaccine Prices." Intercept, 18 March 2021. https://theintercept.com/2021/03/18/covid-vaccine-price-pfizer-moderna.

Farber, D.A., and S. Sherry. 1997. *Beyond All Reason: The Radical Assault on Truth in American Law*. Oxford: Oxford University Press.

Farooqui, S. 2021. "Working from Home, Canadians Are Saving Thousands. Some Don't Want to Go Back to the Office." *Globe and Mail*, 10 May 2021. https://www.theglobeandmail.com/investing/personal-finance/household-finances/article-working-from-home-canadians-are-saving-thousands-some-dont-want-to-go.

Farrer, M. 2021. "Global Supply Chain Crisis Could Last Another Two Years, Warn Experts." *Guardian*, 18 December 2021. https://www.theguardian.com/business/2021/dec/18/global-supply-chain-crisis-could-last-another-two-years-warn-experts.

Federal Insurance Office. 2020. Report on the Effectiveness of the Terrorism Risk Insurance Program. U.S. Department of the Treasury, June 2020. https://home.treasury.gov/system/files/311/2020-TRIP-Effectiveness-Report.pdf.

Felter, C. 2021. "A Guide to Global COVID-19 Vaccine Efforts." Council on Foreign Relations, 27 December 2021. https://www.cfr.org/backgrounder/guide-global-covid-19-vaccine-efforts.

Ferguson, N.M, D. Laydon, G. Nedgjati-Gilani, N. Imai, K. Ainslie, M. Baguelin, S. Bhatia et al. 2020. *Impact of Non-pharmaceutical Interventions (NPIs) to Reduce COVID-19 Mortality and Healthcare Demand*. Imperial College London, 16 March 2020. https://www.imperial.ac.uk/media/imperial-college/medicine/mrc-gida/2020-03-16-COVID19-Report-9.pdf.

Ferlie, E. 2010. "Public Management 'Reform' Narratives and the Changing Organisation of Primary Care." *London Journal of Primary Care (Abingdon)* 3 (2): 76–80. https://doi.org/10.1080%2F17571472.2010.11493306.

Fernandes, N., and B.G. Spencer. 2010. "The Private Cost of Long-Term Care in Canada: Where You Live Matters." *Canadian Journal on Aging* 29 (3): 307–16. https://doi.org/10.1017/S0714980810000346.

Ferris, J.M., and S.Y. Tang. 1993. "The New Institutionalism and Public Administration: An Overview." *Journal of Public Administration Research and Theory* 3 (1): 4–10. https://www.jstor.org/stable/1181566.

Fierlbeck, K. 2010. "Public Health and Collaborative Governance." *Canadian Public Administration* 53: 1–19. https://doi.org/10.1111/j.1754-7121.2010.00110.x.

Fierlbeck, K., and L. Hardcastle. 2020. "Have the Post-SARS Reforms Prepared Us for COVID-19? Mapping the Institutional Landscape." In *Vulnerable: The Law, Policy and Ethics of COVID-19*, edited by C. Flood, V. MacDonnell, J. Philpott, S. Theriault, and S. Venkatapuram, 31–48. Ottawa, ON: University of Ottawa Press. https://muse.jhu.edu/book/76885.

Fife, R., and A. Willis. 2021. "Ottawa to Take Equity Stake in Air Canada as Part of Multibillion-Dollar Relief Package." *Globe and Mail*, 12 April 2021. https://www.theglobeandmail.com/politics/article-ottawa-to-announce-multibillion-dollar-relief-package-for-air-canada.

Fine, S. 2022. "Federal Government Facing Lawsuits over Emergencies Act." *Globe and Mail*, 23 February 2022. https://www.theglobeand mail.com/canada/article-federal-government-facing-lawsuits-over-emergencies-act.

Fink, S., and M. Baker. 2020. "'It's Just Everywhere Already': How Delays in Testing Set Back the U.S. Coronavirus Response." *New York Times*, 16 March 2020. https://www.nytimes.com/2020/03/10/us/coronavirus-testing-delays.html.

Finucane, M., P. Slovic, C.K. Mertz, J. Flynn, and T. Satterfield. 2000. "Gender, Race, and Perceived Risk: The 'White Male' Effect." *Health, Risk & Society* 2 (2): 59–172. https://doi.org/10.1080/713670162.

Firth-Cozens, J. 2004. "Sharing Workload in Group Practices: Unfairness and Early Experience Colour Perception of Inequality." *BMJ* 329 (7467): 685.

Fiser, A., and G. Hermus. 2019. *Canada's Indigenous Tourism Sector: Insights and Economic Impacts*. The Conference Board of Canada. https://indigenoustourism.ca/wp-content/uploads/2019/05/10266_IndigenousTourismSector_RPT.pdf.

Fjaeran, L, and T. Aven. 2021. "Making Visible the Less Visible – How the Use of an Uncertainty-Based Risk Perspective Affects Risk Attenuation and Risk Amplification." *Journal of Risk Research* 24 (6): 673–91. https://doi.org/10.1080/13669877.2019.1687579.

Flanagan, R. 2021. "How Canada's COVID-19 Death Toll Stacks Up to History." CTV News, 5 January 2021. https://www.ctvnews.ca/health/coronavirus/how-canada-s-covid-19-death-toll-stacks-up-to-history-1.5254420.

Fletcher, R. 2021a. "Keep an Eye on the Numbers – COVID-19 in Alberta." Braceworks, 2 November 2021. https://braceworks.ca/2020/06/18/health-tech/keep-an-eye-on-the-numbers-covid-19-in-alberta.

– 2021b. "Many Assumed Suicides Would Spike in 2020. So Far, the Data Tells a Different Story." CBC News, 10 February 2021. https://www.cbc.ca/news/canada/calgary/suicides-alberta-bc-saskatchewan-canada-2020-no-increase-1.5902908.

Flood, C.M., and B. Thomas. 2016. "Modernizing the Canada Health Act." *Dalhousie Law Journal* 39 (2): 397–411. https://digitalcommons.schulichlaw.dal.ca/dlj/vol39/iss2/4.

– 2020. "The Federal Emergencies Act: A Hollow Promise in the Face of COVID-19?" In *Vulnerable: The Law, Policy and Ethics of COVID-19*, edited by C. Flood, V. MacDonnell, J. Philpott, S. Theriault, and S. Venkatapuram, 105–14. Ottawa, ON: University of Ottawa Press.

Flood, C.M., B. Thomas, and K. Wilson. 2020. "Civil Liberties vs. Public Health." In *Vulnerable: The Law, Policy and Ethics of COVID-19*, edited by C. Flood, V. MacDonnell, J. Philpott, S. Theriault, and S. Venkatapuram, 249–63. Ottawa, ON: University of Ottawa Press.

Flyvbjerg, B. 2020. "The Law of Regression to the Tail: How to Survive COVID-19, the Climate Crisis, and Other Disasters." *Environmental Science & Policy* 114 (December): 614–18. https://dx.doi.org/10.2139/ssrn.3600070.

Folkes, V.S. 1988. "Recent Attribution Research in Consumer Behavior: A Review and New Directions." *Journal of Consumer Research* 14 (4): 548–65.

Forani, J. 2020. "How Canada's COVID-19 Pandemic Modelling Forecasts Compare to Reality." CTV News, 9 December 2020. https://www.ctvnews.ca/health/coronavirus/how-canada-s-covid-19-pandemic-modelling-forecasts-compare-to-reality-1.5222193.

Fostik, A., and N. Galbraith. 2021. "Changes in Fertility Intentions in Response to the COVID-19 Pandemic." StatCan COVID-19: Data Insights for a Better Canada, catalogue no. 45280001. https://www150. statcan.gc.ca/n1/en/pub/45-28-0001/2021001/article/00041-eng. pdf?st=u8MRcXqM.

Frakt, A. 2011. "Health Care Market Failures (And What Can Be Done about Them)." *The Incidental Economist*, 17 February 2011. https:// theincidentaleconomist.com/wordpress/health-care-market-failures-and-what-can-be-done-about-them.

Frampton, P. 2013. "Why Inspections and Audits of Nursing Homes Should Be Posted Online." *Telegram*, 1 November 2013. https://www.thetele gram.com/opinion/why-inspections-and-audits-of-nursing-homes-should-be-posted-online-135123.

Frank, L., T. Concannon, and K. Patel. 2020. *Health Care Resource Allocation Decision-Making during a Pandemic*. Santa Monica, CA: RAND Corporation. https://www.rand.org/pubs/research_reports/ RRA326-1.html.

Fraser, A. 2020. "Online Job Scams on the Rise during Pandemic Year, Fraud Prevention Expert Says." CBC News, 23 December 2020. https:// www.cbc.ca/news/canada/toronto/online-job-scams-on-the-rise-during-pandemic-year-fraud-prevention-expert-says-1.5851667.

Frazer, J. 2019. "How the Gig Economy Is Reshaping Careers for the Next Generation." *Forbes*, 15 February 2019. https://www.forbes.com/sites/ johnfrazer1/2019/02/15/how-the-gig-economy-is-reshaping-careers-for-the-next-generation/?sh=1c082e7d49ad.

Freeman, J. 2021. "'We're Not Gonna Have a Split Society': Doug Ford Rules Out a Provincial 'Vaccine Passport.'" CTV News, 15 July 2021. https://toronto.ctvnews.ca/we-re-not-gonna-have-a-split-society-doug-ford-rules-out-a-provincial-vaccine-passport-1.5510704.

Freeze, C. 2021. "Supply Crunch Coming as Demand for COVID-19 Rapid Testing Soars." *Globe and Mail*, 31 December 2021. https://www.the globeandmail.com/canada/article-supply-crunch-coming-as-demand-for-covid-19-rapid-testing-soars.

French, J. 2021. "Alberta, Federal Governments Giving $1,200 Pandemic Danger Pay to Front-Line Workers." CBC News, 10 February 2021. https://www.cbc.ca/news/canada/edmonton/alberta-critical-worker-benefit-payments-1.5908613.

Friesen, J. 2020a. "Enrolment up at Canadian Universities, Mostly Because of Part-Timers." *Globe and Mail*, 24 November 2020. https://www.the globeandmail.com/canada/article-universities-have-weathered-the-pandemic-without-impact-on-enrolment.

– 2020b. "Universities Raise Tuition despite Moving Online Due to COVID-19." *Globe and Mail*, 1 June 2020. https://www.theglobeandmail.com/canada/article-universities-raise-tuition-despite-moving-online-due-to-covid-19.

– 2021. "Bulk of College Tuition in Ontario Comes from International Students, Auditor-General Says." *Globe and Mail*, 1 December 2021. https://www.theglobeandmail.com/canada/article-bulk-of-college-tuition-in-ontario-comes-from-international-students.

– 2022. "Canadian Universities Have Weathered the COVID-19 Pandemic without Impact on Enrolment or Achievement." *Globe and Mail*, 17 January 2022. https://www.theglobeandmail.com/canada/article-universities-have-weathered-the-pandemic-without-impact-on-enrolment.

Fulton, J.M., and W.T. Stanbury. 1985. "Comparative Lobbying Strategies in Influencing Health Care Policy." *Canadian Public Administration* 28 (2): 269–300. https://doi.org/10.1111/j.1754-7121.1985.tb00514.x.

Fung, I.C., K.W. Fu, C.H. Chan, B.S. Chan, C.N. Cheung, T. Abraham, and Z.T. Tse. 2016. "Social Media's Initial Reaction to Information and Misinformation on Ebola, August 2014: Facts and Rumors." *Public Health Reports* 131 (3): 461–73. https://doi.org/10.1177/003335491613100312.

Fuss, J., J. Clemens, and M. Palacios. 2020. "Canada's Spending and Deficits Higher than Comparable Countries during Pandemic." *Fraser Institute Blog*, 26 October 2020. https://www.fraserinstitute.org/blogs/canadas-spending-and-deficits-higher-than-comparable-countries-during-pandemic.

Gains, F., and P. John. 2010. "What Do Bureaucrats Like Doing? Bureaucratic Preferences in Response to Institutional Reform." *Public Administration Review* 70 (3): 455–63. http://doi.org/10.1111/j.1540-6210.2010.02159.x.

Galea, S. 2023. *Within Reason: A Liberal Public Health for an Illiberal Time*. Chicago: University of Chicago Press. https://press.uchicago.edu/ucp/books/book/chicago/W/bo205394268.html.

Galloway, G., and J. Lewington. 2003. "Lack of Political Leadership on SARS Hurts Tourism, Industry Says." *Globe and Mail*, 16 April 2003. https://www.theglobeandmail.com/news/national/lack-of-political-leadership-on-sars-hurts-tourism-industry-says/article25282718.

Galloway, M. 2021. "The Current – March 1, 2021 Episode Transcript." CBC *Radio*, 1 March 2021. https://www.cbc.ca/radio/thecurrent/the-current-for-march-1-2021-1.5931671/march-1-2021-episode-transcript-1.5932437.

Gamage, B., V. Schall, J. Grant, and PICNet Long-Term Care Needs
Assessment Working Group. 2012. "Identifying the Gaps in Infection
Prevention and Control Resources for Long-Term Care Facilities in British
Columbia." *American Journal of Infection Control* 40 (2): 150–4. https://
doi.org/10.1016/j.ajic.2011.03.026.

Gambrill, D. 2021. "2020 Results: Did Canada's Insurers 'Outrun the Bear'
of Claims Inflation?" *Canadian Underwriter*, 23 March 2021. https://
www.canadianunderwriter.ca/earnings-ratings/2020-results-did-canadas-
insurers-outrun-the-bear-of-claims-inflation-1004205467.

Garner, R., P. Tanuseputro, D.G. Manuel, and C. Sanmartin. 2018.
"Transitions to Long-Term and Residential Care among Older
Canadians." *Health Reports* 29 (5), catalogue no. 82-003-X: 13–23.
https://www150.statcan.gc.ca/n1/en/pub/82-003-x/2018005/arti-
cle/54966-eng.pdf?st=BgbY9RF4.

Garnett, H.A., J.N. Bordeleau, A. Harell, and L. Stephenson. 2021.
*Canadian Provincial Elections during the COVID-19 Pandemic – Case
Study, 17 December 2021*. International Institute for Democracy and
Electoral Assistance. https://www.idea.int/sites/default/files/multimedia_
reports/canadian-provincial-elections-during-the-covid-19-pandemic-en.
pdf.

Gatehouse, J. 2020a. "'An Extreme Last Resort': Police Reluctant to Ticket,
Arrest COVID-19 Rule-Breakers." CBC News, 24 March 2020. https://
www.cbc.ca/news/investigates/police-covid-enforcement-fines-arrests-1.
5508144.

– 2020b. "Ontario Needs to Be More Transparent with COVID-19 Data,
Critics Say." CBC News, 28 May 2020. https://www.cbc.ca/news/health/
ontario-covid-19-transparency-1.5587459.

Georgieva, K., T.A. Ghebreyesus, D. Malpass, and N. Okonjo-Iweala. 2021.
"A New Commitment for Vaccine Equity and Defeating the Pandemic."
World Health Organization, 31 May. https://www.who.int/news-room/
commentaries/detail/a-new-commitment-for-vaccine-equity-and-
defeating-the-pandemic.

Geraghty, J. 2020. "Comprehensive Timeline of China's COVID-19 Lies."
National Review, 23 March 2020. https://www.nationalreview.com/the-
morning-jolt/chinas-devastating-lies.

Ghebreyesus, T.A. 2021. "Vaccine Nationalism Harms Everyone and
Protects No One." *Foreign Policy*, 2 February 2021. https://foreignpolicy.
com/2021/02/02/vaccine-nationalism-harms-everyone-and-protects-
no-one.

Ghoussoub, M. 2020. "B.C. Dentists Say They're Being Denied $36M in
Pandemic Insurance Due to Lack of Order to Close Completely." CBC

News, 14 April 2020. https://www.cbc.ca/news/canada/british-columbia/
bc-dentists-insurance-covid-19-coronavirus-1.5531222.

Giattino, C. 2020. "How Epidemiological Models of COVID-19 Help Us
Estimate the True Number of Infections." Our World in Data, 24 April
2020. https://ourworldindata.org/covid-models.

Gibbard, R. 2017. *Sizing up the Challenge: Meeting the Demand for Long-
Term Care in Canada.* The Conference Board of Canada. https://www.
conferenceboard.ca/e-library/abstract.aspx?did=9228.

Gibson, E. 2020. "Provincial Powers of Quarantine – Presentation for
Roundtable." PowerPoint presentation, 25 March 2020. https://cdn.dal.
ca/content/dam/dalhousie/pdf/dept/maceachen-institute/Quarantine%20
and%20COVID-19%20Slides.pdf.

Giles, D. 2021. "COVID-19 Surge in Saskatchewan Straining Health-Care
System, Organ Donations Paused." Global News, 24 September 2021.
https://globalnews.ca/news/8215933/covid-19-surge-saskatchewan-health-
authority.

Gillespie, N., and G. Dietz. 2009. "Trust Repair after an Organization-Level
Failure." *Academy of Management Review* 34 (1): 127–45. https://doi.
org/10.5465/AMR.2009.35713319.

Gillies, R., and D. Crary. 2022. "As Canada Protests Persist, So Do
Challenges for Trudeau." Associated Press, 15 February 2022. https://
apnews.com/article/coronavirus-pandemic-health-toronto-canada-
ottawa-f6a0fa012909c9f302d1f09883d56b9d.

Gilmore, R. 2021. "Pfizer, Moderna COVID-19 Vaccines Get Full Health
Canada Approval – And New Names." Global News, 16 September
2021. https://globalnews.ca/news/8195443/covid-coronavirus-vaccine-12-
kids-pfizer-moderna.

Gilmore, R., and C. Lord. 2022. "Trucker Protest: Ottawa Police Call for
More Personnel to 'Regain Control' of the City." Global News, 8
February 2022. https://globalnews.ca/news/8600507/ottawa-police-
freedom-convoy-on-offensive.

Gilmour, H. 2018a. "Formal Home Care Use in Canada: Health Brief."
Health Reports 29 (9), catalogue no. 82-003-X: 3–9. https://www150.
statcan.gc.ca/n1/pub/82-003-x/2018009/article/00001-eng.pdf.

– 2018b. "Unmet Home Care Needs in Canada: Research Article." *Health
Reports* 29 (11), catalogue no. 82-003-X: 3–11. https://www150.statcan.
gc.ca/n1/pub/82-003-x/2018011/article/00002-eng.pdf.

Glaeser, E., and D. Cutler. 2021. "You May Get More Work Done at Home.
But You'd Have Better Ideas at the Office." *Washington Post*, 24
September 2021. https://www.washingtonpost.com/outlook/2021/09/24/
working-home-productivity-pandemic-remote.

Global Affairs Canada. 2020a. "Government of Canada Evacuating Canadians from Wuhan, China." Government of Canada, 2 February 2020. https://www.canada.ca/en/global-affairs/news/2020/02/government-of-canada-evacuating-canadians-from-wuhan-china.html.

– 2020b. "Government of Canada Repatriates More Canadians and Their Families from Wuhan, China." Government of Canada, 12 February 2020. https://www.canada.ca/en/global-affairs/news/2020/02/government-of-canada-repatriates-more-canadians-and-their-families-from-wuhan-china.html.

Globe and Mail. 2020a. "Atlantic Canada to Allow Regional 'Bubble' Beginning July 3." 25 June 2020. https://www.theglobeandmail.com/canada/article-interprovincial-travel-restrictions-to-be-eased-in-atlantic-canada.

– 2020b. "COVID-19 Has Further Amplified Economic Inequality in Canada, Report Shows." 14 October 2020. https://www.theglobeandmail.com/business/article-covid-19-has-further-amplified-economic-inequality-in-canada-report.

– 2020c. "Federal Government Says 1,350 Soldiers Will Be Deployed to Quebec Long-Term Care Homes by Mid-May." 8 May 2020. https://www.theglobeandmail.com/canada/article-federal-government-says-1350-soldiers-will-be-deployed-to-quebec-long.

– 2021. "Saskatchewan Suspends Organ Donation Program Due to Lack of Resources from COVID-19." 23 September 2021. https://www.theglobeandmail.com/canada/article-saskatchewan-suspends-organ-donation-program-due-to-lack-of-resources.

Globe and Mail Editorial Board. 2021. "Other Countries Are Making Vaccines. Why Can't Canada?" Globe and Mail, 11 February 2021. https://www.theglobeandmail.com/opinion/editorials/article-other-countries-are-making-vaccines-why-cant-canada.

– 2022a. "The Biggest Issue in Canada's Long-Term Care Homes? A Desperate Lack of Beds." Globe and Mail, 31 January 2022. https://www.theglobeandmail.com/opinion/editorials/article-the-biggest-issue-in-canadas-long-term-care-homes-a-desperate-lack-of.

– 2022b. "Canada is Beating Omicron. But the Game's Still On." Globe and Mail, 22 January 2022. https://www.theglobeandmail.com/opinion/editorials/article-canada-is-beating-omicron-but-the-games-still-on.

Globe Staff. 2022. "Police Are Arresting and Clearing the Ottawa Convoy Protesters. Here's What You Need to Know." Globe and Mail, 21 February 2022. https://www.theglobeandmail.com/canada/article-ottawa-convoy-protest-police-make-arrests.

Globe Staff and Wire Services. 2022. "Updates: Officials Condemn 'Desecration' of Monuments, Hateful Signs on Display at Trucker Convoy Protest." *Globe and Mail*, 30 January 2022. https://www. theglobeandmail.com/politics/article-truck-freedom-convoy-ottawa-live-update.

GoFundMe. 2022. "Update: GoFundMe to Refund All Freedom Convoy 2022 Donations (2/5/2022)." *Medium*, 4 February 2022. https://medium. com/gofundme-stories/update-gofundme-statement-on-the-freedom-convoy-2022-fundraiser-4ca7e9714e82.

Goldman, E. 2020. "Exaggerated Risk of Transmission of COVID-19 by Fomites." *Lancet Infectious Diseases* 20 (8): 892–3. https://doi.org/ 10.1016/S1473-3099(20)30561-2.

Goldstein, B. 2001. "The Precautionary Principle Also Applies to Public Health Actions." *American Journal of Public Health* 91 (9): 1358–61. https://dx.doi.org/10.2105%2Fajph.91.9.1358.

Gollum, M. 2020. "Why Attitudes toward Mask Wearing Are Quickly Changing in Canada and the U.S." CBC News, 18 May 2020. https://www. cbc.ca/news/canada/mask-wearing-attitudes-coronavirus-1.5569515.

– 2022. "Ottawa's Police Chief Says the Response to the Protest Has Been a Success. Not Everyone Agrees." CBC News, 2 February 2022. https:// www.cbc.ca/news/canada/ottawa/ottawa-protest-convoy-police-success-reaction-1.6334976.

Gonzalo, J.D., A. Chang, and D.R. Wolpaw. 2019. "New Educator Roles for Health Systems Science: Implications of New Physician Competencies for U.S. Medical School Faculty." *Academic Medicine* 94 (4): 501–6. https://doi.org/10.1097/acm.0000000000002552.

Gooding, M., and D. Moro. 2020. "Accelerating Shifts Driving a Radical Rethink of the Customer Journey: Canadian Consumer Insights 2020." PwC Canada. https://www.pwc.com/ca/en/industries/retail-consumer/consumer-insights-2020.html.

Gorman, M. 2020. "The Powers of N.S.'s Health Protection Act and What Can Happen If You Don't Listen." CBC News, 17 March 2020. https:// www.cbc.ca/news/canada/nova-scotia/robert-strang-public-health-protection-legislation-covid-19-1.5499546.

Goudge, A. 2021. "Balancing Legality and Legitimacy in Canada's COVID-19 Response." *National Journal of Constitutional Law* 41 (2): 153–83. https://ssrn.com/abstract=3890443.

Gouvernement du Québec. 1999. *La complémentarité du secteur privé dans la pousuite des objectifs fondamentaux du système public de santé au Québec*. https://publications.msss.gouv.qc.ca/msss/fichiers/1999/99_653/ rapport.pdf.

Government of Alberta. 2020a. "Expanded Child Care For Essential Workers." 1 April 2020. https://www.alberta.ca/release. cfm?xID=699762C5E7F0F-EC8E-6B55-76C0AA7217CB6409.

– 2020b. *Ministerial Order No. SA:006/2020*. 27 March 2020. https://open. alberta.ca/publications/ministerial-order-006-2020-service-alberta.

– 2020c. "New Mandatory Provincewide Measures to Protect Lives." 8December2020.https://www.alberta.ca/release.cfm?xID=75859ADEA5D5E-045D-2386-0CB140C175A800DD.

– 2020d. "Update 20: COVID-19 Pandemic in Alberta (April 2 at 5 p.m.)." 2 April 2020. https://www.alberta.ca/release.cfm?xID=6999065 88AA0F-F424-1274-777C4D263DE727B6.

– 2020e. "Update 32: COVID-19 Pandemic in Alberta (April 14 at 5:30 p.m.)." 14 April 2020. https://www.alberta.ca/release.cfm?xID=70097 CEC6D814-B62F-2EDC-5CD2C42B460B0E53.

– 2020f. "Update 132: COVID-19 Pandemic in Alberta (Oct. 20, 4 p.m.)." 20 October 2020. https://www.alberta.ca/release.cfm?xID=74513D0250 8C-C6E2-13BA-1827FB54CB6F0918.

– 2023. "Improving Alberta's Response to Public Health Emergencies." 19January2023.https://www.alberta.ca/release.cfm?xID=86404F47300F9-D122-5701-9E14BBC5D4AAFF3E.

– n.d.a. "COVID-19 Alberta Statistics." Accessed December 2020. https:// www.alberta.ca/stats/covid-19-alberta-statistics.htm.

– n.d.b. "Vaccine Incentives – Alberta's Vaccine Lottery." Accessed 22 February 2022. https://www.alberta.ca/open-for-summer-lottery.aspx.

Government of British Columbia. 2020a. "Joint Statement on B.C.'s COVID-19 Response, Latest Updates." 8 December 2020. https://news. gov.bc.ca/releases/2020HLTH0064-002017.

– 2020b. "Province Allows Strata Corporations to Hold Meetings Electronically." 17 April 2020. https://news.gov.bc.ca/ releases/2020MAH0051-000710.

– 2020c. "Province Extends State of Emergency to Support COVID-19 Response." 31 March 2020. https://news.gov.bc.ca/releases/2020 PREM0018-000607.

– 2020d. "Province Supports Local Governments to Hold Public Hearings Electronically." 1 May 2020. https://news.gov.bc.ca/releases/2020 MAH0025-000802.

– 2022a. "B.C. Takes Next Step in Balanced Plan to Life COVID-19 Restrictions." 10 March 2022. https://news.gov.bc.ca/releases/2022 HLTH0081-000324.

– 2022b. *Community Care and Assisted Living Act – Residential Care Regulation*. Amended 17 January 2020 by BC Reg. 7/2022. https://www. bclaws.gov.bc.ca/civix/document/id/complete/statreg/96_2009.

– n.d. "Apply for or Renew a Property Tax Deferment Program Application – Province of British Columbia." Accessed 24 January 2022. https://www2.gov.bc.ca/gov/content/taxes/property-taxes/annual-property-tax/defer-taxes.

Government of Canada. 2006. "Influenza Outbreak in an Ontario Long-Term Care Home – January 2005." *Canada Communicable Disease Report* 32 (21). https://www.canada.ca/en/public-health/services/reports-publications/canada-communicable-disease-report-ccdr/monthly-issue/2006-32/influenza-outbreak-ontario-long-term-care-home-january-2005.html.

– 2008. *Lobbying Act.* RSC 1985, c. 44 (4th supp.). Amended 2 July 2008. https://laws-lois.justice.gc.ca/PDF/L-12.4.pdf.

– 2011a. "Canada Health Transfer." Modified 19 December 2011. https://www.canada.ca/en/department-finance/programs/federal-transfers/canada-health-transfer.html.

– 2011b. "Harper Government Launches the Next Phase of Canada's Economic Action Plan – A Low-Tax Plan for Jobs and Growth." https://www.canada.ca/en/news/archive/2011/03/harper-government-launches-next-phase-canada-economic-action-plan-low-tax-plan-jobs-growth.html.

– 2015. *When Work and Caregiving Collide: How Employers Can Support Their Employees Who Are Caregivers.* http://publications.gc.ca/collections/collection_2015/edsc-esdc/Em12-8-2015-eng.pdf.

– 2016. "Canada's Health Care System." Modified 10 October 2023. https://www.canada.ca/en/health-canada/services/canada-health-care-system.html.

– 2019a. *Creating Middle Class Jobs: A Federal Tourism Growth Strategy.* https://www.ic.gc.ca/eic/site/134.nsf/vwapj/Tourism_Strategy_eng_v8.pdf/$file/Tourism_Strategy_eng_v8.pdf.

– 2019b. *Investing in the Middle Class – Budget 2019.* Modified 19 March 2019. https://www.budget.gc.ca/2019/docs/plan/toc-tdm-en.html.

– 2019c. "National Emergency Strategic Stockpile." Modified 28 November 2019. https://www.canada.ca/en/public-health/services/emergency-preparedness-response/national-emergency-strategic-stockpile.html.

– 2020a. "Applications to Date – Canada Emergency Student Benefit (CESB)." Modified 14 October 2020. https://www.canada.ca/en/revenue-agency/services/benefits/emergency-student-benefit/cesb-statistics.html.

– 2020b. *Bank of Canada Act.* RSC 1985, c. B-2. Amended 31 January 2020. https://laws-lois.justice.gc.ca/PDF/B-2.pdf.

– 2020c. *Quarantine Act.* SC 2005, c. 20. Amended 17 March 2020. https://laws-lois.justice.gc.ca/PDF/Q-1.1.pdf.

– 2020d. "Report a Lead on Suspected Tax or Benefit Cheating in Canada

– Overview." Modified 10 September 2020. https://www.canada.ca/en/
revenue-agency/programs/about-canada-revenue-agency-cra/suspected-
tax-cheating-in-canada-overview.html.

– 2020e. "Support for Students and Recent Graduates Impacted by
COVID-19." Modified 22 April 2020. https://www.canada.ca/en/
department-finance/news/2020/04/support-for-students-and-recent-
graduates-impacted-by-covid-19.html.

– 2021a. "Addressing Vaccine Hesitancy in the Context of COVID-19: A
Primer for Health Care Providers." Modified 7 May 2021. https://www.
canada.ca/en/public-health/services/diseases/2019-novel-coronavirus-
infection/health-professionals/vaccines/vaccine-hesitancy-primer.html.

– 2021b. *Canada Border Services Agency Act.* SC 2005, c. 35. Amended
15 January 2021. https://laws-lois.justice.gc.ca/PDF/C-1.4.pdf.

– 2021c. "Canada Emergency Response Benefit (CERB): Closed." Modified
30 April 2021. https://www.canada.ca/en/services/benefits/ei/cerb-
application.html.

– 2021d. Canada Labour Code. RSC 1985, c. L–2. Amended 29 December
2021. https://laws-lois.justice.gc.ca/PDF/L-2.pdf.

– 2021e. "Canadian Manufacturing Sector Gateway." Modified 12 October
2021. https://www.ic.gc.ca/eic/site/mfg-fab.nsf/eng/home.

– 2021f. *A Consolidation of the Constitution Acts 1867 to 1982.*
https://laws-lois.justice.gc.ca/PDF/CONST_TRD.pdf.

– 2021g. "COVID-19 and Deaths in Older Canadians: Excess Mortality and
the Impacts of Age and Comorbidity." Modified 14 December 2021.
https://www.canada.ca/en/public-health/services/diseases/coronavirus-
disease-covid-19/epidemiological-economic-research-data/excess-
mortality-impacts-age-comorbidity.html.

– 2021h. "Employment Insurance (EI) Program Statistics." Modified 15
August 2021. https://www.canada.ca/en/employment-social-development/
programs/ei/statistics.html.

– 2021i. "Federal Government Launched Tourism Relief Fund to Help
Tourism Businesses and Organizations Recover and Grow." Modified
12 July 2021. https://www.canada.ca/en/innovation-science-economic-
development/news/2021/07/federal-government-launches-tourism-
relief-fund-to-help-tourism-businesses-and-organizations-recover-and-
grow.html.

– 2021j. "Interim Report on Social and Economic Determinants of App
Adoption, Retention and Use." Modified 17 March 2021. https://www.
ic.gc.ca/eic/site/icgc.nsf/eng/07716.html.

– 2021k. *Part 1: Finishing the Fight against COVID-19.* Modified 19 April
2021. https://budget.gc.ca/2021/report-rapport/p1-en.html.

– 2021l. *A Recovery Plan for Jobs, Growth, and Resilience – Budget 2021*. https://www.budget.gc.ca/2021/pdf/budget-2021-en.pdf.

– 2021m. "Rights in the Workplace." Modified 27 October 2021. https:// www.canada.ca/en/canadian-heritage/services/rights-workplace.html.

– 2021n. "Trade and Investment Agreements." Modified 17 November 2021. https://www.international.gc.ca/trade-commerce/trade-agreements-accords-commerciaux/agr-acc/index.aspx?lang=eng&_ga=2. 72952723.1023786849.1594221372-1318896293.1593525759.

– 2022a. *Budget 2022 – A Plan to Grow Our Economy and Make Life More Affordable*. https://www.budget.canada.ca/2022/report-rapport/ toc-tdm-en.html.

– 2022b. "Canada Emergency Wage Subsidy (CEWS)." Modified 22 April 2022. https://www.canada.ca/en/revenue-agency/services/wage-rent-subsidies/emergency-wage-subsidy.html.

– 2022c. *Canada Health Act*. RSC 1985, c. C-6. Amended 12 December 2017. https://laws-lois.justice.gc.ca/PDF/C-6.pdf.

– 2022d. "Canada Recovery Sickness Benefit (CRSB)." Modified 17 January 2022. https://www.canada.ca/en/revenue-agency/services/benefits/ recovery-sickness-benefit.html#shr-pg-pnlShrPg.

– 2022e. "Canada's *Emergencies Act*." Modified 25 February 2022. https://www.canada.ca/en/department-justice/news/2022/02/canadas-emergencies-act.html.

– 2022f. "The Canadian Tourism Sector." Modified 17 January 2022. https://www.ic.gc.ca/eic/site/134.nsf/eng/home.

– 2022g. "Claims to Date – Canada Emergency Wage Subsidy (CEWS)." Modified 7 February 2022. https://www.canada.ca/en/revenue-agency/ services/subsidy/emergency-wage-subsidy/cews-statistics.html.

– 2022h. "COVID Alert Performance Metrics." Modified 16 June 2022. https://www.canada.ca/en/public-health/services/diseases/coronavirus-disease-covid-19/covid-alert/performance-metrics.html.

– 2022i. "COVID-19 Epidemiology Update." Modified 21 November 2023. https://health-infobase.canada.ca/covid-19/.

– 2022j. "COVID-19: Outbreak Update." Modified 16 February 2022. https://www.canada.ca/en/public-health/services/diseases/2019-novel-coronavirus-infection.html?topic=tilelink.

– 2022k. "COVID-19 Vaccination in Canada." Modified 25 March 2022. https://health-infobase.canada.ca/covid-19/vaccination-coverage/archive/ 2022-03-25/.

– 2022l. "Oil Pricing." https://www.nrcan.gc.ca/our-natural-resources/ energy-sources-distribution/clean-fossil-fuels/crude-oil/oil-pricing/ 18087.

– 2022m. "One-Time Payment to Persons with Disabilities." Modified 27 July 2022. https://www.canada.ca/en/services/benefits/one-time-payment-persons-disabilities.html.

– 2022n. "Public Health Ethics Framework: A Guide for Use in Response to the COVID-19 Pandemic in Canada." Modified 12 August 2022. https://www.canada.ca/en/public-health/services/diseases/2019-novel-coronavirus-infection/canadas-reponse/ethics-framework-guide-use-response-covid-19-pandemic.html.

– 2022o. "Social Inequalities in COVID-19 Deaths in Canada." Modified 26 August 2022. https://health-infobase.canada.ca/covid-19/inequalities-deaths.

– 2022p. "Testing for COVID-19: Importance." Modified 4 February 2022. https://www.canada.ca/en/public-health/services/diseases/2019-novel-coronavirus-infection/symptoms/testing.html.

– 2022q. "Testing for COVID-19: Roles and Responsibilities across Canada." Modified 15 August 2022. https://www.canada.ca/en/public-health/services/diseases/2019-novel-coronavirus-infection/symptoms/testing/roles-responsibilities.html.

– 2023a. COVID-19 Vaccine: Canadian Immunization Guide. Modified 2 February 2023. https://www.canada.ca/en/public-health/services/publications/healthy-living/canadian-immunization-guide-part-4-active-vaccines/page-26-covid-19-vaccine.html.

– 2023b. "Hire a Temporary Worker as an In-Home Caregiver: Overview." 2 May 2023. https://www.canada.ca/en/employment-social-development/services/foreign-workers/caregiver.html.

– 2023c. "Work-Sharing Program: Overview." Modified 30 June 2023. https://www.canada.ca/en/employment-social-development/services/work-sharing.html.

Government of Manitoba. 2020a. "Manitoba Provides Update on Child-Care Options for Families during COVID-19." 9 April 2020. https://news.gov.mb.ca/news/index.html?item=47466&posted=2020-04-09.

– 2020b. "Province Extends Public Health Orders Ahead of the Holidays, with Minor Adjustments." 8 December 2020. https://news.gov.mb.ca/news/index.html?item=50003&posted=2020-12-08.

– 2020c. "Restoring Safe Services Together: Manitoba's Phased Approach." 4 May 2020. https://www.gov.mb.ca/covid19/restoring/approach.html.

– n.d. "Information for Manitobans – COVID-19 Testing." Accessed June 2020. https://www.gov.mb.ca/covid19/testing/index.html.

Government of New Brunswick. 2020a. "COVID-19 Job Protection Measures Put in Place; No Active Cases in Hospital." 30 April 2020. https://www2.gnb.ca/content/gnb/en/news/news_release.2020.04.0240.html.

– 2020b."Zone 4 Moving to Orange / Eighth Death Related to COVID-19 / Eight New Cases / Case at Saint Mary's Academy in Edmundston / Changes to Mandatory Order / Exposure Notification." 11 December 2020. https://www2.gnb.ca/content/gnb/en/news/news_release.2020. 12.0679.html.

– n.d. "About COVID-19." Accessed June 2020. https://www2.gnb.ca/content/gnb/en/corporate/promo/covid-19/about-covid-19.html#testing.

Government of Newfoundland and Labrador. n.d. "Symptoms." Accessed June 2020. https://www.gov.nl.ca/covid-19/public-health-guidance/covid-19/symptoms.

Government of Northwest Territories. 2020a. "GNWT to Support Child Care For Essential Workers Responding to COVID-19." 24 April 2020. https://www.gov.nt.ca/en/newsroom/gnwt-support-child-care-essential workers-responding-covid-19.

– 2020b. "New Temporary Regulation Allows Tenants to Defer Their Rent with Landlord's Knowledge." 15 April 2020. https://www.gov.nt.ca/en/newsroom/new-temporary-regulation-allows-tenants-defer-their-rent-landlords-knowledge.

Government of Nova Scotia. 2020a. "Atlantic Canada Bubble Border Crossing." 2 July 2020. https://novascotia.ca/news/release/?id=20200 702003.

– 2020b. "New Restrictions to Reduce Spread of COVID-19." 20 November 2020. https://novascotia.ca/news/release/?id=20201120003.

– 2020c. "Province Announces Mandatory Masks in Indoor Public Places." 24 July 2020. https://novascotia.ca/news/release/?id=20200724004.

– 2020d. "Restrictions Extended, More Asymptomatic Testing Rolls Out across the Province." 4 December 2020. https://novascotia.ca/news/release/?id=20201204004.

– 2021a. *Guide to the Nova Scotia Labour Standards Code.* https://nova scotia.ca/lae/employmentrights/docs/labourstandardscodeguide.pdf.

– 2021b. "News Release – Update to Vaccine Mandate." 4 October 2021. https://novascotia.ca/news/release/?id=20211004006.

– 2022. "COVID-19 Restrictions Easing Next Week, Fully Lifted on March 21." 23 February 2022. https://novascotia.ca/news/release/?id=20220223008.

– n.d. "Coronavirus (COVID-19): Symptoms, Testing and How to Self-Isolate." Accessed October 2020. https://novascotia.ca/coronavirus/ symptoms-and-testing/#who-can-be-tested.

Government of Ontario. 2020a. "Ontario Expanding Data Collection to Help Stop Spread of COVID-19." 15 June 2020. https://news.ontario.ca/en/release/57217/ontario-expanding-data-collection-to-help-stop-spread-of-covid-19.

– 2020b. "Ontario Investing $52.5 Million to Recruit, Retain and Support More Health Care Workers." 28 September 2020. https://news.ontario.ca/en/release/58580/ontario-investing-525-million-to-recruit-retain-and-support-more-health-care-workers.

– 2020c. "Ontario Moving Regions to New Levels with Stronger Public Health Measures." 11 December 2020. https://news.ontario.ca/en/release/59603/ontario-moving-regions-to-new-levels-with-stronger-public-health-measures.

– 2020d. "Province Launching Recruitment Program to Support Long-Term Care Sector." 9 November 2020. https://news.ontario.ca/en/release/59108/province-launching-recruitment-program-to-support-long-term-care-sector.

Government of Prince Edward Island. 2020a. "Province Announces Rental Support Measures." 30 March 2020. https://www.princeedwardisland.ca/en/news/province-announces-rental-support-measures.

– 2020b. "Province Outlines Plans to 'Renew PEI, Together.'" 28 April 2020. https://www.princeedwardisland.ca/en/news/province-outlines-plans-renew-pei-together.

– 2022. "PEI COVID-19 Testing and Case Data." Accessed August 2020. https://www.princeedwardisland.ca/en/information/health-and-wellness/covid-19-testing-and-case-data.

Government of Quebec. n.d. "Testing for COVID-19." Accessed June 2020. https://www.quebec.ca/en/health/health-issues/a-z/2019-coronavirus/testing-for-covid-19.

Government of Saskatchewan. 2020. "Province Announces Re-open Saskatchewan Plan." 23 April 2020. https://www.saskatchewan.ca/government/news-and-media/2020/april/23/reopen-saskatchewan-plan.

– n.d. "Testing and Treatment Information." Accessed August 2020. https://www.saskatchewan.ca/government/health-care-administration-and-provider-resources/treatment-procedures-and-guidelines/emerging-public-health-issues/2019-novel-coronavirus/testing-information.

Government of Yukon. 2020a. "Online Meetings Now Supported for Annual General Meetings under the Civil Emergency Measures Act." 13 May 2020. https://yukon.ca/en/news/online-meetings-now-supported-annual-general-meetings-under-civil-emergency-measures-act.

– 2020b. "Tenants Continue to Receive Protection during COVID-19 Pandemic." 12 June 2020. https://yukon.ca/en/news/tenants-continue-receive-protection-during-covid-19-pandemic.

Graefe, P., and M. Ferdosi. 2021. "CERB Was Luxurious Compared to Provincial Social Assistance." *The Conversation*, 2 May 2021. https://theconversation.com/cerb-was-luxurious-compared-to-provincial-social-assistance-158501.

Graham-Harrison, E., and T. Lindeman. 2022. "Freedom Convoys: Legitimate COVID Protest or Vehicle for Darker Beliefs?" *Guardian*, 13 February 2022. https://www.theguardian.com/world/2022/feb/13/freedom-convoys-legitimate-covid-protest-or-vehicle-for-darker-beliefs.

Grant, K. 2014. "Ottawa to Limit Power of Canada's Top Doctor." *Globe and Mail*, 12 November 2014. https://www.theglobeandmail.com/news/politics/ottawa-to-limit-power-of-canadas-top-doctor-the-chief-public-health-officer/article21550260.

Grant, K., and T.T. Ha. 2020. "How Shoring up Hospitals for COVID-19 Contributed to Canada's Long-Term Care Crisis." *Globe and Mail*, 21 May 2020. https://www.theglobeandmail.com/canada/article-how-shoring-up-hospitals-for-covid-19-contributed-to-canadas-long.

Grant, K., and K. Howlett. 2020. "Proposed Class-Action Lawsuit Filed against Owner of Several Ontario Seniors' Homes." *Globe and Mail*, 26 April 2020. https://www.theglobeandmail.com/canada/article-proposed-class-action-lawsuit-filed-against-owner-of-several-ontario.

Grant, K., and L. Stone. 2020. "Care Homes across Canada Desperate for Staff amid COVID-19 Outbreak Turn to Librarians, Museum Workers." *Globe and Mail*, 3 April 2020. https://www.theglobeandmail.com/canada/article-care-homes-across-canada-desperate-for-staff-amid-covid-19-outbreak.

Grant, M. 2022. "4 Alberta Border Protesters Charged with Conspiring to Murder RCMP Officers." CBC News, 24 February 2022. https://www.cbc.ca/news/canada/calgary/coutts-protest-charges-laid-court-appearance-bail-1.6352482.

Grant, T. 2021. "Multiple Amazon Facilities Face Scrutiny from Ontario for COVID-19, Other Health and Safety Concerns." *Globe and Mail*, 24 March 2021. https://www.theglobeandmail.com/canada/article-multiple-amazon-facilities-face-scrutiny-from-ontario-for-covid-19.

Gray, J. 2020. "To Spare the Homeless from COVID-19, Some Cities Look to Hotels." *Globe and Mail*, 10 April 2020. https://www.theglobeandmail.com/canada/article-to-spare-the-homeless-from-covid-19-some-cities-look-to-hotels.

Green, A. 2020. "Li Wenliang." *Lancet* 395 (10225): 682. https://doi.org/10.1016/S0140-6736(20)30382-2.

Greenard, K. 2020. "Take Advantage of the Property Tax Deferment Program." *Times Colonist*, 26 June 2020. https://www.timescolonist.com/business/kevin-greenard-take-advantage-of-the-property-tax-deferment-program-1.24160741.

Greenslade, B. 2022. "Manitoba Spent More than $40M with Private Nursing Agencies Last Year." Global News, 17 August 2022. https://globalnews.ca/news/9066971/manitoba-private-nursing-agencies-cost.

GreenStep Sustainable Tourism. n.d. "Let's Change the World through Tourism." Accessed 14 July 2021. https://greensteptourism.com.

Grenier, E. 2020a. "A Crisis Can Boost a Leader's Popularity – But It Doesn't Always Last." CBC News, 19 April 2020. https://www.cbc.ca/news/politics/grenier-crisis-popularity-history-1.5536566.

– 2020b. "What National COVID-19 Modelling Can Tell Us – And What It Can't." CBC News, 9 April 2020. https://www.cbc.ca/news/politics/grenier-covid19-models-1.5525478.

– 2021. "COVID-19 and N.L.'s Election Results Probably Killed the Idea of a Spring Federal Election." CBC News, 1 April 2021. https://www.cbc.ca/news/politics/grenier-spring-election-nl-1.5971687.

Grose, J. 2021. "The Primal Scream: America's Mothers Are in Crisis." New York Times, 4 February 2021. https://www.nytimes.com/2021/02/04/parenting/working-moms-mental-health-coronavirus.html.

Guardian. 2019. "The Guardian View on the Gig Economy: Stop Making Burnout a Lifestyle." 30 December 2019. https://www.theguardian.com/commentisfree/2019/dec/30/the-guardian-view-on-the-gig-economy-stop-making-burnout-a-lifestyle.

Ha, T.T. 2020. "How Quebec's Long-Term Care Homes Became Hotbeds for the COVID-19 Pandemic." Globe and Mail, 7 May 2020. https://www.theglobeandmail.com/canada/article-how-quebecs-long-term-care-homes-became-hotbeds-for-the-covid-1.

Haas-Wilson, D. 2001. "Arrow and the Information Market Failure in Health Care: The Changing Content and Sources of Health Care Information." Journal of Health Politics, Policy and Law 26 (6): 1031–44. doi.org/10.1215/03616878-26-5-1031.

Habermas, J. 1971. Knowledge and Human Interests. Boston: Beacon Press.

– 1984. The Theory of Communicative Action. Vol. 1, Reason and the Rationalization of Society. Translated by T.A. McCarthy. Boston: Beacon Press.

– 1987. The Theory of Communicative Action. Vol. 2, Lifeworld and Systems, a Critique of Functionalist Reason. Translated by T.A. McCarthy. Boston: Beacon Press.

Habib, J. 2021. "This Expert Says Medical Racism Is Interfering with Canada's COVID-19 Response." Global Citizen, 29 April 2021. https://www.globalcitizen.org/en/content/worlds-best-shot-krishana-sankar.

Habibi, R., and J. Lexchin. 2021. "The COVID-19 Vaccination Race." Open Canada, 9 March 2021. https://opencanada.org/canada-isntin-a-covid-19-vaccination-race-against-other-countries-were-all-in-a-race-against-time.

Hagan, S. 2021. "Canada Returns to Pre-pandemic Employment Levels." BNN Bloomberg, 8 October 2021. https://www.bnnbloomberg.ca/canada-returns-to-pre-pandemic-employment-levels-1.1663595.

Hager, M., and A. Woo. 2020. "How the Coronavirus Took North Vancouver's Lynn Valley Care Centre." *Globe and Mail*, 21 March 2020. https://www.theglobeandmail.com/canada/article-how-the-coronavirus-took-north-vancouvers-lynn-valley-care-centre.

Hager, M., and J. Keller. 2021. "B.C. Reports Low COVID-19 Transmissions in Schools as Kenney Defends Not Prioritizing Teachers for Vaccines." *Globe and Mail*, 16 April 2021. https://www.theglobeandmail.com/canada/british-columbia/article-bc-reports-low-virus-transmissions-in-schools-as-kenney-defends-not.

Haldane, V., C.D. Foo, S.M. Abdalla, A.S. Jung, M. Tan, S. Wu, A. Chua et al. 2021. "Health Systems Resilience in Managing the COVID-19 Pandemic: Lessons from 28 Countries." *Nature Medicine* 27: 964–80. https://www.nature.com/articles/s41591-021-01381-y.

Hall, C. 2021. "The House: Can Canadian Federalism Cope with 21st Century Threats?" CBC News, 3 July 2021. https://www.cbc.ca/radio/the-house/federal-provincial-pandemic-climate-change-1.6084889.

Hall, J. 2020. "Insurers Are under the Gun as COVID-19 Claims Mount – But Will Those Claims Be Covered?" *Toronto Star*, 31 March 2020. https://www.thestar.com/business/2020/03/30/a-toronto-dentist-who-pays-10000-a-year-for-insurance-that-includes-pandemic-coverage-cant-collect-and-he-is-not-alone.html.

Hall, M. 2019. "The Greatest Wealth Transfer in History: What's Happening and What Are the Implications." *Forbes*, 11 November 2019. https://www.forbes.com/sites/markhall/2019/11/11/the-greatest-wealth-transfer-in-history-whats-happening-and-what-are-the-implications.

Halpin, D.R., and B. Fraussen. 2019. "Laying the Groundwork: Linking Internal Agenda-Setting Processes of Interest Groups to Their Role in Policy Making." *Administration & Society* 51 (8): 1337–59. https://doi.org/10.1177/0095399717728094.

Halpin, D.R., B. Fraussen, and A.J. Nownes. 2017. "The Balancing Act of Establishing a Policy Agenda: Conceptualizing and Measuring Drivers of Issue Prioritization within Interest Groups." *Governance* 31 (2): 215–37. https://doi.org/10.1111/gove.12284.

Hameleers, M. 2020. "Prospect Theory in Times of a Pandemic: The Effects of Gain versus Loss Framing on Policy Preferences and Emotional Responses during the 2020 Coronavirus Outbreak – Evidence from the

US and the Netherlands." *Mass Communication and Society* 24 (4): 479–99. https://doi.org/10.1080/15205436.2020.1870144.

Hansen, G., and A. Cyr. 2020. "Canada's Decentralized 'Human-Driven' Approach during the Early COVID-19 Pandemic." *JMIR Public Health and Surveillance* 6 (4): e2043. https://doi.org/10.2196/20343.

Hardin, R. 2006. *Trust*. Cambridge: Polity Press.

Harrington, C., F.F. Jacobsen, J. Panos, A. Pollock, S. Sutaria, and M. Szebehely. 2017. "Marketization in Long-Term Care: A Cross-Country Comparison of Large For-Profit Nursing Home Chains." *Health Services Insights* 10: 1–23. https://doi.org/10.1177/1178632917710533.

Harris, K. 2020a. "Canadians Have Returned 830,000 Pandemic Benefit Payments." CBC News, 4 October 2020. https://www.cbc.ca/news/politics/cra-cerb-repayments-1.5748334.

– 2020b. "Canadians Should Wear Masks as an 'Added Layer of Protection,' Says Tam." CBC News, 20 May 2020. https://www.cbc.ca/news/politics/masks-covid-19-pandemic-public-health-1.5576895.

Harris, S. 2020. "2 Canadian Insurance Companies Stop Covering Coronavirus-Related Trip Cancellations." CBC News, 5 March 2020. https://www.cbc.ca/news/business/coronavirus-manulife-tugo-travel-insurance-1.5486117.

– 2022. "Ottawa Dropping Pre-arrival PCR Test for Travellers as of Feb. 28." CBC News, 16 February 2022. https://www.cbc.ca/news/business/pcr-test-arrival-travel-drop-1.6350469.

Harrison Warren, T. 2021. "The Limits of 'My Body, My Choice.'" *New York Times*, 26 September 2021. https://www.nytimes.com/2021/09/26/opinion/choice-liberty-freedom.html.

Harun, R., and M. Walton-Roberts. 2022. "Assessing the Contribution of Immigrants to Canada's Nursing and Health Care Support Occupations: A Multi-Scalar Analysis." *Human Resources for Health* 20 (1): 53. https://doi.org/10.1186/s12960-022-00748-7.

Harvey, A. 2020. "Canadian Food Banks Struggle to Stay Open, Just as Demand for Their Services Skyrockets." *Globe and Mail*, 11 April 2020. https://www.theglobeandmail.com/canada/toronto/article-canadian-food-banks-struggle-to-stay-open-just-as-demand-for-their.

Harvey, L. 2020. "Praised by Doug Ford, Vilified by Critics – But Is Dr. David Williams Misunderstood?" *Toronto Star*, 29 November 2020. https://www.thestar.com/news/canada/2020/11/29/he-will-never-throw-you-under-the-bus-but-is-dr-david-williams-in-over-his-head-or-just-a-good-man-in-an-impossible-job.html.

Hassan, Y. 2022. "Health-Care Workers Call for Government Help as Burnout Worsens and Staff Shortages Increase." CBC News, 18 June

2022. https://www.cbc.ca/news/politics/healthcare-workers-burnout-1.
6492889.

Hay, L.J. 2020. "COVID-19: The Global Insurance Response." KPMG
International, April 2020. https://home.kpmg/xx/en/home/insights
2020/04/covid-19-global-insurance-response.html.

Health Canada. 2003. *Learning from SARS: Renewal of Public Health in
Canada – Report of the National Advisory Committee of SARS and Public
Health*. https://www.canada.ca/content/dam/phac-aspc/migration/phac-
aspc/publicat/sars-sras/pdf/sars-e.pdf.

– 2021. *Priority Strategies to Optimize Testing and Screening for COVID-19
in Canada: Report*. https://www.canada.ca/content/dam/hc-sc/documents/
services/drugs-health-products/covid19-industry/medical-devices/test-
ing-screening-advisory-panel/reports-summaries/priority-strategies/
priority-strategies-eng.pdf/.

Health Quality Ontario. n.d. "Wait Times for Long-Term Care Homes."
Accessed 4 March 2022. https://www.hqontario.ca/System-Performance/
Long-Term-Care-Home-Performance/Wait-Times.

Health Standards Organization. 2021. "Public Notice of Intent: Long-Term
Care Services." 16 March 2021. https://healthstandards.org/standards/
notices-of-intent/long-term-care-services.

Healy, P. 2016. "Economically Speaking: Market Failure and the NHS."
NHS Confederation, 26 October 2016. https://www.nhsconfed.org/
articles/economically-speaking-market-failure-and-nhs.

Helland, S.S., and E.R. Morrison. 2021. "The Healthcare System and
Pandemics: Where Is the Market Failure?" *Ohio State Law Journal* 82
(5): 833–44. https://scholarship.law.columbia.edu/faculty_scholarship/
3180.

Helliwell, J.F., R. Layard, J.D. Sachs, J.E. De Neve, L.B. Aknin, and S.
Wang. 2021. *2021 World Happiness Report*. https://happiness-report.
s3.amazonaws.com/2021/WHR*21.pdf.

Hendry, L. 2020. "Could Private Seniors' Residences Be the Next Weak
Link in the Fight against COVID-19?" CBC News, 22 September 2020.
https://www.cbc.ca/news/canada/montreal/private-seniors-residences-rpas-
key-to-next-wave-1.5732867.

Hendry, L., and B. Shingler. 2020. "The Growing Toll of Quebec's Second
Wave of COVID-19." CBC News, 11 November 2020. https://www.cbc.
ca/news/canada/montreal/quebec-covid-19-second-wave-1.5796847.

Henig, R.M. 2020. "Experts Warned of a Pandemic Decades Ago. Why
Weren't We Ready?" *National Geographic*, 8 April 2020. https://www.
nationalgeographic.com/science/article/experts-warned-pandemic-decades-ago-
why-not-ready-for-coronavirus.

Herhalt, C. 2020. "Ford Government Spending $1 Billion to Boost COVID-19 Testing, Tracing." CP24 News, 24 September 2020. https://www.cp24.com/news/ford-government-spending-1-billion-to-boost-covid-19-testing-tracing-1.5117968?cache=dkorkzbx.

Herring, J. 2021. "Alberta Asks Provinces for Help as ICU Capacity Nears Breaking Point." *Calgary Herald*, 17 September 2021. https://calgary herald.com/news/local-news/alberta-could-run-out-of-staffed-icu-beds-sooner-than-reported.

Hess, S., E. Brocklehurst, T. Brauch, and I. Volkmer. 2021. "Social Media and COVID: A Global Study of Digital Crisis Interaction among Gen Z and Millennials." COVID-19 Infodemic. https://covid19infodemic.com/?fbclid=IwAR22xPcTI8WzUhmgW3AzHXfOelabFJx92_tMHN-8bYnpgB8ZsotJCQ9vnZQI#contact.

Heyland, D.K., P. Dodek, G. Rocker, D. Groll, A. Gafni, D. Pichora, S. Shortt et al. 2006. "What Matters Most in End-of-Life Care: Perceptions of Seriously Ill Patients and Their Family Members." *Canadian Medical Association Journal* 174 (5): 627–33. https://doi.org/10.1503/cmaj.050626.

HHS Office of Inspector General. 2020. *Audit of HHS's Production and Distribution of COVID-19 Lab Test Kits*. US Department of Health and Human Services. https://oig.hhs.gov/reports-and-publications/workplan/summary/wp-summary-0000462.asp.

Hill, B., and J. Pazzano. 2020. "20 Million Canadians Still Don't Have Full Access to the COVID Alert App. Why?" Global News, 2 October 2020. https://globalnews.ca/news/7369875/canadians-access-covid-alert-app.

Hill, B., and A. Russell. 2021. "Experts Warned of New COVID-19 Variants. Why Did Ottawa Wait for Stricter Travel Rules?" Global News, 4 February 2021. https://globalnews.ca/news/7614338/canada-covid-19-travel-rules.

Hilton, S., and E. Smith. 2010. "Public Views of the UK Media and Government Reaction to the 2009 Swine Flu Pandemic." *BMC Public Health* 10 (1): 697. http://dx.doi.org/10.1186/1471-2458-10-697.

Hiremath, P., C.S. Suhas Kowshik, M. Manjunath, and M. Shettar. 2020. "COVID 19: Impact of Lock-down on Mental Health and Tips to Overcome." *Asian Journal of Psychiatry* 51 (June): 102088. https://doi.org/10.1016/j.ajp.2020.102088.

History of Vaccines. n.d. "All Timelines Overview." The College of Physicians of Philadelphia. Accessed 17 February 2022. https://www.historyofvaccines.org/timeline/all.

Ho, J., S. Hussain, and O. Sparagano. 2021. "Did the COVID-19 Pandemic Spark a Public Interest in Pet Adoption." *Frontiers in Veterinary Science* 8: 647308. https://doi.org/10.3389/fvets.2021.647308.

Ho, S. 2020. "Nobody Died in These Nursing Homes – What Did They Do Right?" CTV News, 25 June 2020. https://www.ctvnews.ca/health/coronavirus/nobody-died-in-these-nursing-homes-what-did-they-do-right-1.4998204.

Hockaday, J. 2022. "Cost of Living: How Does UK Inflation Compare to Other G7 Countries?" *Yahoo News*, 1 December 2022. https://ca.news.yahoo.com/cost-of-living-how-does-uk-inflation-compare-to-other-g-7-countries-155224597.html.

Hoffman, S.J., M.I. Creatore, A. Klassen, A.M. Lay, and P Fafard. 2019. "Building the Political Case for Investing in Public Health and Public Health Research." *Canadian Journal of Public Health* 110: 270–4. https://dx.doi.org/10.17269%2Fs41997-019-00214-3.

Hoffmann, S.J., and P. Fafard. 2020a. "Border Closures: A Pandemic of Symbolic Acts in the Time of COVID-19." In *Vulnerable: The Law, Policy and Ethics of COVID-19*, edited by C. Flood, V. MacDonnell, J. Philpott, S. Theriault, and S. Venkatapuram, 555–70. Ottawa, ON: University of Ottawa Press.

– 2020b. "Why Pandemic-Era Border Closures Are about Symbolism, Not Science." *Policy Options*, 27 August 2020. https://policyoptions.irpp.org/magazines/august-2020/why-pandemic-era-border-closures-are-about-symbolism-not-science.

Hogan, S., and M. Glanz. 2020. "Oncologist Fears 'Tsunami of Cancer' after COVID-19 Lockdowns Limited Screening." CBC News, 17 December 2020. https://www.cbc.ca/news/health/cancer-tsunami-screening-delays-covid-1.5844708.

Holder, J. 2022. "Tracking Coronavirus Vaccinations around the World." *New York Times*, 28 February 2022. https://www.nytimes.com/interactive/2021/world/covid-vaccinations-tracker.html.

Holman, C., and W. Luneburg. 2012. "Lobbying and Transparency: A Comparative Analysis of Regulatory Reform." *Interest Groups & Advocacy* 1: 75–104. https://doi.org/10.1057/iga.2012.4.

Homeland Security Council. 2005. *National Strategy for Pandemic Influenza*. https://www.cdc.gov/flu/pandemic-resources/pdf/pandemic-influenza-strategy-2005.pdf.

Honderich, H. 2021. "Canada Election: How Vaccine Mandates Became an Issue." BBC, 19 August 2021. https://www.bbc.com/news/world-us-canada-58264006.

Hood, C. 1991. "A Public Management for All Seasons?" *Public Administration* 69 (1): 3–19. https://doi.org/10.1111/j.1467-9299.1991.tb00779.x.

– 1998. *The Art of the State: Culture, Rhetoric and Public Management*. Oxford: Clarendon Press.

Hood, C., H. Rothstein, and R. Baldwin. 2001. *The Government of Risk: Understanding Risk Regulation Regimes*. Oxford: Oxford University Press.

House of Assembly Newfoundland and Labrador. n.d. "Parliamentary Calendar." Accessed 2021. https://www.assembly.nl.ca/HouseBusiness/ParliamentaryCalendar.aspx.

Howard, J., A. Huang, Z. Li, Z. Tufekci, V. Zdimal, H.M. van der Westhuizen, A. von Delft, A. Price, L. Fridman, L.H. Tang et al. 2021. "An Evidence Review of Face Masks against COVID-19." *Proceedings of the National Academy of Sciences of the United States of America* 118 (4): e2014564118. https://doi.org/10.1073/pnas.2014564118.

Howlett, K. 2020. "Ontario Says Owners Must Pay for Emergency Pandemic Costs Associated with Their Seniors' Homes." *Globe and Mail*, 11 June 2020. https://www.theglobeandmail.com/canada/article-ontario-tells-hospitals-they-must-pay-for-emergency-pandemic-costs.

Howlett, K., and T.T. Ha. 2021. "COVID-19 Hit Long-Term Care Homes Harder in Second Wave." *Globe and Mail*, 3 March 2021. https://www.theglobeandmail.com/canada/article-covid-19-hit-long-term-care-homes-harder-in-second-wave.

Howlett, M. 2019. "Procedural Policy Tools and the Temporal Dimensions of Policy Design: Resilience, Robustness and the Sequencing of Policy Mixes." *International Review of Public Policy* 1 (1): 27–45. https://doi.org/10.4000/irpp.

Hristova, B. 2022. "Ontario Waiting On More than $1.5m in Unpaid COVID-19 Fines." CBC News, 21 April 2022. https://www.cbc.ca/news/canada/hamilton/ontario-unpaid-covid-19-fines-1.6425690.

Huang, Y. 2020. "Refining the Precautionary Principle in Public International Law." *US-China Law Review* 17 (3): 75–91. https://doi.org/10.17265/1548-6605/2020.03.001.

Huang, Y., M. Sun, and Y. Sui. 2020. "How Digital Contact Tracing Slowed COVID-19 in East Asia." *Harvard Business Review*, 15 April 2020. https://hbr.org/2020/04/how-digital-contact-tracing-slowed-covid-19-in-east-asia.

Huck, A., J. Monstadt, and P. Driessen. 2020. "Building Urban and Infrastructure Resilience through Connectivity: An Institutional Perspective on Disaster Risk Management in Christchurch, New Zealand." *Cities* 98 (3): 102573. https://doi.org/10.1016/j.cities.2019.102573.

Hunter, A. 2022. "How Sask. Premier Moe's Messaging on Unvaccinated People Has Shifted since the Delta Wave." CBC News, 12 February 2022. https://www.cbc.ca/news/canada/saskatchewan/sask-covid-measures-1.6345397.

Hunter, J. 2020. "B.C. Offers Limited COVID-19 Lawsuit Immunity, Long-Term Care Homes Not Protected." *Globe and Mail*, 22 June 2020. https://www.theglobeandmail.com/canada/british-columbia/article-bc-offers-limited-covid-lawsuit-immunity-long-term-care-homes-not.

– 2021. "B.C. Urged to Change Course, Use COVID-19 Rapid Tests in Care Homes." *Globe and Mail*, 19 January 2021. https://www.theglobeand mail.com/canada/british-columbia/article-bc-urged-to-change-course-use-covid-19-rapid-tests-in-care-homes.

Hurst, D., and B. Butler. 2020. "Australian Government to Pay Qantas and Virgin to Keep Flying during COVID-19 Pandemic." *Guardian*, 16 April 2020. https://www.theguardian.com/australia-news/2020/apr/16/australian-government-to-pay-qantas-and-virgin-to-keep-flying.

Hussain, W. 2020. "Role of Social Media in COVID-19 Pandemic." *International Journal of Frontier Sciences* 4 (2): 59–60. https://doi.org/10.37978/tijfs.v4i2.144.

Ibbitson, J. 2021. "Who Would Refuse the COVID-19 Vaccine? New Research Sheds Some Light." *Globe and Mail*, 4 November 2021. https://www.theglobeandmail.com/politics/article-who-would-refuse-the-covid-19-vaccine-maybe-someone-who-feels.

IBC (Insurance Bureau of Canada). 2020a. "Insurers Support Small Businesses with Business Insurance Action Team." http://www.ibc.ca/on/resources/media-centre/media-releases/insurers-support-small-businesses-with-business-insurance-action-team.

– 2020b. *2020 Facts of the Property and Casualty Insurance Industry in Canada*. http://assets.ibc.ca/Documents/Facts%20Book/Facts_Book/2020/IBC-2020-Facts.pdf.

ILO (International Labour Organization). 2017. *ILO Guidelines on Decent Work and Socially Responsible Tourism*. https://www.ilo.org/wcmsp5/groups/public/---ed_dialogue/---sector/documents/normativeinstrument/wcms_546337.pdf.

– 2022. *The Future of Work in the Tourism Sector: Sustainable and Safe Recovery and Decent Work in the Context of the COVID-19 Pandemic*. https://www.ilo.org/wcmsp5/groups/public/---ed_dialogue/---sector/documents/meetingdocument/wcms_840403.pdf.

Independent Panel for Pandemic Preparedness and Response. 2021. *COVID-19: Make It the Last Pandemic*. https://theindependentpanel.org/wp-content/uploads/2021/05/COVID-19-Make-it-the-Last-Pandemic_final.pdf.

Institute of Medicine (US) Forum on Microbial Threats. 2007. "3. Strategies for Disease Containment." In *Ethical and Legal Considerations in Mitigating Pandemic Disease: Workshop Summary*, 76–154. Washington, DC: National Academies Press (US). https://doi.org/10.17226/11917.

Interlandi, J. 2021. "COVID Proved the C.D.C. Is Broken. Can It Be Fixed?" *New York Times*, 18 October 2021. https://www.nytimes. com/2021/06/16/magazine/cdc-covid-response.html.

International Energy Agency. 2020. *Oil Market Report – April 2020*. Paris: IEA. https://www.iea.org/reports/oil-market-report-april-2020.

Ipsos. 2015. *Three in Five Canadians (63%) Aren't Prepared to Care For Family Members Who Require Long-Term Care*. https://www.ipsos.com/ sites/default/files/publication/2015-08/6959.pdf.

– 2017. *CLAC Long-Term Care Omnibus Research*. https://www.ipsos.com/ sites/default/files/2017-05/7612-pr.pdf.

– 2019. *Global Views on Air Travel and Its Environmental Impact*. https:// www.ipsos.com/sites/default/files/ct/news/documents/2019-09/ipsos-wef_survey_report_-_global_views_on_air_travel_and_its_environmental_impact_v2.pdf.

Ipsos, and Canadian Medical Association. 2019. *2019 Election National Listening Tour: An Aging Population*. https://www.ipsos.com/sites/ default/files/ct/news/documents/2019-05/cma_-_2019_election_-_an_aging_population_v2.pdf.

Ipsos, and Royal College of Physicians. 2009. *Trust in Doctors 2009 – Annual Survey of Public Trust in Professions*. https://www.ipsos. com/sites/default/files/publication/9200-03/sri-trust-in-professions-2009.pdf.

Ireland, N. 2021. "With Most Long-Term Care Residents Vaccinated, Restoring Their Quality of Life Is Urgent, Experts Say." CBC News, 11 March 2021. https://www.cbc.ca/news/canada/toronto/long-term-care-residents-covid-vaccinated-quality-of-life-1.5944683.

ISED (Innovation, Science and Economic Development Canada). 2021. "Interim Report on Social and Economic Determinants of App Adoption, Retention and Use." Government of Canada, modified 17 March 2021. https://www.ic.gc.ca/eic/site/icgc.nsf/eng/07716.html.

ITAC (Indigenous Tourism Association of Canada). 2020. *Forward Together – A Strategic Recovery Plan for the Indigenous Tourism Association of Canada, 2020–2024*. https://indigenoustourism.ca/wp-content/uploads/ 2020/06/ITAC-Strategic-Recovery-Plan-2020-24.pdf.

– 2022. *Making Canada the World Leader in Indigenous Tourism*. https:// indigenoustourism.ca/wp-content/uploads/2022/08/Making-Canada-the-World-Leader-in-Indigenous-Tourism.pdf.

Jabakhanji, S. 2020. "Toronto Food Banks See Big Increase in Demand amid COVID-19 Pandemic." CBC News, 16 November 2020. https:// www.cbc.ca/news/canada/toronto/daily-bread-food-bank-report-2020-covid-1.5802510.

Jabakhanji, S., and J. Knope. 2022. "Ontario to Drop Most Mask Mandates on March 21, Remaining Pandemic Rules to Lift by End of April." CBC News, 10 March 2022. https://www.cbc.ca/news/canada/toronto/covid19-ontario-march-9-mask-mandates-1.6378148.

Jackman, M. 2022. "Canada's Charter Is Not the U.S. Bill of Rights." *Globe and Mail*, 23 February 2022. https://www.theglobeandmail.com/opinion/article-protesters-need-to-understand-canadas-charter-is-not-the-us-bill-of.

Jacobs, J.C., A. Laporte, C.H. Van Houtven, and P.C. Coyte. 2014. "Caregiving Intensity and Retirement Status in Canada." *Social Science & Medicine* 102 (February): 74–82. https://doi.org/10.1016/j.socscimed.2013.11.051.

Jacobs, J.C., M.B. Lill, C. Ng, and P Coyte. 2013. "The Fiscal Impact of Informal Caregiving to Home Care Recipients in Canada: How the Intensity of Care Influences Costs and Benefits to Government." *Social Science & Medicine* 81 (March): 102–9. https://doi.org/10.1016/j.socscimed.2012.12.015.

Jaeger, C., O. Renn, E.A. Rosa, and T. Webler. 2001. Risk, Uncertainty, and Rational Action. London: Earthscan.

Jaeger, G. 2022. "Pandemic Pets Ending Up in Shelters as Owners Return to Office, Struggle with Rising Costs." CBC News, 4 July 2022. https://www.cbc.ca/news/canada/toronto/toronto-animal-services-pet-surrender-increase-1.6507394.

James, O. 1995. "Explaining the Next Steps in the Department of Social Security: The Bureau-Shaping Model of Central State Reorganization." *Political Studies* 43 (4): 614–29. https://doi.org/10.1111/j.1467-9248.1995.tb01722.x.

Janes, S. 2023. "Survey Finds 44% of Canadian Pre-retirees Have Less than $5,000 in Savings." Benefits Canada, 16 June 2023. https://www.benefitscanada.com/pensions/retirement/survey-finds-44-of-canadian-pre-retirees-have-less-than-5000-in-savings.

Jasanoff, S. 1990. *The Fifth Branch: Science Advisors as Policy Makers*. Cambridge, MA: Harvard University Press.

Jedwab, J. 2020a. "Canadian Opinion on the Coronavirus – N°16: Masking or Unmasking? Canadians Increasingly Wearing Protective Mask in Public Spaces as COVID-19 Crisis Evolves." Association for Canadian Studies, 24 April 2020. https://acs-aec.ca/wp-content/uploads/2020/04/ACS-Coronavirus-16-Unmasked-Canadians-in-the-land-of-Covid-19-April-2020.pdf.

– 2020b. "Mask-O-Meter: Tracking Mask Wearing Shows That in Selected City Settings They Have Gone from the Exception to the Rule in Most

Public Spaces." Association for Canadian Studies, 12 July 2020. https://acs-aec.ca/wp-content/uploads/2020/07/ACS-Mask-o-meter-July-2020.pdf.

Jeffcott, S., N. Pidgeon, A. Weyman, and J. Walls. 2006. "Risk, Trust, and Safety Culture in U.K. Train Operating Companies." *Risk Analysis* 26 (5): 1105–21.

Jenni, K.E., and G. Loewenstein. 1997. "Explaining the 'Identifiable Victim Effect.'" *Journal of Risk and Uncertainty* 14: 235–57. https://www.cmu.edu/dietrich/sds/docs/loewenstein/identifiableVictim.PDF.

Jeon, S.H., H. Lius, and Y. Ostrovsky. 2019. "Measuring the Gig Economy in Canada Using Administrative Data." Analytical Studies Branch Research Paper Series 437, catalogue no. 11F0019M. https://www150.statcan.gc.ca/n1/en/pub/11f0019m/11f0019m2019025-eng.pdf?st=0OXY21hZ.

Jeon, S.H., and Y. Ostrovsky. 2020. "The Impact of COVID-19 on the Gig Economy: Short- and Long-Term Concerns." StatCan COVID-19: Data to Insights for a Better Canada, catalogue no. 45280001. https://www150.statcan.gc.ca/n1/en/pub/45-28-0001/2020001/article/00021-eng.pdf?st=d-N5u3Qu.

Jiménez, J. 2021. "Washington State Allows for Free Marijuana with COVID-19 Vaccine." *New York Times*, 7 June 2021. https://www.nytimes.com/2021/06/07/us/washington-marijuana-covid-vaccine.html.

Joffe, A.R. 2020. "Rethinking Lockdowns: The Risks and Trade-Offs of Public Health Measures to Prevent COVID-19 Infections." MacDonald-Laurier Institute. https://macdonaldlaurier.ca/files/pdf/20201209_Rethinking_lockdowns_Joffe_COMMENTARY_FWeb.pdf.

Johns Hopkins Center for Health Security, and the Nuclear Threat Initiative. 2019. *Global Health Security Index*. https://www.ghsindex.org/wp-content/uploads/2019/10/2019-Global-Health-Security-Index.pdf.

Johnson, B.B., and V.T. Covelo. 1987. *The Social and Cultural Construction of Risk*. Dordrecht, Netherlands: Reidel.

Jonas, S. 2021a. "New Visitation Rules for Long-Term Care Homes Fall Short amid High Vaccination Rates: Advocates." CBC News, 22 May 2021. https://www.cbc.ca/news/canada/toronto/relaxed-visitation-rules-for-long-term-care-fall-short-1.6036779.

– 2021b. "Younger, Unvaccinated People Plugging up Quebec's Beleaguered Hospitals amid 4th Wave." CBC News, 19 September 2021. https://www.cbc.ca/news/canada/montreal/quebec-4th-wave-plugging-up-hospitals-1.6179626.

Jones, A. 2020. "Ontario Allows Auto Insurance Companies to Provide Rebates Due to the Pandemic." CBC News, 16 April 2020. https://www.cbc.ca/news/canada/toronto/covid-ontario-automotive-insurance-1.5534887.

Jones, A.M. 2021. "Vaccine Passports: Where and How Could They Be Used in Canada?" CTV News, 16 July 2021. https://www.ctvnews.ca/health/coronavirus/vaccine-passports-where-and-how-could-they-be-used-in-canada-1.5507750.

Jones, B., and F.R. Baumgartner. 2005. *The Politics of Attention: How Government Prioritizes Problems*. Chicago: University of Chicago Press.

Jones, C., W.S. Hesterly, and S.P. Borgatti. 1997. "A General Theory of Network Governance: Exchange Conditions and Social Mechanisms." *Academy of Management Review* 22 (4): 911–45. https://doi.org/10.2307/259249.

Jones, E. 2021. "Sustainable Travel Survey 2021 – Importance & Sentiment to Fight Climate Change When Booking Travel." *The Vacationer*, 30 September 2021. https://thevacationer.com/sustainable-travel-survey-2021.

Jones, J.H., and M. Salathé. 2009. "Early Assessment of Anxiety and Behavioral Response to Novel Swine-Origin Influenza A (H1N1)." *PLOS ONE* 4 (12): e8032. https://doi.org/10.1371/journal.pone.0008032.

Jones, R.P. 2020. "Health Canada Approves Moderna COVID-19 Vaccine." CBC News, 23 December 2020. https://www.cbc.ca/news/politics/canada-approves-moderna-vaccine-1.5852848.

– 2021a. "Federal Government, Air Canada Reach Deal on Relief Package That Includes Customer Refunds." CBC News, 13 April 2021. https://www.cbc.ca/news/politics/air-canada-financial-relief-1.5984543.

– 2021b. "Here's the Latest on the Review of Canada's Assisted Dying Law." CBC News, 16 May 2021. https://www.cbc.ca/news/politics/mature-minors-advance-requests-mental-illness-maid-assisted-death-1.6021717.

Jordan, T. 2020. "News Conference – Introductory Remarks by Thomas Jordan." Swiss National Bank, 17 December 2020. https://www.snb.ch/en/mmr/speeches/id/ref_20201217_tjn/source/ref_20201217_tjn.en.pdf.

Kachulis, E., and M. Perez-Leclerc. 2020. "Temporary Foreign Workers in Canada (Background Paper)." Library of Canada, publication no. 2019-36-E. https://lop.parl.ca/staticfiles/PublicWebsite/Home/ResearchPublications/BackgroundPapers/PDF/2019-36-e.pdf.

Kaimann, D., and I. Tanneberg. 2021. "What Containment Strategy Leads Us through the Pandemic Crisis? An Empirical Analysis of the Measures against the COVID-19 Pandemic." *PLOS ONE* 16 (6): e0253237. https://doi.org/10.1371/journal.pone.0253237.

Kane, L.D. 2021. "Little Mountain Place Care Home Allowed Group Activities to Continue after Positive Test, Family Says." CBC News, 13 January 2021. https://www.cbc.ca/news/canada/british-columbia/little-mountain-care-home-vancouver-1.5871349.

Kaplan, S. 2021. "Ex-C.D.C. Chief on Challenge of Serving Trump during Pandemic." *New York Times*, 20 January 2021. https://www.nytimes.com/2021/01/20/health/covid-CDC-redfield.html.

Karantzas, G. 2020. "Online Dating in a COVID-19 World." *Psychology Today*, 21 April 2020. https://www.psychologytoday.com/us/blog/the-science-love/202004/online-dating-in-covid-19-world.

Karp, P. 2020. "Australian Airline Industry to Receive $715M Rescue Package." *Guardian*, 17 March 2020. https://www.theguardian.com/australia-news/2020/mar/18/australian-airline-industry-to-receive-715m-rescue-package.

Kashte, S., A. Gulbake, S.F. El-Amin III, and A. Gupta. 2021. "COVID-19 Vaccines: Rapid Development, Implications, Challenges and Future Prospects." *Human Cell* 34 (3): 711–33. https://dx.doi.org/10.1007%2Fs13577-021-00512-4.

Kasperson, R.E., N. Jhaveri, and J.X. Kasperson. 2005. "Stigma and the Social Amplification of Risk: Towards a Framework of Analysis." In *Publics, Risk Communication and the Social Amplification of Risk*, 1st ed., 161–80. Vol. 1 of *The Social Contours of Risk*. London: Routledge.

Kasperson, R.E., and J.X. Kasperson. 1996. "The Social Amplification and Attenuation of Risk." *The Annals of the American Academy of Political and Social Science* 545 (May): 95–105. http://www.jstor.org/stable/1047896.

Kasperson, R.E., O. Renn, P. Slovic, H.S. Brown, J. Emel, R. Goble, J.X. Kasperson, and S. Ratick. 1988. "The Social Amplification of Risk: A Conceptual Framework." *Risk Analysis* 8 (2): 177–87. https://doi.org/10.1111/j.1539-6924.1988.tb01168.x.

Kearney, J. 2013. "Perceptions of Non-accidental Child Deaths as Preventable Events: The Impact of Probability Heuristics and Biases on Child Protection Work." *Health, Risk & Society* 15 (1): 51–66. https://doi.org/10.1080/13698575.2012.749451.

Kearney, M., and P. Levine. 2020a. "The Coming COVID-19 Baby Bust: Update." Brookings, 17 December 2020. https://www.brookings.edu/blog/up-front/2020/12/17/the-coming-covid-19-baby-bust-update.

– 2020b. "Half a Million Fewer Children? The Coming COVID Baby Bust." Brookings, 15 June 2020. https://www.brookings.edu/research/half-a-million-fewer-children-the-coming-covid-baby-bust.

Keefe, J., L. MacEachern, and P. Fancey. 2017. "An Overview of Residential Long Term Care in New Brunswick, Nova Scotia, and Prince Edward Island." Nova Scotia Centre on Aging. https://www.msvu.ca/wpcontent/uploads/2020/05/Overview20of20LTC20in20Maritimes_June202017.pdf.

Keller, J. 2021. "Alberta to Offer $100 Incentive to Encourage Vaccination as COVID Cases Continue to Surge." *Globe and Mail*, 3 September 2021.

https://www.theglobeandmail.com/canada/alberta/article-alberta-to-offer-100-incentive-to-encourage-vaccination-as-covid-cases.

Keller, T. 2023. "How Working from Home Gave Canadians a Big Pay Raise – And Why Nobody Wants to Give It Up." *Globe and Mail*, 25 April 2023. https://www.theglobeandmail.com/business/commentary/article-how-working-from-home-gave-canadians-a-big-pay-raise-and-why-nobody.

Kelly, C. 2017. "Exploring Experiences of Personal Support Worker Education in Ontario, Canada." *Health and Social Care in the Community* 25 (4): 1430–38. https://doi.org/10.1111/hsc.12443.

Kemper, P. 2003. "Long-Term Care Research and Policy." *The Gerontologist* 43 (4): 436–46. https://doi.org/10.1093/geront/43.4.436.

Kerr, J. 2021. "Law Firms Embrace COVID-19 Vaccine Mandates." *Globe and Mail*, 26 October 2021. https://www.theglobeandmail.com/business/article-law-firms-embrace-covid-19-vaccine-mandates.

Kids Help Phone. n.d. "Insights." Accessed 3 March 2022. https://kidshelpphone.ca/get insights/home/#tour.

King, A., and M. Gollum. 2021. "Resident Isolation, Staffing Remain Significant Concerns in Ontario Long-Term Care Centres." CBC News, 30 April 2021. https://www.cbc.ca/news/canada/toronto/long-term-care-ontario-year-later-1.6006725.

Kingdon, J.W. 1984. *Agendas, Alternatives, and Public Policies*. Boston: Little, Brown.

Kirka, D. 2021. "UK Opts Not to Vaccinate Most under 18 against COVID-19." *PBS*, 19 July 2021. https://www.pbs.org/newshour/world/uk-opts-not-to-vaccinate-most-under-18-against-covid-19.

Kirkey, S. 2021. "Why NACI Went Dark: Canada's Expert Panel on Vaccines Stops COVID Briefings, Interviews." *National Post*, 15 October 2021. https://nationalpost.com/news/canada/national-advisory-committee-on-immunization.

Kitroeff, N., and I. Austen. 2022. "After Trucker Protest, Canada Grapples with a Question: Was It a Blip, or Something Bigger?" *New York Times*, 21 February 2022. https://www.nytimes.com/2022/02/21/world/americas/canada-protest.html.

Klaiber, P., J.H. Wen, A. DeLongis, and N.L. Sin. 2021. "The Ups and Downs of Daily Life during COVID-19: Age Differences in Affect, Stress, and Positive Events." *Journals of Gerontology, Series B* 76 (2): 30–7. https://doi.org/10.1093/geronb/gbaa096.

Klein, E. 2022. "The COVID Policy That Really Mattered Wasn't a Policy." *New York Times*, 6 February 2022. https://www.nytimes.com/2022/02/06/opinion/covid-pandemic-policy-trust.html.

Kleinfeld, R. 2022. "The Rise in Political Violence in the United States and Damage to Our Democracy: Testimony before the Select Committee to Investigate the January 6th Attack on the United States Capitol." Carnegie Endowment for International Peace, 31 March 2022. https://carnegieendowment.org/files/2022-Rachel%20Kleinfeld%20Jan%20 6%20Committee%20Testimony.pdf.

Kleinman, R.A., and C. Merkel. 2020. "Digital Contact Tracing for COVID-19." *Canadian Medical Association Journal* 192 (24): 653–6. https://doi.org/10.1503/cmaj.200922.

Knell, Y. 2015. "Egypt Tourism Teeters after Sinai Plane Crash." BBC, 12 November 2015. https://www.bbc.com/news/world-europe-34797165.

Knight, J., and J. Johnson. 1999. "Inquiry into Democracy: What Might a Pragmatist Make of Rational Choice Theories?" *American Journal of Political Science* 43 (2): 566–89. https://doi.org/10.2307/2991807.

Kolata, G. 2021. "How Pandemics End." *New York Times*, 22 December 2021. https://www.nytimes.com/2020/05/10/health/coronavirus-plague-pandemic-history.html.

Kottke, J. 2020. "The Paradox of Preparation." Kottke.org, 16 March 2020. https://kottke.org/20/03/the-paradox-of-preparation.

Kramer, F.A. 1983. "Public Management in the 1980s and Beyond." *Annals of the American Academy of Political and Social Science* 466:91–102. http://www.jstor.org/stable/1044740.

Kramer, R M. 1999. "Trust and Distrust in Organizations: Emerging Perspectives, Enduring Questions." *Annual Review of Psychology* 50 (February): 569–98. https://doi.org/10.1146/annurev.psych.50.1.569.

Kriebel, D., J. Tickner, P. Epstein, J. Lemons, R. Levins, E.L. Loechler, M. Quinn, R. Rudel, T. Schettler, and M. Stoto. 2001. "The Precautionary Principle in Environmental Science." *Environmental Health Perspectives* 109 (9): 871–6. https://dx.doi.org/10.1289%2Fehp.01109871.

Kugler Kandestin. 2020. "Kugler Kandestin Files Class Action to Seek Compensation for the Residents, and Their Family Members, of CHSLD Herron." 17 April 2020. https://kklex.com/class-actions/pandemic-class-action.

Kumar, S., S. Crouse Quinn, K.H. Kim, L.H. Daniel, and V.S. Freimuth. 2012. "The Impact of Workplace Policies and Other Social Factors on Self-Reported Influenza-Like Illness Incidence during the 2009 H1N1 Pandemic." *American Journal of Public Health* 102 (1): 134–40. https://dx.doi.org/10.2105%2FAJPH.2011.300307.

Kuncl, M., A. McWhirter, and A. Ueberfeldt. 2021. "The Uneven Economic Consequences of COVID-19: A Structural Analysis." Bank of Canada, 6

August 2021. https://www.bankofcanada.ca/wp-content/uploads/2021/08/san2021-17.pdf.

Kunreuther, H.C., M.V. Pauly, and S. McMorrow. 2013a. "An Introduction to Insurance in Practice and Theory." In *Insurance and Behavioral Economics: Improving Decisions in the Most Misunderstood Industry*, 11–32. Cambridge: Cambridge University Press.

– 2013b. "Strategies for Dealing with Insurance-Related Anomalies." In *Insurance and Behavioral Economics: Improving Decisions in the Most Misunderstood Industry*, 208–28. Cambridge: Cambridge University Press.

Kupfer, M. 2021. "Should Ontario Make the COVID-19 Vaccine Mandatory for School?" CBC News, 14 July 2021. https://www.cbc.ca/news/canada/ottawa/covid-19-vaccine-ontario-students-1.6099579.

Kwon, J., and H. Lee. 2020. "Why Travel Prolongs Happiness: Longitudinal Analysis Using a Latent Growth Model." *Tourism Management* 76 (February): 103944. https://doi.org/10.1016/j.tourman.2019.06.019.

Lacoursière, A. 2021. "COVID-19 Led to an Explosion in the Use of Private Agencies in the Health Care Sector." *Toronto Star*, 15 September 2021. https://www.thestar.com/news/canada/2021/09/15/covid-19-led-to-an-explosion-in-the-use-of-private-agencies-in-the-health-care-sector.html.

Lafrance-Cooke, A. 2021. *Changes in Employment by Businesses during the COVID-19 Pandemic: New Insights on the Experimental Series of Monthly Business Openings and Closures*. Economic and Social Reports 1 (3), catalogue no. 36-28-0001. https://doi.org/10.25318/36280001202100300002-eng.

Lafrance-Cooke, A., R. Macdonald, and M. Willox. 2020. *Monthly Business Openings and Closures: Experimental Series for Canada, the Provinces and Territories, and Census Metropolitan Areas*. Economic Insights 16, catalogue no. 11-626-X. https://www150.statcan.gc.ca/n1/en/pub/11-626-x/11-626-x2020014-eng.pdf?st=PhxQf6h-.

LaFraniere, S., and N. Weiland. 2022. "Walensky, Citing Botched Pandemic Response, Calls for C.D.C. Reorganization." *New York Times*, 17 August 2022. https://www.nytimes.com/2022/08/17/us/politics/cdc-rochelle-walensky-covid.html.

La Grassa, J. 2022. "Ambassador Bridge Blockade Stalled Billions in Trade – And There Could Be Other Effects: Expert." CBC News, 15 February 2022. https://www.cbc.ca/news/canada/windsor/ambassador-bridge-protest-cost-1.6351312.

Lahey, L. 2020. "Nervous about Coronavirus? Don't Forget to Buy Travel Insurance." RatesDotCa, 3 March 2020. https://rates.ca/resources/nervous-about-coronavirus-dont-forget-to-buy-travel-insurance.

Lalancette, M., and M. Lamy. 2020. "COVID-19 and the Total Eclipse of the News." *Policy Options*, 3 April 2020. https://policyoptions.irpp.org/magazines/april-2020/covid-19-and-the-total-eclipse-of-the-news/.

Lalancette, M., and V. Raynauld. 2020. "How Political Leaders in North America Have Used COVID-19 to Improve Their Polls." *Policy Options*, 6 May 2020. https://policyoptions.irpp.org/magazines/may-2020/how-political-leaders-in-north-america-have-used-covid-19-to-improve-their-polls.

LaMattina, J. 2021. "Taxpayer Funded Research and the COVID-19 Vaccine." *Forbes*, 31 March 2021. https://www.forbes.com/sites/john-lamattina/2021/03/31/taxpayer-funded-research-and-the-covid-19-vaccine.

Lancet. 2020. "Global Burden of Disease 2019." *Lancet* 396 (10258):1129–306. https://www.thelancet.com/journals/lancet/issue/vol396no10258/PIIS0140-6736(20)X0042-0.

– 2021. "Editorial: COVID-19 and Cancer: 1 Year On." *Lancet Oncology* 22 (4): 411. https://doi.org/10.1016/S1470-2045(21)00148-0.

Landen, X. 2014. "Doctors a 'Death Sentence'? Patient Mistrust Aggravates Ebola Treatment." *PBS*, 13 July 2014. http://www.pbs.org/newshour/rundown/mistrust-doctors-west-africa-makes-harder-fight-ebola.

Lang, E. 2021. "The COVID-19 Pandemic and the *Emergencies Act*: If Not Now, When?" Canadian Global Affairs Institute, March 2021. https://www.cgai.ca/the_covid_19_pandemic_and_the_emergencies_act_if_not_now_when.

Langer, E.J. 1975. "The Illusion of Control." *Journal of Personality and Social Psychology* 32 (2): 311–28.

Lansbury, L.E., C.S. Brown, and J.S. Nguyen-Van-Tam. 2017. "Influenza in Long-Term Care Facilities." *Influenza and Other Respiratory Viruses* 11 (5): 356–66. https://dx.doi.org/10.1111%2Firv.12464.

Lanthier, N. 2021. "Amid Grim Times, Canadian Hotel Industry Eyes Recovery." *Globe and Mail*, 16 June 2021. https://www.theglobeandmail.com/business/industry-news/property-report/article-amid-grim-times-canadian-hotel-industry-eyes-recovery.

Lao, D. 2021a. "Feds Announce $5.9b Aid Package to Air Canada to Help Customer Refunds, Jobs." Global News, 12 April 2021. https://globalnews.ca/news/7753623/air-canada-aid-package-feds.

– 2021b. "Majority of COVID-19 Infections, Deaths Now among Unvaccinated People in Canada: Data." Global News, 26 June 2021. https://globalnews.ca/news/7981772/covid-19-infections-death unvaccinated.

– 2021c. "Most Canadians Unsympathetic to Unvaccinated Who Get Sick with COVID-19, Poll Finds." Global News, 19 August 2021. https://globalnews.ca/news/8122893/canadians-unsympathetic-covid-vaccine.

Lapierre, M. 2022. "Ottawa Police Chief Peter Sloly Resigns amid Criticism over Handling of Convoy Protests." *Ottawa Citizen*, 16 February 2022. https://ottawacitizen.com/news/local-news/ottawa-police-chief-peter-sloly-resigns-amid-criticism-over-handling-of-convoy-protests.

La Porte, T.R. 1996. "High Reliability Organizations: Unlikely, Demanding and at Risk." *Journal of Crisis and Contingency Management* 4 (2): 60–71.

La Porte, T.R., and P. Consolini. 1991. "Working in Practice but Not in Theory: Theoretical Challenges of High Reliability Organizations." *Journal of Public Administration Research and Theory* 1:19–47.

Lata, C., and L. Stevenson. 2020. *Executive Summary & Recommendations Submitted to the Minister of Health and Wellness by the Northwood Quality-Improvement Review Committee.* https://novascotia.ca/dhw/ccs/infection-control-ltc/Northwood-QIIPA-Report-Executive-Summary-Recommendations.pdf.

Lau, R. 2021. "What You Need to Know as a Modified Atlantic Bubble Opens." Global News, 23 June 2021. https://globalnews.ca/news/7970808/atlantic-bubble-travel-restrictions-june-23.

Lavoie-Tremblay, M., G. Cyr, T. Aubé, and G. Lavigne. 2022. "Lessons from Long-Term Care Facilities without COVID-19 Outbreaks." Special issue, *Healthcare Policy* 17:40–52. https://www.longwoods.com/content/26855/healthcare-policy-lessons-from-long-term-care-facilities-without-covid-19-outbreaks.

Law Library of Congress. 2009. "Medical Liability in Selected Countries: Canada." https://www.loc.gov/item/2015372201.

Law Society of Saskatchewan. 2020. "Remote Execution of Certain Documents by Electronic Means." https://lsslib.wpcomstaging.com/2020/03/26/remote-executive-of-certain-documents-by-electronic-means.

Lawson, T., L. Nathans, A. Goldenberg, M. Fimiani, D. Boire-Schwab, J.S. Castonguay, G. Waschuk et al. 2022. "COVID-19: Emergency Measures Tracker." McCarthy Tetrault. https://www.mccarthy.ca/en/insights/articles/covid-19-emergency-measures-tracker.

Lee, H. 2022. "More 'Pandemic Pets' Are Ending Up in Shelters. Is There a Fix? Experts Weigh In." Global News, 24 July 2022. https://globalnews.ca/news/9011043/pandemic-pets-canada-shelters-fix.

Lee, Y., and F. Tang. 2013. "More Caregiving, Less Working: Caregiving Roles and Gender Difference." *Journal of Applied Gerontology* 34 (4): 465–83. https://doi.org/10.1177%2F0733464813508649.

Leech, G., C. Rogers-Smith, J. Teperowski Monrad, J.B. Sandbrink, B. Snodin, R. Zinkov, B. Rader, J.S. Brownstein, Y. Gal, S. Bhatt et al. 2022. "Mask Wearing in Community Settings Reduces Sars-Cov-2 Transmission." *Proceedings of the National Academy of Sciences of the United States of America* 119 (23): e2119266119. https://doi. org/10.1073/pnas.2119266119.

Lee Kong, S. 2023. "Nature-Focused Vacations a Growing Trend That Connects Travellers to Their Destination." *Globe and Mail*, 21 March 2023. https://www.theglobeandmail.com/life/article-nature-focused-vacations-a-growing-trend-that-connects-travellers-to.

Leffler, C.T., E. Ing, J.D. Lykins, M.C. Hogan, C.A. McKeown, and A. Grzybowski. 2020. "Association of Country-Wide Coronavirus Mortality with Demographics, Testing, Lockdowns, and Public Wearing of Masks." *American Journal of Tropical Medicine and Hygiene* 103 (6): 2400–11. https://doi.org/10.4269/ajtmh.20-1015.

Legal Information Institute. n.d. "Tort." Accessed 1 November 2021. https://www.law.cornell.edu/wex/tort.

Leger, and ACS (Association for Canadian Studies). 2020a. *Report: COVID-19 Tracking Survey Results – March 30, 2020.* https://leger360.com/concerns-about-covid-19-march-31-2020/.

– 2020b. *Report: COVID-19 Tracking Survey Results – April 13, 2020.* https://leger360.com/concerns-about-covid-19-april-14-2020/.

– 2020c. *Report: COVID-19 Tracking Survey Results – April 20, 2020.* https://leger360.com/concerns-about-covid-19-april-21-2020/.

– 2020d. *Report: Leger's Weekly Survey – August 17, 2020.* https://leger360.com/legers-weekly-survey-august-18-2020/.

– 2020e. *Report: Weekly Pandemic Tracker – May 11, 2020.* https://leger360.com/weekly-covid-19-pandemic-tracker-may-12-2020/.

– 2020f. *Report: Weekly Pandemic Tracker – July 13, 2020.* https://leger360.com/legers-weekly-survey-july-14-2020/.

Leger, Canadian Press, and ACS (Association for Canadian Studies). 2021a. *Leger's North American Tracker – January 18, 2021.* https://leger360.com/legers-north-american-tracker-january-19-2021/.

– 2021b. *Leger's North American Tracker – February 22, 2021.* https://leger360.com/legers-north-american-tracker-february-23-2021/.

– 2021c. *Leger's North American Tracker – April 12, 2021.* https://leger360.com/legers-north-american-tracker-april-13-2021/.

– 2021d. *Leger's North American Tracker – May 3, 2021.* https://leger360.
com/legers-north-american-tracker-may-4-2021/.

– 2022a. *Leger's North American Tracker – February 10, 2022.* https://
leger360.com/legers-north-american-tracker-february-10-2022/.

– 2022b. *Leger's North American Tracker – April 14, 2022.* https://
leger360.com/legers-north-american-tracker-april-13-2022/.

Legislative Assembly of Alberta. n.d. "Assembly Online – Audio and Video
Assembly/Committee Proceedings." Accessed 2021. http://assemblyonline.
assembly.ab.ca/Harmony/en/View/UpcomingEvents.

Legislative Assembly of British Columbia. n.d. "Parliamentary Calendar."
Accessed 2021. https://www.leg.bc.ca/parliamentary-business/
parliamentary-calendar.

Legislative Assembly of Manitoba. n.d. "Broadcast Archives." Accessed
2021. https://gov.mb.ca/legislature/business/broadcast_archives.html.

Legislative Assembly of New Brunswick. n.d.a. "House Business." Accessed
2021. https://www.legnb.ca/en/house-business.

– n.d.b. "Webcasts." Accessed 2021. https://www.legnb.ca/en/webcasts?
startdate=2020-01-01&enddate=2020-12-31&type=HouseDaily
Sitting&page=1#webcast-filters.

Legislative Assembly of the Northwest Territories. n.d. "Hansard Archive."
Accessed 2021. https://www.ntassembly.ca/documents-proceedings/
hansard.

Legislative Assembly of Nunavut. n.d. "Hansard." Accessed 2021. https://
www.assembly.nu.ca/hansard.

Legislative Assembly of Ontario. n.d.a. "House Documents." Accessed
2021. https://www.ola.org/en/legislative-business/house-documents.

– n.d.b. "Parliamentary Calendars." Accessed 2021. https://www.ola.org/en/
legislative-business/parliamentary-calendars.

Legislative Assembly of Prince Edward Island. n.d.a. "Debates." Accessed
2021. https://www.assembly.pe.ca/legislative-business/house-records/
debates#/service/LegislativeAssemblyDebates/
LegislativeAssemblyDebateSearch;search=sitting;general_assembly=
null;session=null;sitting=null;year=2018;keyword=null;wdf_url_
query=true;wdf_submission_removed=true.

– n.d.b. "Rules, Parliamentary Calendar, and Daily Routine." Accessed
2021. https://www.assembly.pe.ca/index.php/legislative-business/
rules-parliamentary-calendar-and-daily-routine.

Legislative Assembly of Saskatchewan. n.d. "Legislative Meeting Archive."
Accessed 2021. https://www.legassembly.sk.ca/Archive?page=1
&start=2018-01-01&end=2021-09-30&context=280140000.

Leiter, M.P., and C. Maslach. 2009. "Nurse Turnover: The Mediating Role of Burnout." *Journal of Nursing Management* 17 (3): 331–9. https://doi.org/10.1111/j.13652834.2009.01004.x.

Lemmens, T., and L. Krakowitz-Broker. 2020. "Why the Federal Government Should Rethink Its New Medical Assistance in Dying Law." CBC News, 10 November 2020. https://www.cbc.ca/news/opinion/opinion-medical-assistance-in-dying-maid-legislation-1.5790710.

Lennox, A. 2011. "NZ Quakes Raise a Number of Issues for Reinsurers." Bryan Cave Leighton Paisner, 10 November 2011. https://www.bclplaw.com/en-US/insights/nz-quakes-raise-a-number-of-issues-for-reinsurers.html.

Leo, G. 2020. "Depleted National Stockpile Leaves Canada Reliant on China for Masks, Gowns and Other Supplies." CBC News, 6 May 2020. https://www.cbc.ca/news/canada/saskatchewan/ppe-import-china-shortage-1.5552426.

Leonhardt, D. 2021a. "Bad News Bias." *New York Times*, 22 April 2021. https://www.nytimes.com/2021/03/24/briefing/boulder-shooting-george-segal-astrazeneca.html.

– 2021b. "Red Covid." *New York Times*, 1 October 2021. https://www.nytimes.com/2021/09/27/briefing/covid-red-states-vaccinations.html.

– 2022. "Follow the Science?" *New York Times*, 11 February 2022. https://www.nytimes.com/2022/02/11/briefing/covid-cdc-follow-the-science.html.

Levasseur, J. 2021. "Families Sue Revera, Winnipeg Health Authority of COVID-19 Deaths at Maples Care Home." CBC News, 12 May 2021. https://www.cbc.ca/news/canada/manitoba/families-lawsuit-maples-care-home-covid-19-deaths-1.6022707.

Levitt, H. 2020. "Howard Levitt: Note to Companies and Their Staff – COVID-19 Has Not Changed Employment Law." *Financial Post*, 24 July 2020. https://financialpost.com/executive/careers/howard-levitt-note-to-companies-and-their-staff-covid-19-has-not-changed-employment-law.

Lewis, D. 2021. "Why Indoor Spaces Are Still Prime COVID Hotspots." *Nature*, 30 March 2021. https://www.nature.com/articles/d41586-021-00810-9.

Lexchin, J. 1993. "Pharmaceuticals, Patients, and Politics: Canada and Bill C-22." *International Journal of Health Services* 23 (1): 147–60. https://doi.org/10.2190/UCWG-YBR3-X3L0-NWYT.

– 2016. *Private Profits versus Public Policy: The Pharmaceutical Industry and the Canadian State*. Toronto: University of Toronto Press.

Lilley, B. 2020. "Lilley: Feds Quarantined Some, Not All, Air Passengers from Virus Epicentre." *Toronto Sun*, 8 April 2020. https://torontosun.

com/opinion/columnists/lilley-feds-quarantined-some-not-all-air-passengers-
from-virus-epicentre.

Lindsay, B. 2022. "Doctor's Appeal over Right to Pay for Private Health
Care Dismissed by B.C. Court." CBC News, 15 July 2022. https://www.
cbc.ca/news/canada/british-columbia/cambie-surgeries-case-trial-court-
of-appeal-judgment-1.6521746.

Ling, J. 2020. "Where Canada Is Falling Short on Its Coronavirus
Communications." *Maclean's*, 19 March 2020. https://www.macleans.ca/
news/canada/canadas-mixed-messages-on-the-coronavirus-outbreak.

Ling, P., and R. Barton. 2020. "The Coronavirus Crisis Is Driving a Sudden
Thaw in Canada-China Relations." CBC News, 15 February 2020.
https://www.cbc.ca/news/politics/coronavirus-china-canada-meng-
wanzhou-1.5465011.

Litton, E., T. Bucci, S. Chavan, Y.Y. Ho, A. Holley, G. Howard, S. Huckson
et al. 2020. "Surge Capacity of Intensive Care Units in Case of Acute
Increase in Demand Caused by COVID-19 in Australia." *Medical Journal
of Australia* 212 (10): 463–7. https://doi.org/10.5694/mja2.50596.

Llewellyn, R., C. Jaye, R. Egan, W. Cunningham, J. Young, and P. Radue.
2016. "Cracking Open Death: Death Conversations in Primary Care."
Journal of Primary Health Care 8 (4): 303–11. https://doi.org/10.1071/
HC15058.

Lloyd, E. 2021. "Divorce Rates up 30% Due to COVID-19 Pandemic: B.C.
Group." CTV News, 19 January 2021. https://vancouverisland.ctvnews.
ca/divorce-rates-up-30-due-to-covid-19-pandemic-b-c-group-1.5273859.

Lloyd, L., A. Banerjee, C. Harrington, F.F. Jacobsen, and M. Szebehely.
2014. "It Is a Scandal! Comparing the Causes and Consequences of
Nursing Home Media Scandals in Five Countries." *International Journal
of Sociology and Social Policy* 34 (1/2): 2–18. https://doi.org/10.1108/
IJSSP-03-2013-0034.

Loblaw Companies Limited. 2021. *2020 Annual Report – Financial Review.*
https://www.loblaw.ca/en/investors-reports.

Locke, W., A. Parker, P. Boucher, and F. Rahimi. 2020. "Ontario
Government Issues Emergency Order Providing Flexibility with Respect
to Shareholder and Director Meetings." *McCarthy Tetrault* (blog), 1 April
2020. https://www.mccarthy.ca/en/insights/blogs/canadian-securities-
regulatory-monitor/ontario-government-issues-emergency-order-providing-
flexibility-respect-shareholder-and-director-meetings.

Long, S. 2021. "Nova Scotia to Take 'Cautious Approach' in Final Phase of
Reopening; Mandates Vaccines for Health-Care Workers, Teachers." CTV

News, 30 September 2021. https://atlantic.ctvnews.ca/nova-scotia-to-take-cautious-approach-in-final-phase-of-reopening-mandates-vaccines-for-health-care-workers-teachers-1.5605331.

Longo, J., and K. McNutt. 2018. "From Policy Analysis to Policy Analytics." In *Policy Analysis in Canada*, edited by L. Dobuzinskis and M. Howlett, 369–91. Bristol, UK: Policy Press.

Lord, C. 2023. "Many Canadian Offices Are Empty. It Could Be the Economy's 'Canary in the Coal Mine.'" Global News, 4 May 2023. https://globalnews.ca/news/9671226/canada-office-covid-economy-risk-recession.

Loriggio, P. 2021. "Group of Active, Retired Police Officers File Constitutional Challenge over Ontario's COVID-19 Rules." Global News, 6 May 2021. https://globalnews.ca/news/7832846/covid-ontario-pandemic-orders-police.

Loubergé, H. 2013. "Developments in Risk and Insurance Economics: The Past 40 Years." In *Handbook of Insurance*, edited by G. Dionne, 1–40. New York: Springer. http://dx.doi.org/10.1007/978-1-4614-0155-1_1.

Lowe, K. 2020. "Labour Issues and COVID-19: Roundtable Discussion." MIPP COVID-19 Research Briefing, March 2020. https://cdn.dal.ca/content/dam/dalhousie/pdf/dept/maceachen-institute/Employment%20and%20COVID-19.pdf.

Lowndes, R., and J. Struthers. 2016. "Changes and Continuities in the Workplace of Long-Term Residential Care in Canada, 1970–2015." *Journal of Canadian Studies* 50 (2): 368–95. https://utpjournals.press/doi/10.3138/jcs.50.2.368.

Lowrance, W. 1976. *Of Acceptable Risk: Science and the Determination of Safety*. Los Altos, CA: William Kaufman.

Lu, M. 2020. "This Chart Shows How Debt-to-GDP Is Rising around the World." World Economic Forum, 14 December 2020. https://www.weforum.org/agenda/2020/12/global-debt-gdp-covid19.

Lu, Y. 2020. "The Distribution of Temporary Foreign Workers across Industries in Canada." StatCan COVID-19: Data to Insights for a Better Canada, catalogue no. 45280001. https://www150.statcan.gc.ca/n1/en/pub/45-28-0001/2020001/article/00028-eng.pdf?st=eGbeVDiE.

Luck, S. 2020. "Who's Getting Sick (and Who's Not) in Nova Scotia's Second Wave." CBC News, 28 November 2020. https://www.cbc.ca/news/canada/nova-scotia/covid-coronavirus-second-wave-nova-scotia-1.5817213.

Lundy, M., and M. Rendell. 2023. "Ottawa's COVID-19 Spending Had Small Impact on Inflation, Larger Effect on Interest Rates: Report." *Globe and Mail*, 25 January 2023. https://www.theglobeandmail.com/business/article-ottawa-covid-19-spending-impact-interest-rates.

Luz, C., and K. Hanson. 2015. "Training the Personal and Home Care Aide Workforce: Challenges and Solution." *Home Health Care Management & Practice* 27 (3): 150–3. https://doi.org/10.1177%2F1084822314566301.

Lysyk, B. 2021. *COVID-19 Preparedness and Management: Special Report on Pandemic Readiness and Response in Long-Term Care*. Office of the Auditor General of Ontario. https://www.auditor.on.ca/en/content/specialreports/specialreports/COVID-19_ch5readinessresponseLTC_en202104.pdf.

Ma, S., and M. Popp. 2021. "New Employment Standards Leaves for COVID-19 & Their Impact on Pension & Benefits Plans." *Lawson Lundell Labour and Employment Law Blog*, 4 May 2021. https://www.lawsonlundell.com/labour-and-employment-law-blog/new-employment-standards-leaves-for-covid-19.

Mabry, P.L., D.H. Olster, G.D. Morgan, and D.B. Abrams. 2008. "Interdisciplinarity and Systems Science to Improve Population Health: A View from the NIH Office of Behavioral and Social Sciences." *American Journal of Preventive Medicine* 35 (2S): s211–24. https://dx.doi.org/10.1016%2Fj.amepre.2008.05.018.

MacDonald, F. 2022. "The 'Freedom Convoy' Protesters Are a Textbook Case of 'Aggrieved Entitlement.'" *The Conversation*, 16 February 2022. https://theconversation.com/the-freedom-convoy-protesters-are-a-textbook-case-of-aggrieved-entitlement-176791.

MacDonald, G. 2020. "Patience Is Essential When Trying to Get a Refund on Booked Travel." *Globe and Mail*, 7 April 2020. https://www.theglobeandmail.com/life/travel/article-patience-is-essential-when-trying-to-get-a-refund-on-booked-travel.

MacDonald, J., N. Edwards, B. Davies, P. Marck, and J.R. Guernsey. 2012. "Priority Setting and Policy Advocacy by Nursing Associations: A Scoping Review and Implications Using a Socio-ecological Whole System Lens." *Health Policy* 107 (1): 31–43. https://doi.org/10.1016/j.healthpol.2012.03.017.

Macdonald, J.M. 1995. "Appreciating the Precautionary Principle as an Ethical Evolution in Ocean Management." *Ocean Development & International Law* 26 (3): 255–86. https://doi.org/10.1080/00908329509546062.

Macdougall, C.W., D. Kirsch, B. Schwartz, and R.B. Deber. 2014. "Looking For Trouble: Developing and Implementing a National Network for Infectious Disease Surveillance in Canada." In *Case Studies in Canadian*

Health Policy and Management, edited by R. Deber and C. Mah, 179–205. Toronto: University of Toronto Press.

MacKinnon, B.J. 2021a. "COVID-19 Vaccine Mandatory for New Brunswick Health-Care Workers Sept. 7, Memo Says." CBC News, 31 August 2021. https://www.cbc.ca/news/canada/new-brunswick/mandatory-vaccines-health-care-workers-new-brunswick-covid-19-1.6159793.

– 2021b. "Vitalité Hospitals at 96.4% Capacity, Some of Horizon's at or over 100% as COVID Cases Spike." CBC News, 23 September 2021. https://www.cbc.ca/news/canada/new-brunswick/new-brunswick-hospital-capacity-vitalite-horizon-covid-1.6186794.

MacKinnon, M., N. Vanderklippe, and G. Robertson. 2020. "Flattery and Foot Dragging: China's Influence over the WHO under Scrutiny." *Globe and Mail*, 25 April 2020. https://www.theglobeandmail.com/world/article-flattery-and-foot-dragging-chinas-influence-over-the-who-under.

Macklem, T. 2021. "Release of the Financial System Review." Bank of Canada, 20 May 2021. https://www.bankofcanada.ca/2021/05/opening-statement-200521.

– 2022. "Speech: Halifax Chamber of Commerce." Bank of Canada. Video, 43:46. https://www.bankofcanada.ca/multimedia/speech-halifax-chamber-of-commerce.

MacLean, C. 2021a. "Grief on Pause: Family Has Waited More than a Year to Hold Funeral amid COVID-19 Restrictions." CBC News, 2 May 2021. https://www.cbc.ca/news/canada/manitoba/manitoba-funeral-families-delayed-grief-1.6007242.

– 2021b. "Manitoba to Give Nearly \$2M in Prizes to People Who Get Vaccinated." CBC News, 9 June 2021. https://www.cbc.ca/news/canada/manitoba/manitoba-covid-19-vaccine-incentives-1.6058815.

– 2021c. "Vaccine and Mask Mandates Coming for Many Provincial Workers, Indoor Spaces in Manitoba." CBC News, 24 August 2021. https://www.cbc.ca/news/canada/manitoba/pallister-roussin-vaccine-initiatives-1.6151268.

MacLellan, A. 2020. "Quebec Vows to Dramatically Boost COVID-19 Testing, as Deconfinement Begins." CBC News, 28 April 2021. https://www.cbc.ca/news/canada/montreal/covid-19-quadrupling-testing-quebec-1.5547051.

Macrotrends. n.d. "Taiwan Population, 1950–2022." Accessed 21 March 2022. https://www.macrotrends.net/countries/TWN/taiwan/population.

Madhi, S. 2022. "New COVID Data: South Africa Has Arrived at the Recovery Stage of the Pandemic." *The Conversation*, 1 March 2022. https://theconversation.com/new-covid-data-south-africa-has-arrived-at-the-recovery-stage-of-the-pandemic-177933.

Madhi, S., G. Kwatra, J. Myers, W. Jassat, N. Dhar, K. Mukendi, A. Nana et al. 2022. "Population Immunity and COVID-19 Severity with Omicron Variant in South Africa." *New England Journal of Medicine* 386 (14): 1314–26. https://doi.org/10.1056/NEJMoa2119658.

Magee, S. 2021. "Reassessed Property Value for Hotels, Offices, Retail Brings Budget Risks in Moncton." CBC News, 30 March 2021. https://www.cbc.ca/news/canada/new-brunswick/moncton-covid-assessment-downtown-property-values-1.5968168.

Maher, D. 2020. "COVID-19 Testing in Newfoundland and Labrador Expanding to Focus More on Vulnerable Populations." *Telegram*, 6 April 2020. https://www.thetelegram.com/news/local/covid-19-testing-in-newfoundland-and-labrador-expanding-to-focus-more-on-vulnerable-populations-433898.

Maher, S. 2021. "Year One: The Untold Story of the Pandemic in Canada." *Maclean's*, 24 March 2021. https://www.macleans.ca/longforms/covid-19-pandemic-canada-year-one.

Mahmud, S.M., L.H. Thompson, D.L. Nowicki, and P.J. Plourde. 2013. "Outbreaks of Influenza-Like Illness in Long-Term Care Facilities in Winnipeg, Canada." *Influenza and Other Respiratory Viruses* 7 (6): 1055–61. https://doi.org/10.1111/irv.12052.

Major, D. 2022a. "Emergencies Act Passes Crucial House of Commons Vote with NDP Support." CBC News, 22 February 2022. https://www.cbc.ca/news/politics/trudeau-emergencies-act-vote-1.6359243.

– 2022b. "Thousands of Canadians Still on the Hook for Pandemic Benefit Repayments." CBC News, 19 November 2022. https://www.cbc.ca/news/politics/thousands-canadians-expected-to-repay-pandemic-benefits-1.6656937.

Maldonato, M., and S. Dell'Orco. 2011. "How to Make Decisions in an Uncertain World: Heuristics, Biases, and Risk Perception." *World Futures* 67 (8): 569–77.

Malone, K. 2021. "Provinces Consider COVID-19 Vaccine Incentives to Reach Those Not Getting Shots." *Toronto Sun*, 3 June 2021. https://torontosun.com/news/national/provinces-consider-covid-19-vaccine-incentives-to-reach-those-not-getting-shots.

– 2022a. "Canada Is Past Peak of Omicron-Fuelled Wave of COVID-19, Dr. Tam Says." *Globe and Mail*, 18 February 2022. https://www.theglobeandmail.com/canada/article-tam-says-canada-is-past-peak-of-omicron-fuelled-wave-of-covid-19.

– 2022b. "More Provinces Preparing to Loosen COVID-19 Restrictions in Coming Weeks." CTV News, 2 February 2022. https://www.ctvnews.ca/

health/coronavirus/more-provinces-preparing-to-loosen-covid-19-restrictions-in-coming-weeks-1.5764194.

Manguvo, A., and B. Mafuvadze. 2015. "The Impact of Traditional and Religious Practices on the Spread of Ebola in West Africa: Time for a Strategic Shift." *Pan African Medicine Journal* 22 (9): 1–4. https://dx.doi.org/10.11694%2Fpamj.supp.2015.22.1.6190.

Manuel, D.G., A. Bader Eddeen, R.C. Colley, M. Tjepkema, R. Garner, C. Bennett, and J. Bernier. 2021. "The Effect of COVID-19 on Physical Activity among Canadians and the Future Risk of Cardiovascular Disease." StatCan COVID-19: Data to Insights for a Better Canada, catalogue no. 45280001. https://www150.statcan.gc.ca/n1/en/pub/45-28-0001/2021001/article/00019-eng.pdf?st=7snnohSx.

March, J.G., and J.P. Olsen. 1989. *Rediscovering Institutions: The Organizational Basis of Politics*. New York: Free Press.

Marchitelli, R. 2020. "Why Many Passengers Grounded by COVID-19 Aren't Getting Refunds for Cancelled Flights." CBC News, 26 March 2020. https://www.cbc.ca/news/business/passengers-grounded-covid-19-air-canada-westjet-sunwing-1.5510105.

Marotta, S. 2020. "The Paid Sick Days Conundrum: Pandemic Revives Debate over Who Should Foot the Bill." *Globe and Mail*, 17 December 2020. https://www.theglobeandmail.com/canada/article-canadian-businesses-lobby-for-paid-sick-days-as-covid-19-rips-through.

Marsh, D.M., M.J. Smith, and D. Richards. 2000. "Bureaucrats, Politicians and Reform in Whitehall: Analysing the Bureau-Shaping Model." *British Journal of Political Science* 30 (3): 461–82. https://www.jstor.org/stable/194004.

Martin, C. 2022. "Don Martin: Trudeau Feels Our Pandemic Pain – And Deflects the Blame." CTV News, 5 January 2022. https://www.ctvnews.ca/politics/don-martin-trudeau-feels-our-pandemic-pain-and-deflects-the-blame-1.5729044.

Maru Blue. 2021. *Public Opinion Poll: Support for Pandemic Lockdown Rules*. https://static1.squarespace.com/static/5a17333e-b0786935ac112523/t/603ec3e66f138e15aa1d11fd/1614726118707/Lockdown*Rules*Jan*9*2021*F.pdf.

Maru Public Opinion. 2022. *The Emergencies Act*. 17 February 2022. https://static1.squarespace.com/static/5a17333eb0786935ac112523/t/620d9994ac49674e50dd99d6/1645058455817/Emergencies*17*02*22.pdf.

Masket, S. 2021. "Seth Masket: The Great Vaccine Divide Puts Republican Leaders in a Moral Quandary." *Denver Post*, 25 June 2021. https://www.

denverpost.com/2021/06/25/covid-19-vaccine-rates-donald-trump-joe-biden.

Mauracher, J. 2021. "First Nations Communities Are Disproportionately Impacted by COVID-19. Here's Why." Global News, 1 October 2021. https://globalnews.ca/news/8234102/first-nations-communities-covid.

McArthur, J. 2020. "How Governments Can Make Public Health Decisions When Some Information about Coronavirus Is Missing." The Conversation, 4 May 2020. https://theconversation.com/how-governments-can-make-public-health-decisions-when-some-information-about-coronavirus-is-missing-137368.

McCann, N. 2020. "Coronavirus: No Wake, No Funeral, Just Prayers in a Cemetery." BBC, 1 April 2020. https://www.bbc.com/news/uk-northern-ireland-52106863.

McCarthy, N. 2021. "Which Companies Received the Most COVID-19 Vaccine R&D Funding [Infographic]." Forbes, 6 May 2021. https://www.forbes.com/sites/niallmccarthy/2021/05/06/which-companies-received-the-most-covid-19-vaccine-rd-funding-infographic.

McDonald, S.M., L.M. Wagner, and A. Gruneir. 2015. "Accreditation and Resident Safety in Ontario Long-Term Care Homes." Healthcare Quarterly 18 (1): 54–9. https://doi.org/10.12927/hcq.2015.24214.

McGilton, K.S., V.M. Boscart, M. Brown, and B. Bowers. 2014. "Making Tradeoffs between the Reasons to Leave and Reasons to Stay Employed in Long-Term Care Homes: Perspectives of Licensed Nursing Staff." International Journal of Nursing Studies 51 (6): 917–26. http://dx.doi.org/10.1016/j.ijnurstu.2013.10.015.

McGrail, K.M., M.J. McGregor, M. Cohen, R.B. Tate, and L.A. Ronald. 2007. "For-Profit versus Not-for-Profit Delivery of Long-Term Care." Canadian Medical Association 176 (1): 57–8. https://doi.org/10.1503/cmaj.060591.

McKay, M., M.R. Lavergne, A.P. Lea, M. Le, A. Grudniewicz, D. Blackie, L.J. Goldsmith et al. 2022. "Government Policies Targeting Primary Care Physician Practice from 1998–2018 in Three Canadian Provinces: A Jurisdictional Scan." Health Policy 126 (6): 565–75. https://doi.org/10.1016/j.healthpol.2022.03.006.

McKeen, A. 2022. "Amid Shortage of Family Doctors across Canada, Med School Grads Increasingly Don't Want the Jobs." Toronto Star, 27 April 2022. https://www.thestar.com/news/canada/2022/04/27/amid-shortages-of-family-doctors-across-canada-med-school-grads-increasingly-dont-want-the-jobs.html.

McKenna, K. 2020. "How Quebec's Desperate Attempt to Fill Staffing Holes Is Spreading COVID-19 in Hospitals and Nursing Homes." CBC

News, 6 May 2020. https://www.cbc.ca/news/canada/montreal/quebec-covid-cross-contamination-1.5556946.

McKenzie, K. 2020. "Race and Ethnicity Data Collection during COVID-19 in Canada: If You Are Not Counted You Cannot Count on the Pandemic Response." Royal Society of Canada, 12 November 2020. https://rsc-src.ca/en/race-and-ethnicity-data-collection-during-covid-19-in-canada-if-you-are-not-counted-you-cannot-count.

McKenzie-Sutter, H. 2020. "'We Have No Other Choice': How Funerals Are Adapting to COVID-19 Measures." CTV News, 3 April 2020. https://www.ctvnews.ca/health/coronavirus/we-have-no-other-choice-how-funerals-are-adapting-to-covid-19-measures-1.4873083.

– 2021. "Ontario to Introduce Policies Requiring COVID-19 Vaccinations or Regular Tests for Staff in Health-Care, Education." *Globe and Mail*, 17 August 2021. https://www.theglobeandmail.com/canada/article-ontario-set-to-introduce-vaccination-policies-in-education-health-care.

McKercher, B., and S. Darcy. 2018. "Re-conceptualizing Barriers to Travel by People with Disabilities." *Tourism Management Perspectives* 26: 59–66. https://doi.org/10.1016/j.tmp.2018.01.003.

McLaughlin, E.C. 2020. "CDC Official Warns It's Not a Question of If Coronavirus Will Spread, but When." CNN, 26 February 2020. https://www.cnn.com/2020/02/25/health/coronavirus-us-american-cases/index.html.

McLeod, M. 2022. "International, Canadian Experts Warn Right-Wing Extremism Is Becoming Increasingly Mainstream." *Globe and Mail*, 14 September 2022. https://www.theglobeandmail.com/politics/article-international-canadian-experts-warn-right-wing-extremism-is-becoming.

McLeod Macey, J. 2020. "Two-Thirds of Canadians Think, Long Term, Climate Change Is as Serious of a Problem as Coronavirus." Ipsos, 22 April 2020. https://www.ipsos.com/en-ca/news-and-polls/Two-Thirds-Of-Canadians-Think--In-The-Long-Term-Climate-Change-Is-As-Serious-Of-A-Problem-As-Coronavirus.

McPhail, C. 2020. "New Brunswick Progressive Conservatives Win Majority in Pandemic Vote." CBC News, 15 September 2020. https://www.cbc.ca/news/canada/new-brunswick/new-brunswick-election-day-results-2020-1.5722438.

McSheffrey, E. 2020. "Premier Faces Backlash for Singling Out African Nova Scotian Communities during COVID-19." Global News, 8 April 2020. https://globalnews.ca/news/6793768/premier-faces-backlash-for-singling-out-african-nova-scotian-communities-during-covid-19.

Meckbach, G. 2020a. "COVID BI Coverage Dispute Lawsuit Arises over 'Civil Authority' Order Clause." *Canadian Underwriter*, 8 May 2020. https://www.canadianunderwriter.ca/legal/covid-bi-coverage-dispute-lawsuit-arises-over-civil-authority-order-clause-1004178036.

– 2020b. "The Liability of Long-Term Care Facilities: Covid-19's Projected Impact." *Canadian Underwriter*, 24 April 2020. https://www.canadian underwriter.ca/insurance/the-liability-of-long-term-care-facilities-covid-19s-projected-impact-1004177364.

– 2020c. "More Class Actions Headed to Court over Pandemic Business Interruption." *Canadian Underwriter*, 7 July 2020. https://www.canadian underwriter.ca/insurance/more-class-actions-headed-to-court-over-pandemic-business-interruption-1004194079.

– 2020d. "Where the Federal Government Sits with Its National Flood Insurance Review." *Canadian Underwriter*, 20 May 2020. https://www.canadianunderwriter.ca/catastrophes/where-the-federal-government-sits-with-its-national-flood-insurance-review-1004178465.

Mehrabi, K.A. 2022. "Police Spent $7.6 Million Preparing for Potential 'Freedom Convoy' in Toronto." *BlogTO*. https://www.blogto.com/city/2022/08/toronto-police-spent-76m-preparing-potential-trucker-convoy.

Mendelson, M., F. Venter, M. Moshabela, G. Gray, L. Blumberg, T. de Oliveira, and S.A. Madhi. 2021. "The Political Theatre of the UK's Travel Ban on South Africa." *Lancet* 398 (10318): 2211–13. https://doi.org/10.1016/S0140-6736(21)02752-5.

Menec, V.H., L. MacWilliam, and F.Y. Aoki. 2002. "Hospitalizations and Deaths Due to Respiratory Illnesses during Influenza Seasons: A Comparison of Community Residents, Senior Housing Residents, and Nursing Home Residents." *Journals of Gerontology: Series A* 57 (10): 629–35. https://doi.org/10.1093/gerona/57.10.M629.

Mercuri, M. 2020. "Just Follow the Science: A Government Response to a Pandemic." *Journal of Evaluation in Clinical Practice* 26 (6): 1575–8. https://doi.org/10.1111/jep.13491.

Mercury. 2020. "Italian Doctor's Emotional Response to Coronavirus Crisis: 'I Cry Inside.'" Filmed 19 March 2020. Video, 1:25. https://www.themercury.com.au/news/world/italian-doctors-emotional-response-to-coronavirus-crisis-i-cry-inside/video/032185621db41140f38785a2db9b66cd.

Merino, D., and G. Ware. 2021. "Planet Pharma: What the Industry Got Out of COVID – Podcast." *The Conversation*, 2 December 2021. https://theconversation.com/planet-pharma-what-the-industry-got-out-of-covid-podcast-172990.

Mertz, E. 2021. "Support for Private Health-Care Options Has Grown since Start of Pandemic: Survey." Global News, 7 December 2021. https://globalnews.ca/news/8428767/canada-health-care-reform-private-pandemic.

Messacar, D., R. Morissette, and Z. Deng. 2020. "Inequality in the Feasibility of Working from Home during and after COVID-19." StatCan COVID-19: Data to Insights for a Better Canada, catalogue no. 45280001. https://www150.statcan.gc.ca/n1/en/pub/45-28-0001/2020001/article/00029-eng.pdf?st=bn-7pyjh.

MHCC (Mental Health Commission of Canada). 2017. *Strengthening the Case for Investing in Canada's Mental Health System: Economic Considerations.* March 2017. https://www.mentalhealthcommission.ca/wp-content/uploads/drupal/2017-03/case_for_investment_eng.pdf.

– 2021. *COVID-19 and Suicide.* https://www.mentalhealthcommission.ca/sites/default/files/2021-02/covid_and_suicide_tip_sheet_eng.pdf.

Mignacca, F. 2020. "Thousands Send in Applications to Work in Quebec Long-Term Care Homes." CBC News, 2 June 2020. https://www.cbc.ca/news/canada/montreal/chsld-orderlies-training-program-announced-1.5595010.

Migone, A.R. 2020. "Trust, but Customize: Federalism's Impact on the Canadian COVID-19 Response." *Policy and Society* 39 (3): 382–402. https://doi.org/10.1080/14494035.2020.1783788.

Mikles, N. 2021. "Indians Are Forced to Change Rituals for the Dead as COVID-19 Rages." *The Conversation,* 4 May 2021. https://theconversation.com/indians-are-forced-to-change-rituals-for-their-dead-as-covid-19-rages-through-cities-and-villages-160076.

Miller, A. 2021a. "A Canadian COVID-19 Study That Turned Out to Be Wrong Has Spread like Wildfire among Anti-vaxxers." CBC News, 25 September 2021. https://www.cbc.ca/news/health/covid-19-vaccine-study-error-anti-vaxxers-1.6188806.

– 2021b. "Why Canada's Vaccine Rollout Is Slower than Other Countries' – And What Can Be Done to Fix It." CBC News, 6 January 2021. https://www.cbc.ca/news/health/canada-slow-vaccine-rollout-covid-19-1.5862358.

– 2022. "Canada's Abandoning of COVID-19 Testing Leaves Us Vulnerable to Future Variants, Experts Say." CBC News, 26 February 2022. https://www.cbc.ca/news/health/canada-covid-19-testing-omicron-variants-1.6365133.

Miller, A., and B. Shingler. 2022. "Would More Privatization in Canadian Health Care Solve the Current Crisis?" CBC News, 20 August 2022. https://www.cbc.ca/news/health/canada-healthcare-privatization-debate-second-opinion-1.6554073.

Miller, C.C. 2021. "Out of Office: The Office Will Never Be the Same." *New York Times*, 22 September 2021. https://www.nytimes.com/ 2020/08/20/style/office-culture.html.

Miller, H.E., and K.J. Engemann. 2019. "Resilience and Sustainability in Supply Chains." In *Revisiting Supply Chain Risk*, edited by G. Zsidisin and M. Henke, 251–63. Springer Series in Supply Chain Management 7. Cham, Switzerland: Springer. https://doi.org/10.1007/978-3-030-03813-7_15.

Miller, M. 2021. "Female Workers Could Take Another Pandemic Hit: To Their Retirements." *New York Times*, 28 June 2021. https://www. nytimes.com/2020/12/11/business/women-retirement-covid-social-security.html.

Milstead, D. 2021. "Long-Term Care Home Operators Paid 2020 Bonuses to Top Executives amid COVID-19 Pandemic." *Globe and Mail*, 4 May 2021. https://www.theglobeandmail.com/business/article-long-term-care-home-operators-pay-2020-performance-bonuses-to-top.

Ministry of Justice. n.d. "Coronavirus (COVID-19): Justice System Measures." Government of Quebec. Accessed January 2021. https://www. justice.gouv.qc.ca/en/coronavirus.

Mitchell, D.E. 2021. "Taxpayers Fund Research and Drug Companies Make a Fortune." *New York Times*, 24 March 2021. https://www.nytimes. com/2021/03/24/opinion/coronavirus-vaccine-cost-pfizer-moderna.html.

MNP LLP. 2021. *Improving Quality of Life for Residents in Facility-Based Continuing Care*. https://open.alberta.ca/dataset/f680d1a6-bee5-4862-8ea4-e78d98b7965d/resource/22092c9c-99bb-4fee-9929-7ce06e71bbd1/ download/health-improving-quality-life-residents-facility-based-continuing-care-2021-04-30.pdf.

Modjeski, M. 2020. "Cab Drivers Call for Insurance Break during Pandemic." CBC News, 3 April 2020. https://www.cbc.ca/news/canada/ saskatoon/cab-driver-ask-sgi-1.5519693.

Montpetit, J. 2020. "Why Are Quebec's Nursing Homes So Understaffed, and What's Being Done about It?" CBC News, 15 April 2020. https:// www.cbc.ca/news/canada/montreal/quebec-nursing-homes-understaffed-1. 5531997.

Moody, R. 2021. "Netflix Subscribers and Revenue by Country." Comparitech, 10 September 2021. https://www.comparitech.com/ tv-streaming/netflix-subscribers.

Moore, M. 1995. *Creating Public Value: Strategic Management in Government*. Cambridge, MA: Harvard University Press.

Morawetz, B. 2020. "Update Regarding the Suspension of Superior Court of Justice Regular Operations." Ontario Superior Court of Justice, 2 April

2020. https://www.ontariocourts.ca/scj/notices-and-orders-covid-19/
notices-no-longer-in-effect/notice-to-the-profession-the-public-and-the-
media-regarding-civil-and-family-proceedings-update.

Morgan, M.G., B. Fischhoff, A. Bostrom, and C.J. Atman. 2001. *Risk
Communication*. New York: Cambridge University Press.

Moriarty, L.F., M.M. Plucinski, B.J. Marston, E.V. Kurbatova, B. Knust,
E.L. Murray, N. Pesik et al. 2020. "Public Health Responses to COVID-
19 Outbreaks on Cruise Ships – Worldwide, February–March 2020."
Morbidity and Mortality Weekly Report 69 (12): 347–52. http://dx.doi.
org/10.15585/mmwr.mm6912e3.

Morissette, R., M. Turcotte, A. Bernard, and E. Olson. 2021. "Workers
Receiving Payments from the Canada Emergency Response Benefit
Program in 2020." StatCan COVID-19: Data to Insights for a Better
Canada, catalogue no. 45280001. https://www150.statcan.gc.ca/n1/en/
pub/45-28-0001/2021001/article/00021-eng.pdf?st=TFXKsTPP.

Morneau, B. 2023. *Where to from Here: A Path to Canadian Prosperity*.
Toronto: ECW Press.

Morrison, J. 2004. "Development of a Resource Model for Infection
Prevention and Control Programs in Acute, Long Term, and Home Care
Settings: Conference Proceedings of the Infection Prevention and Control
Alliance." *American Journal of Infection Control 32* (1): 2–6. https://doi.
org/10.1016/j.ajic.2003.10.002.

Moscrop, D. 2022. "Opinion: Canada Must Confront the Toxic 'Freedom
Convoy' Head-On." *Washington Post*, 28 January 2022. https://www.
washingtonpost.com/opinions/2022/01/28/canada-must-confront-toxic-
protest-freedom-convoy.

Moura, A., C. Eusébio, and E. Devile. 2023. "The 'Why' and 'What For' of
Participation in Tourism Activities: Travel Motivations of People with
Disabilities." *Current Issues in Tourism 26* (6): 941–57. https://doi.org/10
.1080/13683500.2022.2044292.

Mueller, D.C. 1976. "Public Choice: A Survey." *Journal of Economic
Literature 14* (2): 395–433. https://www.jstor.org/stable/2722461.

Mulholland, E., A. Bucik, and V. Odu. 2020. *Roadblock to Recovery:
Consumer Debt of Low- and Moderate-Income Canadian Households in
the Time of COVID-19*. Prosper Canada. https://prospercanada.org/get
attachment/901099d6-03fc-4550-9102-6f9fe91b94a3/Roadblock-to-
recovery_Consumer-debt-report.aspx.

Murdoch, B. 2020. "The Downsides of Vaccine Passports Have Been
Exaggerated." *Globe and Mail*, 21 July 2020. https://www.theglobeand
mail.com/opinion/article-the-downsides-of-vaccine-passports-have-been-
exaggerated.

Murdoch, B., and T. Caulfield. 2023. "COVID-19 Lockdown Revisionism." *Canadian Medical Association Journal* 195 (15): E552–4. https://doi. org/10.1503/cmaj.221543.

Murphy, G.T., L.B. Bearskin, N. Cashen, G. Cummings, A.E. Rose, J. Etowa, D. Grinspun, E.W. Jones, M. Lavoi-Tremblay, K. MacMillan et al. 2022. "Investing in Canada's Nursing Workforce Post-Pandemic: A Call to Action." *Facets* 7 (1): 1051–120. https://doi.org/10.1139/facets-2022-0002.

Murphy, J. 2020. "WE Charity Scandal – A Simple Guide to the New Crisis for Trudeau." BBC News, 20 August 2020. https://www.bbc.com/news/world-us-canada-53494560.

Murphy, S.L., K.D. Kochanek, J.Q. Xu, and E. Arias. 2021. "Mortality in the United States, 2020." National Center for Health Statistics Data Brief 427 (2021). Hyattsville, MD. https://dx.doi.org/10.15620/cdc:112079 external icon.

Murray, W.C. 2017. "Human Resource Challenges in Canada's Hospitality and Tourism Industry: Finding Innovative Solutions." *Worldwide Hospitality and Tourism Themes* 9 (4): 1–11. http://dx.doi.org/10.1108/WHATT-04-2017-0022.

Mwachofi, A., and A.F. Al-Assaf. 2011. "Health Care Deviations from the Ideal Market." *Sultan Qaboos University Medical Journal.* 11 (3): 328–37. https://www.ncbi.nlm.nih.gov/pmc/articles/PMC3210041.

Nardi, C. 2020. "Growing Number of Canadians Furious That Airlines Won't Reimburse for Travel Cancelled Due to COVID-19." *National Post,* 20 May 2020. https://nationalpost.com/news/politics/growing-number-of-canadians-furious-that-airlines-wont-reimburse-cancelled-travel-due-to-covid-19.

National Advisory Committee on SARS and Public Health. 2003. *Learning from SARS: Renewal of Public Health in Canada.* https://www.canada.ca/content/dam/phac-aspc/migration/phac-aspc/publicat/sars-sras/pdf/sars-e.pdf.

National Assembly of Quebec. 2021. "Assembly Proceedings." Government of Quebec. http://www.assnat.qc.ca/en/recherche/recherche-avancee.html.

National Audit Office. 2002. *The 2001 Outbreak of Foot and Mouth Disease.* Report by the Comptroller and Auditor General, HC 939 Session 2001–02.

National Center for Health Statistics. 2022. "COVID-19 Mortality Overview." Centers for Disease Control and Prevention, last reviewed 16 May 2022. https://www.cdc.gov/nchs/covid19/mortality-overview.htm.

National Collaborating Centre for Aboriginal Health. 2016. *Pandemic Planning in Indigenous Communities: Lessons Learned from the 2009*

H1N1 Influenza Pandemic in Canada. https://www.ccnsa-nccah.ca/docs/other/FS-InfluenzaPandemic-EN.pdf.

National Commission on Terrorist Attacks. 2004. *The 9/11 Commission Report.* https://govinfo.library.unt.edu/911/report/911Report_Exec.pdf.

National Expert Commission. 2012. "A Nursing Call to Action." http://zweb-s3.uploads.s3.amazonaws.com/carp/2012/08/NEC_Report_e.pdf.

National Institute of Public Health Quebec. 2021. "Données COVID-19 au Québec." https://www.inspq.qc.ca/covid-19/donnees.

National Institute of Statistics and Economic Studies. 2021. "Demographic Balance Sheet, 2020." Government of France. https://www.insee.fr/en/statistiques/5015919?sommaire=5015923.

National Institute on Ageing. 2019. "Enabling the Future Provision of Long-Term Care in Canada." https://static1.squarespace.com/static/5c2fa7b03917eed9b5a436d8/t/5d9de15a38dca21e46009548/15706279 31078/Enabling*the*Future*Provision*of*Long-Term*Care*in*Canada.pdf.

– 2021. "Pandemic Perspectives on Long-Term Care: Insights from Canadians in Light of COVID-19." 9 March 2021. https://www.cma.ca/sites/default/files/pdf/Activities/National-Institute-on-Ageing-CMA-Report-EN.pdf.

National Institutes of Health. n.d. "COVID-19 Vaccine Development: Behind the Scenes." Accessed 17 February 2022. https://covid19.nih.gov/news-and-stories/vaccine-development.

National Post. 2020. "COVID-19 Full Text: Read Public Health Ontario's Modelling Report on the Coronavirus Outbreak." 3 April 2020. https://nationalpost.com/news/canada/public-health-ontario-covid19-modelling-technical-briefing-full-text.

– 2022. "Liberal MP Joël Lightbound's Full Remarks: 'It's Time to Choose Positive, Not Coercive Methods.'" 8 February 2022. https://nationalpost.com/news/politics/joel-lightbound-full-transcript.

National Research Council. 2013. *Subjective Well-Being – Measuring Happiness, Suffering, and Other Dimensions of Experience.* Panel of Measuring Subjective Well-Being in a Policy-Relevant Framework, National Research Council. Washington, DC: National Academies Press. https://www.ncbi.nlm.nih.gov/books/NBK179225.

National Statistics Institute. 2021. "Population Figures, Latest Data." Government of Spain. https://www.ine.es/dyngs/INEbase/en/operacion.htm?c=Estadistica_C&cid=1254736176951&menu=ultiDatos&idp=1254735572981.

National WWII Museum. n.d. "Research Starters: Worldwide Deaths in World War II." Accessed 9 March 2022. https://www.nationalww2

museum.org/students-teachers/student-resources/research-starters/ research-starters-worldwide-deaths-world-war.

Natural Resources Canada. 2018. *Energy Fact Book, 2018–2019.* https://www.nrcan.gc.ca/sites/www.nrcan.gc.ca/files/energy/pdf/ energy-factbook-oct2-2018%20(1).pdf.

Netherlands (National Institute for Public Health and the Environment). 2021. "Vaccines Very Effective against Hospital and ICU Admissions, Also for Delta Variant." 28 August 2021. https://www.rivm.nl/en/news/ vaccines-very-effective-against-hospital-and-icu-admissions-also-for-delta-variant.

Neustadt, R.E., and H.V. Fineberg. 1983. *The Epidemic That Never Was: Policy-Making and the Swine Flu Scare.* New York: Vintage Books.

Neustaeter, B. 2020. "Majority of Canadians' Work Refusal Claims Being Denied amid COVID-19." CTV News, 25 June 2020. https://www. ctvnews.ca/health/coronavirus/majority-of-canadians-work-refusal-claims-being-denied-amid-covid-19-1.4999369.

Newfoundland and Labrador Executive Council. 2020. "Premier Furey Announces Temporary Changes to Atlantic Bubble." Government of Newfoundland and Labrador, 23 November 2020. https://www.gov.nl.ca/ releases/2020/exec/1123n04.

Newfoundland and Labrador Provincial Public Health Laboratory Network. 2020. "The Provincial Public Health Microbiology Laboratory Has a Prioritization Strategy for COVID19 Testing." 9 April 2020. http:// www.nlma.nl.ca/FileManager/coronavirus/April/PHML_Specimen Prioritization_Strategy_Memo_FINAL_Thursday_April_9_2020.pdf.

Newman, A. 2019. "If Seeing the World Helps Ruin It, Should We Stay Home?" *New York Times*, 3 June 2019. https://www.nytimes. com/2019/06/03/travel/traveling-climate-change.html.

Ng, E. 2021. "COVID-19 Deaths among Immigrants: Evidence from the Early Months of the Pandemic." Statistics Canada, 9 June 2021. https:// www150.statcan.gc.ca/n1/pub/45-28-0001/2021001/article/00017-eng. htm.

Niskanen, W.A. 1968. "Nonmarket Decision Making: The Peculiar Economics of Bureaucracy." *American Economic Review* 58 (2): 293–305. https://www.jstor.org/stable/1831817.

– 1994. *Bureaucracy and Public Economics.* Cheltenham, UK: Edward Elgar Publishing.

Nixon, G. 2021. "Rethinking Your Relationship with Work? So Are a Lot of People." CBC News, 6 November 2021. https://www.cbc.ca/news/ opinion/opinion-medical-assistance-in-dying-maid-legislation-1. 5790710.

Normandin, J.M., and M.C. Therrien. 2016. "Resilience Factors Reconciled with Complexity: The Dynamics of Order and Disorder." *Journal of Contingencies and Crisis Management* 24 (2): 107–18. https://doi.org/10.1111/1468-5973.12107.

Norris, S. 2020. "Federal Funding for Health Care (Background Paper)." Parliamentary Information and Research Service, 29 December 2020. https://bdp.parl.ca/sites/PublicWebsite/default/en_CA/Research Publications/201845E.

Nova Scotia Advocate. 2020. "An Open Letter to Premier Stephen McNeil and Chief Medical Health Officer Dr. Robert Strang." 24 April 2020. https://nsadvocate.org/2020/04/24/an-open-letter-to-premier-stephen-mcneil-and-chief-medical-health-officer-dr-robert-strang.

Nova Scotia Department of Health and Wellness. 2023. *Nova Scotia Monthly COVID-19 Epidemiologic Summary: February 08, 2023.* https://novascotia.ca/coronavirus/docs/COVID-19-epidemiologic-summary_2023-02-08.pdf.

Nova Scotia Legislature. n.d. "Calendar." Accessed 2021. https://nslegislature.ca/get-involved/calendar/year/2020 ns_leg_calendar%5B0%5D=house.

Nuriddin, A., G. Mooney, and A.I.R. White. 2020. "The Art of Medicine – Reckoning with Histories of Medical Racism and Violence in the USA." *Lancet* 396 (10256): 949–51. https://doi.org/10.1016/S0140-6736(20)32032-8.

OAG (Office of the Auditor General of Canada). 2008. "Surveillance of Infectious Diseases – Public Health Agency of Canada." Chap. 5 in *Report of the Auditor General of Canada to the House of Commons.* https://www.oag-bvg.gc.ca/internet/docs/aud_ch_oag_200805_05_e.pdf.

– 2021a. *Report 6 – Canada Emergency Response Benefit.* Government of Canada. https://www.oag-bvg.gc.ca/internet/English/parl_oag_202103_01_e_43783.html.

– 2021b. *Report 7 – Canada Emergency Wage Subsidy.* Government of Canada. https://www.oag-bvg.gc.ca/internet/English/parl_oag_202103_02_e_43784.html.

– 2021c. *Report 8 – Pandemic Preparedness, Surveillance, and Border Control Measures.* Government of Canada. https://www.oag-bvg.gc.ca/internet/English/parl_oag_202103_03_e_43785.html.

– 2022. *2022 Reports 9 and 10 of the Auditor General of Canada to the Parliament of Canada.* Government of Canada, 6 December 2022. https://www.oag-bvg.gc.ca/internet/English/parl_oag_202212_10_e_44176.html.

O'Brien, K., M. St-Jean, P. Wood, S. Willbond, O. Phillips, D. Currie, and M. Turcotte. 2020. "COVID-19 Death Comorbidities in Canada."

StatCan COVID-19: Data Insights for a Better Canada, catalogue no. 45280001. https://www150.statcan.gc.ca/n1/en/pub/45-28-0001/2020001/article/00087-eng.pdf?st=hmzXbWGv.

Observatory of Economic Complexity. n.d. "Country Profile – Canada." Accessed 27 January 2022. https://oec.world/en/profile/country/can.

OCL (Office of the Commissioner of Lobbying of Canada). n.d.a. "All Monthly Communication Reports for Air Canada – Don Boudria, Don Boudria Consulting Inc (Consultant)." Accessed January 2022. https://lobbycanada.gc.ca/app/secure/ocl/lrs/do/vwRg?cno=358340&regId=862478#regStart.

– n.d.b. "All Monthly Communication Reports for Air Canada – Michael Rousseau, President and Chief Executive Officer (Corporation)." Accessed January 2022. https://lobbycanada.gc.ca/app/secure/ocl/lrs/do/vwRg?cno=15009&regId=898848#regStart.

– n.d.c. "All Monthly Communication Reports for Tourism Industry Association of Canada." Accessed 11 January 2022. https://lobby canada.gc.ca/app/secure/ocl/lrs/do/vwRg?cno=13771&regId=902737#regStart.

– n.d.d. "Registration – In-House Organization: Tourism Industry Association of Canada." Accessed January 2022. https://lobbycanada.gc.ca/app/secure/ocl/lrs/do/vwRg?cno=13771&regId=881601.

OECD (Organisation for Economic Co-operation and Development). 2017. "Health at a Glance 2017: OECD Indicators." https://doi.org/10.1787/health_glance-2017-en.

– 2019a. "Health at a Glance 2019: OECD Indicators." https://doi.org/10.1787/4dd50c09-en.

– 2019b. "Pensions at a Glance 2019: OECD and G20 Indicators." https://doi.org/10.1787/b6d3dcfc-en.

– 2020a. "Beyond Containment: Health Systems Responses to COVID-19 in the OECD." 16 April 2020. https://read.oecd-ilibrary.org/view/?ref=119_119689-ud5comtf84&title=Beyond_Containment:Health_systems_responses_to_COVID-19_in_the_OECD.

– 2020b. "Income Distribution Database: By Country." https://stats.oecd.org/index.aspx?queryid=66670.

– 2020c. "Intensive Care Beds Capacity." 20 April 2020. https://www.oecd.org/coronavirus/en/data-insights/intensive-care-beds-capacity.

– 2020d. "Job Retention Schemes during the COVID-19 Lockdown and Beyond." OECD Policy Responses to Coronavirus (COVID-19). Paris: OECD Publishing. https://read.oecd-ilibrary.org/view/?ref=135_135415-6bardplc5q&title=Job-retention-schemes-during-the-COVID-19-lockdown-and-beyond.

– 2020e. *OECD Tourism Trends and Policies 2020.* Paris: OECD Publishing. https://doi.org/10.1787/6b47b985-en.

– 2021. "Hospital Beds – Acute Care." https://www.oecd.org/coronavirus/en/data-insights/hospital-beds-acute-care.

– n.d.a. "Quarterly National Accounts: G20 – Quarterly Growth Rates of GDP in Volume." Accessed 25 January 2022. https://stats.oecd.org/index.aspx?queryid=33940.

Office for National Statistics. 2021. "United Kingdom Population Mid-Year Estimate." Government of the United Kingdom, 25 June 2021. https://www.ons.gov.uk/peoplepopulationandcommunity/populationand migration/populationestimates/timeseries/ukpop/pop.

Office of Audit and Evaluation. 2022. *Audit of the Security of National Emergency Strategic Stockpile (NESS) Warehouse Facilities.* Health Canada and the Public Health Agency of Canada. https://www.canada.ca/content/dam/hc-sc/documents/corporate/transparency/corporate-management-reporting/internal-audits/security-national-emergency-strategic-stockpile-warehouse-facilities/security-national-emergency-strategic-stockpile-warehouse-facilities.pdf.

Office of the Assistant Secretary for Planning and Evaluation. 2017. "Guidelines for Regulatory Impact Analysis." US Department of Health and Human Services. https://aspe.hhs.gov/reports/guidelines-regulatory-impact-analysis.

Office of the High Commissioner of Human Rights. 2020. "Human Rights and Access to COVID-19 Vaccines." United Nations Office of Human Rights, 17 December 2020. https://www.ohchr.org/Documents/Events/COVID-19_AccessVaccines_Guidance.pdf.

Office of the Premier of New Brunswick. 2020a. "Ten New Cases of COVID-19; Improved Testing and New Equipment." Government of New Brunswick, 2 April 2020. https://www2.gnb.ca/content/gnb/en/news/news_release.2020.04.0177.html.

– 2020b. "Zone 2 Moves to Orange Level / Nine New Cases / Outbreak at a Nursing Home in Saint John." Government of New Brunswick, 20 November 2020. https://www2.gnb.ca/content/gnb/en/news/news_release.2020.11.0622.html.

Office of the Premier of Ontario. 2020. "Ontario Unveils Guiding Principles to Reopen the Province." Government of Ontario, 27 April 2020. https://news.ontario.ca/en/release/56780/ontario-unveils-guiding-principles-to-reopen-the-province.

– 2021. "Ontario's COVID-19 Vaccination Strategy Targets High-Risk Neighbourhoods." Government of Ontario, 13 April 201. https://news.

ontario.ca/en/release/61124/ontarios-covid-19-vaccination-strategy-targets-high-risk-neighbourhoods.

Office of the Seniors Advocate British Columbia. 2018. *Monitoring Seniors Services.* https://www.seniorsadvocatebc.ca/app/uploads/sites/4/2019/01/MonitoringReport2018.pdf.

– 2020. *A Billion Reasons to Care: A Funding Review of Contracted Long-Term Care in B.C.* https://www.seniorsadvocatebc.ca/app/uploads/sites/4/2020/02/ABillionReasonsToCare.pdf.

Ogden, N.H., P. AbdelMalik, and J.R.C. Pulliam. 2017. "Emerging Infectious Diseases: Prediction and Detection." *Canada Communicable Disease Report* 43 (10): 206–11. https://doi.org/10.14745/ccdr.v43i10a03.

Ogden, N.H, A. Fazil, J. Arino, P. Berthiaume, D.N. Fisman, A.L. Greer, A. Ludwig, V. Ng, A.R. Tuite, P. Turgeon et al. 2020. "Modelling Scenarios of the Epidemic of COVID-19 in Canada." *Canada Communicable Disease Report* 46 (6): 198–204. https://doi.org/10.14745/ccdr.v46i06a08.

O'Kane, J. 2020. "The Urban Atlantic Advantage: Work-from-Home Era Offers Halifax More People and More Wealth, but at a Price." *Globe and Mail,* 19 November 2020. https://www.theglobeandmail.com/business/article-the-urban-atlantic-advantage-work-from-home-era-offers-halifax-more.

Olofsson, A., J.O. Zinn, G. Griffin, K.G. Nygren, A. Cebulla, and K. Hannah-Moffat. 2014. "The Mutual Constitution of Risk and Inequalities: Intersectional Risk Theory." *Health, Risk & Society* 16 (5): 417–30. https://doi.org/10.1080/13698575.2014.942258.

Ombudsman Saskatchewan. 2021. *Caring in Crisis: An Investigation into the Response to the COVID-19 Outbreak at Extendicare Parkside.* https://ombudsman.sk.ca/app/uploads/2021/08/Caring-in-Crisis-Full-Report.pdf.

Ontario COVID-19 Science Advisory Table. 2022. "About Us." https://covid19-sciencetable.ca/about.

Ontario Health Coalition. 2020. "COVID-19 Second Wave Survey of Staff in Long-Term Care Homes with Large Outbreaks." 17 December 2020. https://www.ontariohealthcoalition.ca/wp-content/uploads/Final-large-outbreaks-staff-survey-report.pdf.

Ontario Long-Term Care Association. 2019. *Long-Term Care That Works. For Seniors, for Ontario: 2019 Budget Submission.* https://www.oltca.com/OLTCA/Documents/Reports/2019OLTCABudgetSubmission-LTCthatWorks.pdf.

Ontario Ministry of Health and Long-Term Care. 2020. "Management of Cases and Contacts of COVID-19 in Ontario (Version 9.1)." Government of Ontario, 9 October 2020. https://www.readkong.com/page/management-of-cases-and-contacts-of-covid-19-in-ontario-9605618.

Ontario Ministry of Long-Term Care. 2019. "Long-Term Care Home Quality Inspection Program." Modified 15 January 2019. http://www.health.gov.on.ca/en/public/programs/ltc/31_pr_inspections.aspx.

– 2020. *Long-Term Care Staffing Study.* https://files.ontario.ca/mltc-long-term-care-staffing-study-en-2020-07-31.pdf.

Ontario Nurses' Association. 2020. "ONA Long-Term Care Nurses Pleased with Superior Court Ruling That Forces Four Long-Term Care Homes to Follow Directives." 23 April 2020. https://www.ona.org/news-posts/ona-wins-ltc.

Ontario Solicitor General. 2020. "Ontario Extends COVID-19 Orders." Government of Ontario, 10 December 2020. https://news.ontario.ca/en/release/59551/ontario-extends-covid-19-orders-1.

OPC (Office of the Privacy Commissioner of Canada). 2020a. "Privacy and the COVID-19 Pandemic." Modified 20 March 2020. https://priv.gc.ca/en/privacy-topics/health-genetic-and-other-body-information/health-emergencies/gd_covid_202003.

– 2020b. "Privacy in a Pandemic – Commissioner's Message." https://www.priv.gc.ca/en/opc-actions-and-decisions/ar_index/201920/ar_201920.

Orchard, L., and H. Stretton. 1997. "Public Choice." *Cambridge Journal of Economics* 21 (3): 409–30. https://doi.org/10.1093/oxfordjournals.cje.a013678.

Orîndaru, A., M.F. Popescu, A.P. Alexoaei, S.C. Caescu, M.S. Florescu, and A.C. Orzan. 2021. "Tourism in a Post-COVID-19 Era: Sustainable Strategies for Industry's Recovery." *Sustainability* 13 (12): 1–22. https://doi.org/10.3390/su13126781.

Ormel, I., R. Stalteri, V. Goel, S. Horton, L. Puchalski-Ritchie, N. Muhajarine, K. Milaney, S. Pisheh, R. Plouffe, and S. Law. 2021. "Misinformation and Disinformation in Relation to COVID-19." CanCOVID Issue Note, 1 June 2021. https://cancovid.ca/wp-content/uploads/2021/12/CanCOVID-Issue-Note-Misinformation-EN.pdf.

Ortega, B., S. Bronstein, C. Devine, and D. Griffin. 2020. "How the Government Delayed Coronavirus Testing." CNN, 9 April 2020. https://www.cnn.com/2020/04/09/politics/coronavirus-testing-cdc-fda-red-tape-invs/index.html.

OSB (Office of the Superintendent of Bankruptcy). 2022. "Insolvency Statistics in Canada – 2021." Government of Canada, modified 3 July 2022. https://ised-isde.canada.ca/site/office-superintendent-bankruptcy/en/

statistics-and-research/insolvency-statistics/annual-reports/insolvency-statistics-canada-2021.

– 2023. "Insolvency Statistics in Canada – 2022." Government of Canada, modified 4 July 2023. https://ised-isde.canada.ca/site/office-superintendent-bankruptcy/en/statistics-and-research/insolvency-statistics-canada-2022.

Osman, L. 2020. "Hotels for Homeless People Could Tackle Two Crises at Once: Advocates." *National Post*, 21 April 2020. https://nationalpost.com/pmn/news-pmn/canada-news-pmn/hotels-for-homeless-people-could-tackle-two-crises-at-once-advocates.

– 2023. "Subcontracting ArriveCan Development 'Seems Highly Illogical and Inefficient': Trudeau." CTV News, 23 January 2023. https://www.ctvnews.ca/politics/subcontracting-arrivecan-development-seems-highly-illogical-and-inefficient-trudeau-1.6242290.

O'Sullivan, T., and M. Bourgoin. 2010. "Vulnerability in an Influenza Pandemic: Looking beyond Medical Risk." Public Health Agency of Canada, October 2010. https://www.researchgate.net/publication/282817477_Vulnerability_in_an_Influenza_Pandemic_Looking_Beyond_Medical_Risk.

Ottawa Police Service. 2022. "Chief Peter Sloly Remarks during Media Availability – January 31, 2022." https://www.ottawapolice.ca/Modules/News/index.aspx?newsId=4e505c6b-0e2e-4a69-a9f0-cfccdcb3e542.

Ovens, H, and D. Petrie. 2021. "WTBS 25 COVID-19 Pandemic Exposes the Importance of Resilience in Health System Redesign." Emergency Medicine Cases, 12 January 2021. https://emergencymedicinecases.com/covid-19-pandemic-resilience-health-system-redesign.

Pachur, T., R. Hertwig, and F. Steinmann. 2012. "How Do People Judge Risks: Availability Heuristic, Affect Heuristic, or Both?" *Journal of Experimental Psychology: Applied* 18 (3): 314–30. http://dx.doi.org.ezproxy.library.dal.ca/10.1037/a0028279.

Padron-Regalado, E. 2020. "Vaccines for SARS-COV-2: Lessons from Other Coronavirus Strains." *Infectious Diseases and Therapy* 10 (1): 255–74. https://dx.doi.org/10.1007%2Fs40121-020-00300-x.

Page, H. 2020. "Employment & Human Rights Law in Canada – Ontario's New Infection Disease Emergency Leave." Spring Law, 20 March 2020. https://www.canadaemploymenthumanrightslaw.com/2020/03/ontarios-new-infectious-disease-emergency-leave.

Palmer, A. 2020. "Amazon Says More than 19,000 Workers Got COVID-19." CNBC, 1 October 2020. https://www.cnbc.com/2020/10/01/amazon-says-more-than-19000-workers-got-covid-19.html.

Palmer, D., and M. Maher. 2010. "A Normal Accident Analysis of the Mortgage Meltdown." *Research in the Sociology of Organizations* 30: 219–56. http://dx.doi.org/10.1108/S0733-558X(2010)000030A011.

Pandey, A. 2020. "Coronavirus' Top Winners: From Netflix to Tesla." Deutsche Welle, 17 July 2020. https://www.dw.com/en/coronavirus-top-winners-from-netflix-to-tesla/g-52623562.

Panetta, A. 2022. "In America's Partisan Carnival, Justin Trudeau Is Now on Display." CBC News, 19 February 2022. https://www.cbc.ca/news/world/america-justin-trudeau-partisan-1.6357882.

Panneton, D. 2022. "The Trucker Convoy Shows How Canadians Are Being Sucked into Larger Conspiratorial Narratives." *Globe and Mail*, 11 February 2022. https://www.theglobeandmail.com/opinion/article-the-trucker-convoy-shows-how-canadians-are-being-sucked-into-larger.

Paris, R., and J. Welsh, J. 2021. "The World's Democracies, Including Canada, Face a Historic Choice." *Globe and Mail*, 4 June 2021. https://www.theglobeandmail.com/opinion/article-the-worlds-democracies-including-canada-face-a-historic-choice.

Park, K., B. Chamberlain, Z. Song, H.N. Esfahani, J. Sheen, T. Larsen, V.L. Novack, C. Licon, and K. Christensen. 2022. "A Double Jeopardy: COVID-19 Impacts on Travel Behaviour and Community Living of People with Disabilities." *Transportation Research Part A: Policy and Practice* 156:24–35. https://doi.org/10.1016%2Fj.tra.2021.12.008.

Parker, N., and C. Terhune. 2021. "Special Report: How U.S. CDC Missed Chances to Spot Covid's Silent Spread." Reuters, 22 January 2021. https://www.reuters.com/article/us-health-coronavirus-cdc-response-speci-idUSKBN29R1E7.

Parkin, A., A. Sweetman, V. Rego, and Y. Li. 2021. "Vaccine Hesitancy Is Decreasing in Canada, but It's Too Soon to Celebrate." *The Conversation*, 28 July 2021. https://theconversation.com/vaccine-hesitancy-is-decreasing-in-canada-but-its-too-soon-to-celebrate-165133.

Parkinson, D. 2021. "Atlantic Canada Grapples with Pandemic-Fuelled Population Boom." *Globe and Mail*, 7 October 2021. https://www.theglobeandmail.com/business/commentary/article-atlantic-canada-grapples-with-pandemic-fuelled-population-boom.

– 2022. "There Are No Quick Fixes for Canada's Soaring Inflation." *Globe and Mail*, 16 February 2022. https://www.theglobeandmail.com/business/commentary/article-there-are-no-quick-fixes-for-canadas-soaring-inflation.

Parks Canada. 2021. "Parks Canada Attendance, 2019–20." 22 January 2021. https://www.pc.gc.ca/en/docs/pc/attend#summary.

Parliament of Canada. 2020. *An Act Respecting Certain Measures in Response to COVID-19*. Government of Canada, 25 March 2021. https://

www.parl.ca/DocumentViewer/fr/43-1/projet-loi/C-13/sanction-royal?col=2.

– 2021. "House of Commons Sitting Calendar." Government of Canada. https://www.ourcommons.ca/en/sitting-calendar/2021.

– n.d. "Parlinfo – Sittings by Calendar Year." Accessed 23 March 2022. https://lop.parl.ca/sites/ParlInfo/default/en_CA/Parliament/SittingsByYear.

Patterson, I., and A. Balderas. 2020. "Continuing and Emerging Trends of Senior Tourism: A Review of the Literature." *Population Ageing* 13 (September): 385–99. https://doi.org/10.1007/s12062-018-9228-4.

Pearce, K., 2020. "Distributing a COVID-19 Vaccine Raises Complex Ethical Issues." Hub – Johns Hopkins University, 1 July 2020. https://hub.jhu.edu/2020/07/01/covid-vaccine-ethics-faden.

Pecoraro, V., A. Negro, T. Pirotti, and T. Trenti. 2021. "Estimate False-Negative RT-PCR Rates for SARS-COV-2. A Systematic Review and Meta-Analysis." *European Journal of Clinical Investigation* 52 (2022): e13706. https://doi.org/10.1111/eci.13706.

Pederson, K., M. Mancini, and D. Common. 2020. "Ontario Scaled Back Comprehensive, Annual Inspections of Nursing Homes to Only a Handful Last Year." CBC News, 15 April 2020. https://www.cbc.ca/news/canada/seniors-homes-inspections-1.5532585.

Peesker, S. 2020. "Renovation and Home-Improvement Spending Booms as COVID-19 Changes Consumer Habits." *Globe and Mail*, 1 July 2020. https://www.theglobeandmail.com/investing/personal-finance/house-hold-finances/article-renovation-and-home-improvement-spending-booms-as-covid-19-changes.

Pelley, L. 2021. "How Often Are Canadian Kids Actually Getting Seriously Ill or Dying from COVID-19?" CBC News, 29 April 2021. https://www.cbc.ca/news/health/covid-19-kids-risk-pandemic-1.6006172.

Perkel, C. 2020. "Coronavirus: Firearms and Ammo Sales Spike across Canada amid COVID-19, Gun Law Fears." Global News, 20 March 2020. https://globalnews.ca/news/6706985/coronavirus-firearms-and-ammo-sales-spike-across-canada-amid-covid-19-gun-law-fears.

– 2021. "'It Wasn't Called COVID at the Time': One Year since Canada's First COVID-19 Case." CTV News, 24 January 2021. https://www.ctvnews.ca/health/coronavirus/it-wasn-t-called-covid-at-the-time-one-year-since-canada-s-first-covid-19-case-1.5279999.

Perreaux, L., M. Walsh, and J. Gray. 2020. "Canada Administers Its First COVID-19 Vaccine Shots." *Globe and Mail*, 14 December 2020. https://www.theglobeandmail.com/canada/article-canada-administers-its-first-covid-19-vaccine-shots.

Perrow, C. 1999. *Normal Accidents: Living with High Risk Technologies.* 2nd ed. Princeton, NJ: Princeton University Press.

Perry, B., and R. Scrivens. 2016. "Uneasy Alliances: A Look at the Right-Wing Extremist Movement in Canada." *Studies in Conflict and Terrorism* 39 (9): 819–41. https://doi.org/10.1080/1057610X.2016.1139375.

Peters, R.G., V.T. Covello, and D.B. McCallum. 1997. "The Determinants of Trust and Credibility in Environmental Risk Communication: An Empirical Study." *Risk Analysis* 17 (1): 43–54. https://doi. org/10.1111/j.1539-6924.1997.tb00842.x.

Peterson, B. 2020. "How We Reason about COVID Tradeoffs." *New Atlantis: A Journal of Technology & Society* 62: 69–75. https://www.the newatlantis.com/publications/how-we-reason-about-covid-tradeoffs.

Peterson, M. 2017. "Yes, the Precautionary Principle Is Incoherent." *Risk Analysis* 37 (11): 2035–8. https://doi.org/10.1111/risa.12783.

Petracca, M.P. 1991. "The Rational Choice Approach to Politics: A Challenge to Democratic Theory." *Review of Politics* 53 (2): 289–319. https://www.jstor.org/stable/1407756.

Pew Research Center. 2021. *People in Advanced Economies Say Their Society Is More Divided than before Pandemic.* https://www.pewresearch. org/global/wp-content/uploads/sites/2/2021/06/PG_2021.06.23_Global-COVID_FINAL.pdf.

PHAC (Public Health Agency of Canada). 2005. *Improving Public Health System Infrastructure in Canada: Report of the Strengthening Public Health System Infrastructure Task Group.* https://books.google.ca/books?id=JxH5jwEACAAJ.

– 2010. *Lessons Learned Review: Public Health Agency of Canada and Health Canada Response to the 2009 H1N1 Pandemic.* https://www. canada.ca/content/dam/phac-aspc/migration/phac-aspc/about_apropos/ evaluation/reports-rapports/2010-2011/h1n1/pdf/h1n1-eng.pdf.

– 2011a. "External Advisory Boards: Public Health Agency of Canada's Policy on External Advisory Bodies (2011) Summary." Government of Canada. https://www.canada.ca/en/public-health/corporate/mandate/ about-agency/external-advisory-bodies/policy.html.

– 2011b. "Mandate." https://www.canada.ca/en/public-health/corporate/ mandate/about-agency/mandate.html.

– 2012. "What Is the Population Health Approach?" Government of Canada, 7 February 2012. https://www.canada.ca/en/public-health/ services/health-promotion/population-health/population-health-approach. html.

– 2013a. *The Chief Public Health Officer's Report on the State of Public Health in Canada, 2013: Infectious Disease – The Never-Ending Threat.*

https://www.canada.ca/en/public-health/corporate/publications/chief-public-health-officer-reports-state-public-health-canada/chief-public-health-officer-report-on-state-public-health-canada-2013-infectious-disease-never-ending-threat.html.

– 2013b. *Follow-Up Audit of Emergency Preparedness and Response.* https://www.canada.ca/content/dam/phac-aspc/migration/phac-aspc/about_apropos/asd-dsv/ar-rv/2013/assets/pdf/epr-mid-eng.pdf.

– 2016. *Public Health Agency of Canada 2015–16 Departmental Results Report.* https://www.canada.ca/content/dam/phac-aspc/documents/corporate/transparency/corporate-management-reporting/departmental-performance-reports/2016-2017-departmental-results-report.pdf.

– 2019. *Public Health Agency of Canada 2018–19 Departmental Results Report.* https://www.canada.ca/content/dam/phac-aspc/documents/corporate/transparency/corporate-management-reporting/depart mental-performance-reports/2018-2019/phac_2018-19_drr.pdf.

– 2020a. "COVID-19 in Canada: Modelling Update." Government of Canada, 28 April 2020. https://www.canada.ca/content/dam/phac-aspc/documents/services/diseases/2019-novel-coronavirus-infection/using-data-modelling-inform-eng-04-28.pdf.

– 2020b. "COVID-19 in Canada: Using Data and Modelling to Inform Public Health Action – Technical Briefing for Canadians." Government of Canada, 9 April 2020. https://www.canada.ca/content/dam/phac-aspc/documents/services/diseases/2019-novel-coronavirus-infection/using-data-modelling-inform-eng.pdf.

– 2020c. "Government of Canada Announces New Mandatory Requirements for Travellers to Canada." Government of Canada, 2 November 2020. https://www.canada.ca/en/public-health/news/2020/11/government-of-canada-announces-new-mandatory-requirements-for-travellers-to-canada.html.

– 2020d. "Government of Canada Confirms Support for 32 Community-Based Projects Aimed at Improving Mental Health." Government of Canada, 10 September 2020. https://www.canada.ca/en/public-health/news/2020/09/government-of-canada-supports-projects-aimed-at-improving-the-mental-health-of-vulnerable-communities.html.

– 2020e. "Government of Canada Updates Mandatory Requirements for Travellers Entering Canada." Government of Canada, 14 April 2020. https://www.canada.ca/en/public-health/news/2020/04/government-of-canada-updates-mandatory-requirements-for-travellers-entering-canada.html.

– 2020f. "New Order Makes Self-Isolation Mandatory for Individuals Entering Canada." Government of Canada, 25 March 2020. https://www.

canada.ca/en/public-health/news/2020/03/new-order-makes-self-isolation-mandatory-for-individuals-entering-canada.html.

– 2020g. *Public Health Agency of Canada 2019–2020 Departmental Results Report.* https://www.canada.ca/content/dam/phac-aspc/documents/corporate/transparency/corporate-management-reporting/departmental-performance-reports/2019-2020/phac-drr-eng.pdf.

– 2020h. *Public Health Agency of Canada 2020–21 Departmental Plan.* https://www.canada.ca/content/dam/phac-aspc/documents/corporate/transparency/corporate-management-reporting/reports-plans-priorities/2020-2021-departmental-plan/phac_2020-21_dp_main_report-eng.pdf.

– 2020i. "Update: COVID-19 in Canada." Government of Canada, 4 June 2020. https://www.canada.ca/content/dam/phac-aspc/documents/services/diseases-maladies/coronavirus-disease-covid-19/epidemiological-economic-research-data/mathematical-modelling/mathematical-modelling-en.pdf.

– 2020j. "Update on COVID-19 in Canada: Epidemiology and Modelling." Government of Canada, 28 April 2020. https://www.canada.ca/en/public-health/services/publications/diseases-conditions/covid-19-using-data-modelling-inform-public-health-action-april-28-2020.html.

– 2020k. "Update on COVID-19 in Canada: Epidemiology and Modelling." Government of Canada, 4 June 2020. https://www.canada.ca/en/public-health/services/diseases/coronavirus-disease-covid-19/epidemiological-economic-research-data/mathematical-modelling.html.

– 2020l. "Update on COVID-19 in Canada: Epidemiology and Modelling." Government of Canada, 29 June 2020. https://www.canada.ca/en/public-health/services/diseases/coronavirus-disease-covid-19/epidemiological-economic-research-data/mathematical-modelling.html.

– 2020m. "Update on COVID-19 in Canada: Epidemiology and Modelling." Government of Canada, 8 July 2020. https://www.canada.ca/en/public-health/services/diseases/coronavirus-disease-covid-19/epidemiological-economic-research-data/mathematical-modelling.html.

– 2020n. "Update on COVID-19 in Canada: Epidemiology and Modelling." Government of Canada, 14 August 2020. https://www.canada.ca/en/public-health/services/diseases/coronavirus-disease-covid-19/epidemiological-economic-research-data/mathematical-modelling.html.

– 2020o. "Update on COVID-19 in Canada: Epidemiology and Modelling." Government of Canada, 22 September 2020. https://www.canada.ca/en/public-health/services/diseases/coronavirus-disease-covid-19/epidemiological-economic-research-data/mathematical-modelling.html.

– 2020p. "Update on COVID-19 in Canada: Epidemiology and Modelling." Government of Canada, 8 October 2020. https://www.canada.ca/en/

public-health/services/diseases/coronavirus-disease-covid-19/epidemiologi
cal-economic-research-data/mathematical-modelling.html.

– 2020q. "Update on COVID-19 in Canada: Epidemiology and Modelling."
Government of Canada, 30 October 2020. https://www.canada.ca/en/
public-health/services/diseases/coronavirus-disease-covid-19/epidemiologi
cal-economic-research-data/mathematical-modelling.html.

– 2020r. "Update on COVID-19 in Canada: Epidemiology and Modelling."
Government of Canada, 20 November 2020. https://www.canada.ca/en/
public-health/services/diseases/coronavirus-disease-covid-19/epidemiologi
cal-economic-research-data/mathematical-modelling.html.

– 2020s. "Update on COVID-19 in Canada: Epidemiology and Modelling."
Government of Canada, 11 December 2020. https://www.canada.ca/en/
public-health/services/diseases/coronavirus-disease-covid-19/epidemiologi
cal-economic-research-data/mathematical-modelling.html.

– 2021a. *2021–22 Departmental Plan.* https://www.canada.ca/content/dam/
phac-aspc/documents/corporate/transparency/corporate-management-
reporting/reports-plans-priorities/2021-2022-departmental-plan/
2021-22-departmental-plan-eng.pdf.

– 2021b. "CPHO Sunday Edition: The Impact of COVID-19 on Racialized
Communities." Government of Canada, 21 February 2021. https://www.
canada.ca/en/public-health/news/2021/02/cpho-sunday-edition-the-
impact-of-covid-19-on-racialized-communities.html.

– 2021c. "Government of Canada Announces Adjustments to Canada's
Border Measures." Government of Canada, 19 November 2021. https://
www.canada.ca/en/public-health/news/2021/11/government-of-canada-
announces-adjustments-to-canadas-border-measures.html.

– 2021d. "Mathematical Modelling and COVID-19."
https://www.canada.ca/en/public-health/services/diseases/coronavirus-
disease-covid-19/epidemiological-economic-research-data/mathemati
cal-modelling.html.

– 2021e. "Statement from the Chief Public Health Officer of Canada on
September 3, 2021." Government of Canada, modified 10 September
2021. https://www.canada.ca/en/public-health/news/2021/09/statement-
from-the-chief-public-health-officer-of-canada-on-september-3-2021.html.

– 2021f. "Update on COVID-19 in Canada: Epidemiology and Modelling."
Government of Canada, 15 January 2021. https://www.canada.ca/en/
public-health/services/diseases/coronavirus-disease-covid-19/epidemiologi
cal-economic-research-data/mathematical-modelling.html.

– 2021g. "Update on COVID-19 in Canada: Epidemiology and Modelling."
Government of Canada, 19 February 2021. https://www.canada.ca/en/

public-health/services/diseases/coronavirus-disease-covid-19/epidemiologi
cal-economic-research-data/mathematical-modelling.html.

– 2021h. "Update on COVID-19 in Canada: Epidemiology and Modelling."
Government of Canada, 26 March 2021. https://www.canada.ca/en/
public-health/services/diseases/coronavirus-disease-covid-19/epidemiologi
cal-economic-research-data/mathematical-modelling.html.

– 2021i. "Update on COVID-19 in Canada: Epidemiology and Modelling."
Government of Canada, 23 April 2021. https://www.canada.ca/en/
public-health/services/diseases/coronavirus-disease-covid-19/epidemiologi
cal-economic-research-data/mathematical-modelling.html.

– 2021j. "Update on COVID-19 in Canada: Epidemiology and Modelling."
Government of Canada, 28 May 2021. https://www.canada.ca/en/
public-health/services/diseases/coronavirus-disease-covid-19/epidemiologi
cal-economic-research-data/mathematical-modelling.html.

– 2021k. "Update on COVID-19 in Canada: Epidemiology and Modelling."
Government of Canada, 25 June 2021. https://www.canada.ca/content/
dam/phac-aspc/documents/services/diseases-maladies/coronavirus-
disease-covid-19/epidemiological-economic-research-data/update-covid-
19-canada-epidemiology-modelling-20210625-en.pdf.

– 2021l. "Update on COVID-19 in Canada: Epidemiology and Modelling."
Government of Canada, 8 October 2021. https://www.canada.ca
content/dam/phac-aspc/documents/services/diseases-maladies/coronavirus-
disease-covid-19/epidemiological-economic-research-data/update-covid
19-canada-epidemiology-modelling-20211008-en.pdf.

– 2021m. *A Vision to Transform Canada's Public Health System: The Chief
Public Health Officer of Canada's Report on the State of Public Health in
Canada, 2021.* https://www.canada.ca/content/dam/phac-aspc/documents/
corporate/publications/chief-public-health-officer-reports-state-public-
health-canada/state-public-health-canada-2021/cpho-report-eng.pdf.

– 2022a. "Government of Canada Lightens Border Measures as Part of
Transition of the Pandemic Response." Government of Canada, 15
February 2022. https://www.canada.ca/en/public-health/news/2022/02/
government-of-canada-lightens-border-measures-as-part-of-transition-of-
the-pandemic-response.html.

– 2022b. *Public Health Agency of Canada 2020–2021 Departmental
Results Report.* https://www.canada.ca/content/dam/phac-aspc/
documents/corporate/transparency/corporate-management-reporting/
departmental-performance-reports/2020-2021/departmental-
performance-reports-2020-2021.pdf.

– 2023. "Canada's COVID-19 Border Measures Data." Government of
Canada, 26 June 2023. https://www.canada.ca/en/public-health/services/

diseases/coronavirus-disease-covid-19/testing-screening-contact-tracing/
summary-data-travellers.html#a23.

Phillips, H., and J. Rendall. 2021. "School Vaccine Mandates Aren't New:
A History of Requirements." CNET, 7 October 2021. https://www.
cnet.com/health/school-vaccine-mandates-arent-new-a-history-of-
requirements.

PHO (Public Health Ontario). 2020a. "COVID-19 Laboratory Testing in
Ontario and Ontario Public Health, 2 June, COVID-19 Provincial Testing
Guidance Update." 4 June 2020. https://www.publichealthontario.ca/
en/diseases-and-conditions/infectious-diseases/respiratory-diseases/
novel-coronavirus/lab-testing-ontario.

– 2020b. "COVID-19 Provincial Testing Guidance Update." 2 June 2020.
https://www.publichealthontario.ca/en/diseases-and-conditions/infec
tious-diseases/respiratory-diseases/novel-coronavirus/lab-testing-ontario.

– 2020c. "The Story of COVID-19 Testing in Ontario." 26 May 2020.
https://www.publichealthontario.ca/en/about/blog/2020/story-covid-19-
testing-ontario.

Phua, J., M.O. Faruq, A.P. Kulkarni, I.S. Redjeki, K. Detleuxay, N.
Mendsaikhan, K.K. Sann et al. 2020. "Critical Care Bed Capacity in
Asian Countries and Regions." *Critical Care Medicine* 48 (5): 654–62.
https://doi.org/10.1097/ccm.0000000000004222.

Picard, A. 2020. "In the Stay-at-Home Era, Why Have We So Sorely
Neglected Home Care?" *Globe and Mail*, 15 June 2020. https://www.the
globeandmail.com/opinion/article-in-the-stay-at-home-era-why-have-we-
so-sorely-neglected-home-care.

– 2021. *Neglected No More*. Toronto: Random House Canada.

Pigou, A.C. 1932. *The Economics of Welfare*. London: Macmillan.

Pike, H., F. Khan, and P. Amyotte. 2020. "Precautionary Principle (PP)
versus as Low as Reasonably Practicable (ALARP): Which One to Use and
When." *Process Safety and Environmental Protection* 137: 158–68.
https://doi.org/10.1016/j.psep.2020.02.026.

Piller, T. 2020. "Universal Testing Introduced as Saskatchewan Reports
56 New Coronavirus Cases." Global News, 13 July 2020. https://global
news.ca/news/7171605/universal-coronavirus-testing-introduced-
saskatchewan.

Pinkerton, C. 2021. "Canada Might Learn Soon Whether COVID Alert App
Is a Dud." iPolitics, 11 February 2021. https://ipolitics.ca/2021/02/
11/canada-might-learn-soon-whether-covid-alert-app-is-a-dud.

Pinkesz, M. 2020. "COVID-19 Standard of Care." Top Class Actions, 15
May 2020. https://ca.topclassactions.com/lawsuit-settlements/lawsuit-
news/covid-19-standard-of-care.

Pinto-Bazurco, J.F. 2020. "The Precautionary Principle. Still Only One Earth: Lessons from 50 Years of UN Sustainable Development Policy." International Institute for Sustainable Development, Brief #4. https://www.iisd.org/articles/precautionary-principle.

Pitcavage, M. 2022. "Anti-government Anger Isn't New – But the Source of Today's Anger Is Different." Anti-Defamation League, 28 September 2022. https://www.adl.org/resources/blog/anti-government-anger-isnt-new-source-todays-anger-different.

Pittis, D. 2020. "Bank of Canada Says Economy Will Likely Be Scarred by COVID-19." CBC News, 31 October 2020. https://www.cbc.ca/news/business/bank-canada-economy-covid-19-1.5780703.

– 2021. "Airline Deal Means Taxpayers Once Again Take a Risk on Corporate Canada." CBC News, 14 April 2021. https://www.cbc.ca/news/business/air-canada-bailout-column-don-pittis-1.5985185.

Plunkett, L. 2020. "COVID-19 and the Failure of Business Interruption Insurance." *New York State Dental Journal* 86 (4): 5–7.

Poland, G.A., and R.M. Jacobson. 2001. "Understanding Those Who Do Not Understand: A Brief Review of the Anti-vaccine Movement." *Vaccine* 2001 (19): 2440–5. http://morrisonlucas.com/GL/vaccines/Vaccine_19_2440_anti_vaccine_movement.pdf.

Polat, H.A., and A. Arslan. 2019. "The Rise of Popular Tourism in the Holy Land: Thomas Cook and John Mason Cook's Enterprise Skills That Shaped the Travel Industry." *Tourism Management* 75: 231–44. https://doi.org/10.1016/j.tourman.2019.05.003.

Poloz, S. 2022a. "Former Bank of Canada Governor Says Uncertain Times Are Here to Stay." Hosted by D. Common. *The Sunday Magazine*, 20 February 2022. https://www.cbc.ca/radio/sunday/the-sunday-magazine-for-february-20-2022-1.6357337.

– 2022b. *The Next Age of Uncertainty: How the World Can Adapt to a Riskier Future*. London: Allen Lane.

Pompeo, M.R. 2021. "Ensuring a Transparent, Thorough Investigation of COVID-19's Origin." US Department of State, 15 January 2021. https://2017-2021.state.gov/ensuring-a-transparent-thorough-investigation-of-covid-19s-origin/index.html.

Porter, C. 2020. "From Behind the Scenes to the Forefront: Canada's Public Health Officers." *New York Times*, 10 April 2020. https://www.nytimes.com/2020/04/10/world/canada/coronavirus-bonnie-henry.html.

Pottie, E. 2021. "Why Life under COVID-19 Is Playing into the Hands of Scammers." CBC News, 22 February 2021. https://www.cbc.ca/news/canada/nova-scotia/covid-scams-cost-millions-ns-1.5920568.

Powers, L. 2020. "Personal Support Worker Becomes First Ontarian to Get Dose of COVID-19 Vaccine." CBC News, 14 December 2020. https://www.cbc.ca/news/canada/toronto/covid-19-coronavirus-ontario-december-14-vaccines-arrive-1.5840092.

PricewaterhouseCoopers Canada. 2021. *The Impact of the Pandemic on the Downtown Areas of Canada's Six Major Cities*. 22 March 2021. https://www.pwc.com/ca/en/deals/publications/950628-the-impact-of-the-pandemic-on-the-downtown-areas-of-canada-s-six-major-cities-en.pdf.

Prince Edward Island Health and Wellness. 2020. "Masks to Become Mandatory in Prince Edward Island." Government of Prince Edward Island, 17 November 2020. https://www.princeedwardisland.ca/en/news/masks-become-mandatory-prince-edward-island.

Province of British Columbia. 2020a. *Electronic Attendance at Corporate Meetings (COVID-19) Order*. Ministerial Order no. M116. 21 April 2020. https://www.bclaws.gov.bc.ca/civix/document/id/mo/mo/mo116_2020.

– 2020b. *Electronic Attendance at Credit Union Meetings (COVID-19) Order*. Ministerial Order no. M138. 30 April 2020. https://www.bclaws.gov.bc.ca/civix/document/id/mo/mo/mo138_2020.

Provincial Laboratory Services. 2020. "Testing Guidance for COVID-19: Asymptomatic Testing & New Return to Work Criteria for Health Care Workers." Health Prince Edward Island, 27 July 2020. https://src.health-pei.ca/sites/src.healthpei.ca/files/Laboratory%20Services/Testing_Guidance_for_COVID_19_Asymptomatic_Testing_and_New_Return_to_Work_Criteria_2020-07-27.pdf.

PS (Public Safety Canada). 2020a. "Government Creates Task Force on Flood Insurance and Relocation." Government of Canada, 23 November 2020. https://www.canada.ca/en/public-safety-canada/news/2020/11/government-of-canada-creates-task-force-on-flood-insurance-and-relocation.html.

– 2020b. "Guidance on Essential Services and Functions in Canada during the COVID-19 Pandemic." Government of Canada, 30 April 2020. https://www.publicsafety.gc.ca/cnt/ntnl-scrt/crtcl-nfrstrctr/esf-sfe-en.aspx.

– 2021. "Guidance on Essential Services and Functions in Canada during the COVID-19 Pandemic." Government of Canada, 14 October 2021. https://www.publicsafety.gc.ca/cnt/ntnl-scrt/crtcl-nfrstrctr/esf-sfe-en.aspx.

Public Health Physicians of Canada. 2022. "Public Health Lessons Learned from the COVID-19 Pandemic." https://www.phpc-mspc.ca/resources/Documents/PHPC_Public%20Health%20Lessons%20Learned%20from%20the%20COVID-19%20Pandemic.pdf.

Public Services and Procurement Canada. 2021. "Canada Announces
    Accelerated Delivery of COVID-19 Paediatric Vaccine Pending
    Regulatory Authorization." Government of Canada, 21 October 2021.
    https://www.canada.ca/en/public-services-procurement/news/2021/10/
    canada-announces-accelerated-delivery-of-covid-19-paediatric-vaccine-
    pending-regulatory-authorization.html.
Pyper, W. 2004. "Employment Trends in Nursing." *Perspectives on Labour
    and Income* 16 (4): 39–51. https://www150.statcan.gc.ca/n1/en/pub/75-
    001-x/11104/7611-eng.pdf?st=EOvT4_i.
Quigley, K. 2008. *Responding to Crises in the Modern Infrastructure:
    Policy Lessons from Y2K*. Basingstoke, UK: Palgrave MacMillan.
– 2018. "Grief and the Value of a Statistical Life." *Globe and Mail*, 5 May
    2018. https://www.theglobeandmail.com/opinion/article-grief-and-the-
    value-of-a-statistical-life.
Quigley, K., B. Bisset, and B. Mills. 2017. *Too Critical to Fail: How Canada
    Manages Threats to Critical Infrastructure*. Montreal, QC: McGill-
    Queen's University Press.
Quigley, K., C. Macdonald, and J. Quigley. 2016. "Pre-existing Condition:
    Taking Media Coverage into Account When Preparing for H1N1."
    Canadian Public Administration 59 (2): 267–88. https://doi.org/10.1111/
    capa.12169.
Quon, A. 2021. "Doctor Warns That 200 Surgeries a Day Are Being
    Cancelled in Saskatchewan." CBC News, 8 October 2021. https://www.
    cbc.ca/news/canada/saskatchewan/sha-surgeries-cancelled-saskatchewan-
    1.6200378.
– 2022. "Sask. to End COVID-19 Proof of Vaccination Policy on Feb. 14,
    Mandatory Masking to Remain until End of Month." CBC News, 9
    February 2022. https://www.cbc.ca/news/canada/saskatchewan/
    covid-19-update-feb-8-2022-1.6343563.
Rabin, C.C. 2022. "The C.D.C. Will Undergo a Comprehensive
    Re-evaluation, the Agency's Director Said." *New York Times*, 4 April
    2022. https://www.nytimes.com/2022/04/04/health/cdc-re-evaluation-
    covid.html.
Rabson, M. 2021. "Moderna to Sign Agreement to Build mRNA Production
    Plant in Canada." CBC News, 10 August 2021. https://www.cbc.ca/news/
    politics/moderna-plant-champagne-1.6135759.
– 2022. "Pandemic Fatigue Leaves Canada in 'Tricky Moment,' Freeland
    Says." *Globe and Mail*, 4 February 2022. https://www.theglobeandmail.
    com/canada/article-pandemic-fatigue-leaves-canada-in-tricky-moment-
    freeland-says-2.

Rabson, M., and M. Woolf. 2022. "Emergencies Act Motion Passes after Heated House of Commons Debate." *Canada's National Observer*, 22 February 2022. https://www.nationalobserver.com/2022/02/22/news/emergencies-act-motion-passes-house-commons-debate.

Rappeport, A., and N. Chokshi. 2020. "Crippled Airline Industry to Get $25 Billion Bailout, Part of It as Loan." *New York Times*, 14 April 2020. https://www.nytimes.com/2020/04/14/business/coronavirus-airlines-bailout-treasury-department.html.

Rasmussen, A., B. Carroll, and D. Lowery. 2014. "Representatives of the Public? Public Opinion and Interest Group Activity." *European Journal of Political Research* 53 (2): 250–68. https://doi.org/10.1111/1475-6765.12036.

Rastello, S. 2021. "Air Canada Pleads with Trudeau for Plan to Ease Travel Rules." BNN Bloomberg, 7 May 2021. https://www.bnn-bloomberg.ca/air-canada-pleads-with-trudeau-for-plan-to-relax-travel-rules-1.1600601.

Rauh, J., and K. Warsh. 2022. "The Inflation Message and a Financial Refuge." *Wall Street Journal*, 21 February 2022. https://www.wsj.com/articles/inflation-financial-refuge-price-surge-savings-wages-pandemic-fed-powell-biden-fomc-investment-i-bonds-11645464310.

Raymond, T. 2022. "Ontario Police Watchdog Closes Investigation into Mounted Officers at 'Freedom Convoy.'" CTV News, 4 April 2022. https://ottawa.ctvnews.ca/ontario-police-watchdog-closes-investigation-into-mounted-officers-at-freedom-convoy-1.5847725.

Refinitiv StreetEvents. 2021. *Edited Transcript PFE.EN – Q4 2020 Pfizer Inc Earnings Call*. https://s21.q4cdn.com/317678438/files/doc_financials 2020/q4/PFE-USQ_Transcript_2021-02-02.pdf.

Registry of Lobbyists. 2022a. "Lobbying Statistics." Office of the Commissioner of Lobbying of Canada, modified 24 February 2022. https://lobbycanada.gc.ca/app/secure/ocl/lrs/do/slctRprt.

– 2022b. "Recent Monthly Communication Reports." Office of the Commissioner of Lobbying of Canada, modified 24 February 2022. https://lobbycanada.gc.ca/app/secure/ocl/lrs/do/rcntCmLgs.

– 2022c. "Recent Registrations." Office of the Commissioner of Lobbying of Canada, modified 24 February 2022. https://lobbycanada.gc.ca/app/secure/ocl/lrs/do/rcntRgstrns.

Remuzzi, A., and G. Remuzzi. 2020. "COVID-19 and Italy: What Next?" *Lancet* 395 (10231): 1225–8. https://doi.org/10.1016/s0140-6736(20)30627-9.

Rendell, M. 2022. "Bank of Canada Poised to Lose Money for the First Time on Rising Interest Expenses." *Globe and Mail*, 16 November 2022.

https://www.theglobeandmail.com/business/article-bank-of-canada-losing-money-interest-rates.

Renn, O. 1992. "Concepts of Risk: A Classification." In *Social Theories of Risk*, edited by S. Krimsky and D. Golding, 53–79. Westport, CT: Praeger. http://dx.doi.org/10.18419/opus-7248.

– 2008a. "Concepts of Risk: An Interdisciplinary Review. Part 1: Disciplinary Risk Concepts." *GAJA – Ecological Perspectives for Science and Society* 17 (1): 50–66. http://dx.doi.org/10.14512/gaia.17.1.13.

– 2008b. "White Paper on Risk Governance: Toward an Integrative Framework." In *Global Risk Governance: Concept and Practice Using the IRGC Framework*, edited by O. Renn and K. Walker, 3–73. Dordrecht, Netherlands: Springer.

Renn, O., W.J. Burns, J.X. Kasperson, R.E. Kasperson, and P. Slovic. 1992. "The Social Amplification of Risk: Theoretical Foundations and Empirical Applications." *Journal of Social Issues* 48 (4): 137–60. https://doi.org/10.1111/j.1540-4560.1992.tb01949.x.

Resnik, D.B. 2004. "The Precautionary Principle and Medical Decision Making." *Journal of Medicine and Philosophy* 29 (3): 281–99. https://doi.org/10.1080/03605310490500509.

Reynolds, C. 2020. "Manufacturers Scramble to Find Raw Materials amid 'Desperate' Shortage for PPE." *Globe and Mail*, 24 May 2020. https://www.theglobeandmail.com/business/article-manufacturers-scramble-to-find-raw-materials-amid-desperate-shortage-2.

– 2022. "Emails Raise Questions about Regulator's Independence amid Covid-Related Flight Refunds." CBC News, 2 February 2022. https://www.cbc.ca/news/business/cta-airline-regulator-1.6336687.

Richter, E.D., and R. Laster. 2004. "The Precautionary Principle, Epidemiology and the Ethics of Delay." *International Journal of Occupational Medicine and Environmental Health* 17 (1): 9–16.

Rieger, S. 2020a. "Alberta Health-Care Workers Say New Masks Don't Seal, Cause Rashes and Headaches." CBC News, 18 April 2020. https://www.cbc.ca/news/canada/calgary/mask-issues-alberta-1.5537345.

– 2020b. "3rd Death Linked to Canada's Largest COVID-19 Outbreak at Alberta Slaughterhouse." CBC News, 12 May 2020. https://www.cbc.ca/news/canada/calgary/3rd-covid-19-death-cargill-meat-processing-plant-high-river-1.5565265.

Riker, W.H. 1995. "The Political Psychology of Rational Choice Theory." *Political Psychology* 16 (1): 23–44. https://doi.org/10.2307/3791448.

Ritchie, H., E. Mathieu, L. Rodés-Guirao, C. Appel, C. Giattino, E. Ortiz-Ospina, J. Hasell, B. Macdonald, D. Beltekian, and M. Roser. 2022a. "Coronavirus Pandemic (COVID-19)." https://ourworldindata.org/coronavirus#explore-the-global-situation.

– 2022b. "COVID-19 Data Explorer Vaccinations – Share of People Vaccinated against COVID-19." Our World in Data. https://ourworld indata.org/covid-vaccinations.

Roberts, Z. 2020. "Workplace Safety during COVID-19: The Right to Refuse Unsafe Work." *Canadian Unemployment Law Today* (July): 3, 7.

Robertson, G. 2021a. "Misuse of Pandemic Early Warning System, Inaccurate Risk Assessments Hurt Canada's Response to COVID-19, Auditor-General Says." *Globe and Mail*, 26 March 2021. https://www.theglobeandmail.com/politics/article-misuse-of-pandemic-early-warning-system-inaccurate-risk-assessments.

– 2021b. "Review of Pandemic Early-Warning System Calls on Ottawa to Overhaul Its Approach to Outbreaks." *Globe and Mail*, 12 July 2021. https://www.theglobeandmail.com/canada/article-review-of-pandemic-early-warning-system-calls-on-ottawa-to-overhaul.

– 2021c. "'We Are Not Prepared': The Flaws inside Public Health That Hurt Canada's Readiness for COVID-19." *Globe and Mail*, 3 February 2021. https://www.theglobeandmail.com/canada/article-we-are-not-prepared-the-flaws-inside-public-health-that-hurt-canadas.

Robertson, G., and M. Walsh. 2021. "Tam Criticized for Supporting 'Indefensible' Assessment of COVID-19 Risk." *Globe and Mail*, 29 March 2021. https://www.theglobeandmail.com/canada/article-tam-criticized-for-supporting-indefensible-assessment-of-covid-19-risk.

Robinson, L. 2020. "COVID-19 and Uncertainties in the Value per Statistical Life." *The Regulatory Review*, 5 August 2020. https://www.theregreview.org/2020/08/05/robinson-covid-19-uncertainties-value-statistical-life.

Robinson, R.N.S., A. Martins, D. Solnet, and T. Baum. 2019. "Sustaining Precarity: Critically Examining Tourism and Employment." *Journal of Sustainable Tourism* 27 (7): 1008–25. https://doi.org/10.1080/09669582.2018.1538230.

Rocca, R. 2021. "Vaccine Mandates Permissible as Long as Those with Exemptions Are Accommodated: Ontario Commission." Global News, 22 September 2021. https://globalnews.ca/news/8214207/vaccine-mandates-generally-permissible-ontario-human-rights-commission.

Rocklöv, J., H., Sjödin, and A. Wilder-Smith. 2020. "COVID-19 Outbreak on the Diamond Princess Cruise Ship: Estimating the Epidemic Potential and Effectiveness of Public Health Countermeasures." *Journal of Travel Medicine* 27 (3): 1–7. https://doi.org/10.1093/jtm/taaa030.

Roman, K. 2023. "New Voluntary Standards Released for Long-Term Care Homes Devastated by the Pandemic." CBC News, 1 February 2023. https://www.cbc.ca/news/politics/long-term-care-canada-standards-pandemic-1.6730780.

Romo, V. 2020. "Pence on Coronavirus: 'Risk Remains Low,' Says Treatments on the Horizon." *NPR*, 2 March 2020. https://www.npr.org/2020/03/02/811372994/pence-on-coronavirus-risk-remains-low-says-treatments-on-the-horizon.

Rosenblatt, C. 2020. "Is It Safe to Visit Aging Parents? What You Can Do to Minimize Risks." *Forbes*, 20 May 2020. https://www.forbes.com/sites/carolynrosenblatt/2020/05/20/is-it-safe-to-visit-aging-parents-what-you-can-do-to-minimize-risk.

Ross, S., and J. Lofaro. 2021. "Vaccines Won't Be Mandatory for Existing Quebec Health-Care Workers, Only New Hires." CTV News, 4 November 2021. https://montreal.ctvnews.ca/vaccines-won-t-be-mandatory-for-existing-quebec-health-care-workers-only-new-hires-1.5650001.

Rosselló, J., S. Becken, and M. Santana-Gallego. 2020. "The Effects of Natural Disasters on International Tourism: A Global Analysis." *Tourism Management* 79 (August). https://doi.org/10.1016/j.tourman.2020.104080.

Rothstein, H. 2003. "Neglected Risk Regulation: The Institutional Attenuation Phenomenon." *Health, Risk & Society* 5 (1): 85–103. https://doi.org/10.1080/1369857031000066023.

Rouleau, P.S. 2023. *Report of the Public Inquiry into the 2022 Public Order Emergency. Volume 1: Overview*. https://publicorderemergencycommission.ca/files/documents/Final-Report/Vol-1-Report-of-the-Public-Inquiry-into-the-2022-Public-Order-Emergency.pdf.

Roulet, T. 2020. "To Combat Conspiracy Theories Teach Critical Thinking – And Community Values." *The Conversation*, 9 November 2020. https://theconversation.com/to-combat-conspiracy-theories-teach-critical-thinking-and-community-values-147314.

Rousseau, D, S. Sitkin, R. Burt, and C. Camerer. 1998. "Not So Different after All: A Cross-Discipline View of Risk." *Academy of Management Review* 23 (3): 393–404.

Roxby, P., and N. Triggle. 2021. "COVID: Children Aged 12–17 Unlikely to Be Offered Vaccine in UK." BBC, 16 July 2021. https://www.bbc.com/news/health-57496074.

Royal Society. 1992. *Risk: Analysis, Perception and Management*. 6th ed. London: Royal Society.

Ruan, L., J. Knockel, and M. Crete-Nishihata. 2020. "Censored Contagion: How Information on the Coronavirus Is Managed on Chinese Social Media." Munk School and University of Toronto, 3 March 2020. https://citizenlab.ca/2020/03/censored-contagion-how-information-on-the-coronavirus-is-managed-on-chinese-social-media.

Rusnell, C. 2021. "Alberta's Rising COVID-19 Cases Due to Faulty Modelling and Government Inaction, Experts Say." CBC News, 9 September 2021. https://www.cbc.ca/news/canada/edmonton/alberta-covid-19-modelling-1.6168948.

Russell, A. 2020. "Canadians Have Racked Up $13M in Coronavirus Fines, Racial Profiling Evident: Report." Global News, 24 June 2020. https://globalnews.ca/news/7102217/coronavirus-canada-fines-ccla.

– 2021. "Coronavirus: Ontario Nursing Home Where 81 Died Was Later Cited for 13 Violations." Global News, 22 February 2021. https://global news.ca/news/7651166/tendercare-covid-19-deaths.

Russell, A., C. Jarvis., E. Campanella, and J. Patel. 2021a. "Strategic Missteps, Logistical Hurdles Plague Ontario's Early Vaccine Rollout." Global News, 23 January 2021. https://globalnews.ca/news/7588530/ontario-coronavirus-vaccine-rollout-inside-look.

– 2021b. "'Too Slow, Too Late': Ford Gov. Received Months of Warnings about Long-Term Care before Second Wave." Global News, 3 May 2021. https://globalnews.ca/news/7826134/ford-government-ignored-covid-warnings.

Russell, J. 2020. "After Decades of Systemic Issues, Time to Finally Overhaul Alberta Long-Term Care, Experts Say." CBC News, 12 May 2020. https://www.cbc.ca/news/canada/edmonton/alberta-long-term-care-pandemic-covid-19-1.5562331.

Sagan, S. 1993. *The Limits of Safety: Organizations, Accidents, and Nuclear Weapons*. Princeton, NJ: Princeton University Press.

Saillant, R. 2017. "After the 'Boom': Re-imagining Health Care after a Generation – Policy Matters Panel." Filmed 17 October 2017 at the MacEachen Institute of Public Policy and Governance, Halifax, NS. Video, 1:27:49. https://www.youtube.com/watch?v=RQIxE3a4bVA&ab_channel=MacEachenInstituteforPublicPolicyandGovernance.

Saminather, N., and V. Waldersee. 2020. "FOCUS-Homebound Workers Inject Life into Suburban Malls after Downtowns Empty Out." Reuters, 8 November 2020. https://www.reuters.com/article/health-coronavirus-can-ada-property/focus-homebound-workers-inject-life-into-suburban-malls-after-downtowns-empty-out-idINL4N2H546U.

Sandin, P. 1999. "Dimensions of the Precautionary Principle." *Human and Ecological Risk Assessment: An International Journal* 5 (5): 889–907. https://doi.org/10.1080/10807039991289185.

– 2004. "Better Safe than Sorry: Applying Philosophical Methods to the Debate on Risk and the Precautionary Principle." PhD diss., Royal Institute of Technology, Stockholm.

Saskatchewan Health Authority. 2021. "Saskatchewan Health Authority to Require Proof of Full COVID-19 Vaccination for Health Care Workers." Government of Saskatchewan, 1 October 2021. https://www.saskhealth authority.ca/news-events/news/saskatchewan-health-authority-require-proof-full-covid-19-vaccination-health-care-workers.

Saskatchewan Ministry of Health. 2009. *Design Guidelines and Standards for Long-Term Care Facilities in Saskatchewan.* http://wabenbow.com/wp-content/uploads/2011/06/Sask-Guidlelines-and-Standards-for-Long-Term-Care-2009.pdf.

Savage, M. 2020. "Why the Pandemic Is Causing Spikes in Break-Ups and Divorces." BBC, 6 December 2020. https://www.bbc.com/worklife/article/20201203-why-the-pandemic-is-causing-spikes-in-break-ups-and-divorces.

Scardina, G., L. Ceccarelli, V. Casigliani, S. Mazzilli, M. Napoletano, M. Padovan, A. Petillo et al. 2021. "Evaluation of Flu Vaccination Coverage among Healthcare Workers during a 3 Years' Study Period and Attitude Towards Influenza and Potential COVID-19 Vaccination in the Context of the Pandemic." *Vaccines* 9 (7): 769. https://doi.org/10.3390/vaccines 9070769.

Schembri, L. 2021. "COVID-19, Savings and Household Spending." Bank of Canada, 11 March 2021. https://www.bankofcanada.ca/2021/03/covid-19-savings-and-household-spending.

Schettler, T., and C. Raffensperger. 2004. "Why Is a Precautionary Approach Needed?" In *The Precautionary Principle: Protecting Public Health, the Environment and the Future of Our Children,* edited by M. Martuzzi and J.A. Tickner, 63–84. Copenhagen: World Health Organization Europe.

Schmunk, R. 2020. "B.C. NDP Will Form Decisive Majority Government, CBC News Projects." CBC News, 25 October 2020. https://www.cbc.ca/news/canada/british-columbia/bc-election-results-2020-1.5776058.

Schofield, P. 1996. "Bentham on the Identification of Interests." *Utilitas* 8 (2): 223–34. https://doi.org/10.1017/S095382080000488X.

Schultheis, E., and K. Grieshaber. 2021. "'My Body, My Choice': Thousands Protest Ahead of Austria's COVID-19 Lockdown." Global News, 20 November 2021. https://globalnews.ca/news/8389579/austria-covid-lockdown-protest.

Schwartz, H.M. 1994. "Public Choice Theory and Public Choices: Bureaucrats and State Reorganization in Australia, Denmark, New Zealand, and Sweden in the 1980s." *Administration & Society* 26 (1): 48–77. https://doi.org/10.1177/009539979402600104.

Schwartz, N.S. 2020. "Why Canadians and Americans Are Buying Guns during the Coronavirus Pandemic." The Conversation, 8 April 2020.

https://theconversation.com/why-canadians-and-americans-are-buying-guns-during-the-coronavirus-pandemic-135409.

Semeniuk, I. 2021. "What We've Learned about Omicron So Far, Including How Severe Illness from the Variant Appears to Be." *Globe and Mail*, 20 December 2021. https://www.theglobeandmail.com/canada/article-what-weve-learned-about-omicron-so-far.

Seow, H., K. McMillan, M. Civak, D. Bainbridge, A. van der Wal, C. Haanstra, J. Goldhar, and S. Winemaker. 2021. "#Caremongering: A Community-Led Social Movement to Address Health and Social Needs during COVID-19." *PLOS ONE* 16 (1): e0245483. https://doi.org/10.1371/journal.pone.0245483.

Sethi, A. 2021. "'Death Is the Only Truth.' Watching India's Funeral Pyres Burn." *New York Times*, 30 April 2021. https://www.nytimes.com/2021/04/30/opinion/india-covid-crematorium.html.

Shaban, H. 2021. "The Pandemic's Home-Workout Revolution May Be Here to Stay." *Washington Post*, 7 January 2021. https://www.washingtonpost.com/road-to-recovery/2021/01/07/home-fitness-boom.

Shah, Z. 2021. "Suicide Deaths Have Declined during the Pandemic, but Experts Warn the Toll Might Be Yet to Come." *National Post*, 29 March 2021. https://nationalpost.com/news/postpandemic/suicide-deaths-have-declined-during-the-pandemic-but-experts-warn-the-toll-might-be-yet-to-come.

Shahid, S. 2021. "Low-Income Canadian Households Will Suffer the Most from Soaring Inflation." Conference Board of Canada, 16 September 2021. https://www.conferenceboard.ca/insights/featured/canadian-economics/low-income-canadian-households-will-suffer-the-most-from-soaring-inflation.

Shaman, J. 2022. "What Will Our COVID Future Be Like? Here Are Two Signs to Look Out For." *New York Times*, 4 March 2022. https://www.nytimes.com/2022/03/04/opinion/endemic-covid-future.html.

Sharma, G.D., A. Thomas, and J. Paul. 2021. "Reviving Tourism Industry Post-COVID-19: A Resilience-Based Framework." *Tourism Management Perspectives* 37 (January). https://doi.org/10.1016/j.tmp.2020.100786.

Sharon, K. 2009. "Anatomy of a Pandemic: H1N1 2009; Swine Flu Less Lethal than Expected." *Windsor Star*, 26 December 2009.

Sharot, T. 2011. "The Optimism Bias." *Current Biology* 21 (23): 41–5. https://doi.org/10.1016/j.cub.2011.10.030.

Sharpley, R., and B. Craven. 2001. "The 2001 Foot and Mouth Crisis – Rural Economy and Tourism Policy Implications: A Comment." *Current Issues in Tourism* 4 (6): 527–37. http://dx.doi.org/10.1080/13683500108667901.

Shaw, D. 2021. "Coronavirus: Tinder Boss Says 'Dramatic' Changes to Dating." BBC, 21 May 2021. https://www.bbc.com/news/business-52743454.

Shear, M.D., S. Fink, and N. Weiland. 2020. "Inside Trump Administration, Debate Raged over What to Tell Public." *New York Times*, 9 March 2020. https://www.nytimes.com/2020/03/07/us/politics/trump-coronavirus.html.

Sheps, S. B., and K. Cardiff. 2011. "Patient Safety: A Wake-Up Call." *Clinical Governance: An International Journal* 16 (2): 148–58. https://doi.org/10.1108/14777271111124509.

Shield, D. 2022. "Mayor of Ottawa Demands Apology after Sask. Conservative MPs, Senator Take Picture at Convoy Protest." CBC News, 3 February 2022. https://www.cbc.ca/news/canada/saskatoon/mayor-of-ottawa-demands-apology-after-sask-conservative-mps-senator-take-picture-at-convoy-protest-1.6337951.

Shier, P. 2020. "The Lessons SARS Offers on How to Rebound from a Crisis." *Strategy*, 31 March 2020. https://strategyonline.ca/2020/03/31/the-lessons-sars-offers-on-how-to-rebound-from-a-crisis.

Shih, W.C. 2020. "Global Supply Chains in a Post-Pandemic World." *Harvard Business Review*, September–October 2020. https://hbr.org/2020/09/global-supply-chains-in-a-post-pandemic-world.

Shillington, R. 2016. "An Analysis of the Economic Circumstances of Canadian Seniors." Broadbent Institute. https://d3n8a8pro7vhmx.cloudfront.net/broadbent/pages/4904/attachments/original/1455216659/An_Analysis_of_the_Economic_Circumstances_of_Canadian_Seniors.pdf.

Shingler, B. 2023. "What the Federal Workers' Deal Means for the Future of Remote Work." CBC News, 2 May 2023. https://www.cbc.ca/news/canada/psac-agreement-government-union-remote-work-1.6828427.

Shiraef, M.A., P. Friesen, L. Feddern, M.A. Weiss, and COBAP Team. 2022. "Did Border Closures Slow SARS-COV-2?" *Scientific Reports* 12 (1709). https://doi.org/10.1038/s41598-022-05482-7.

Shoukat, A., C.R. Wells, J.M. Langley, B.H. Singer, A.P. Galvani, and S.M. Moghadas. 2020. "Projecting Demand for Critical Care Beds during COVID-19 Outbreaks in Canada." *Canadian Medical Association Journal* 192 (19): e489–96. https://doi.org/10.1503/cmaj.200457.

Shukman, D. 2020. "Coronavirus: WHO Advises to Wear Masks in Public Areas." BBC, 6 June 2020. https://www.bbc.com/news/health-52945210.

Siatchinov, A., A. De Champlain, and R. Verma. 2020. "Price Trends and Outlook in Key Canadian Housing Markets." StatCan COVID-19: Data to Insights for a Better Canada, catalogue no. 45280001. https://www150.statcan.gc.ca/n1/en/pub/45-28-0001/2020001/article/00053-eng.pdf?st=r85CARHh.

Siegrist, M., and A. Bearth. 2021. "Worldviews, Trust, and Risk Perceptions Shape Public Acceptance of COVID-19 Public Health Measures." *Proceedings of the National Academy of Sciences of the USA* 118 (24): e2100411118. https://doi.org/10.1073%2Fpnas.2100411118.

Silver, J.E. 2022. "Truckers' Protest in Ottawa Splits Tory Caucus." iPolitics, 4 February 2022. https://ipolitics.ca/2022/02/04/truckers-protest-in-ottawa-splits-tory-caucus.

Simard, F. 2004. "Self-Interest in Public Administration: Niskanen and the Budget-Maximizing Argument." *Canadian Public Administration* 47 (3): 406–11. https://doi.org/10.1111/j.1754-7121.2004.tb01872.x.

Simpson, C. 2022. "No Easy Answers: The Complicated and Involved Practice of Ethics in Health Care during Crises." Panel, Policy Matters: Health Care Reconsidered Speaker Series, MacEachen Institute for Public Policy and Governance. https://www.dal.ca/dept/maceachen-institute/events/health-care-reconsidered/Health-Care-Ethics-Panel.html.

Simpson, J. 2012. *Chronic Condition: Why Canada's Health-Care System Needs to Be Dragged into the 21st Century*. Toronto: Allen Lane.

Singh, I. 2020. "More Canadians Are Refusing Work Due to COVID-19 – But It's Tough to Get Authorities to Agree." CBC News, 22 June 2020. https://www.cbc.ca/news/canada/work-refusal-safety-covid-1.5617787.

Sinha, S., C. Feil, and N. Iciaszczyk. 2021. "The Rollout of COVID-19 Vaccines in Canadian Long-Term Care Homes, 30th March Update." International Long-Term Care Policy Network, 1 April 2021. https://ltccovid.org/2021/04/01/the-rollout-of-covid-19-vaccines-in-canadian-long-term-care-homes-30th-march-update.

Sivarajan, S. 2022. "How Worrying about Inflation Can Lead to More Inflation." *Globe and Mail*, 11 February 2022. https://www.theglobeandmail.com/investing/personal-finance/household-finances/article-how-worrying-about-inflation-can-lead-to-more-inflation.

Sjöberg, L. 1998. "Risk Perception: Experts and the Public." *European Psychologist* 3 (1): 1–12.

– 2000. "Factors in Risk Perception." *Risk Analysis* 20 (1): 1–12.

Skochelak, S.E., and R.E. Hawkins. 2017. *Health Systems Science*. St Louis, MO: Elsevier.

Slovic, P., B. Fischhoff, and S. Lichtenstein. 1982. "Why Study Risk Perception?" *Risk Analysis* 2 (2): 83–93. https://doi.org/10.1111/j.1539-6924.1982.tb01369.x.

Smith, C. 2020. "N.B. Students as Young as 13 Fill Lobster Processing Jobs Left by Barred Temporary Foreign Workers." Global News, 18 May 2020. https://globalnews.ca/news/6956295/coronavirus-n-b-s-student-lobster-jobs.

Smith, M. 2022. "No Easy Answers: The Complicated and Involved Practice of Ethics in Health Care during Crises." Panel, Policy Matters: Health Care Reconsidered Speaker Series, MacEachen Institute for Public Policy and Governance. https://www.dal.ca/dept/maceachen-institute/events/health-care-reconsidered/Health-Care-Ethics-Panel.html.

Smith, M.J., A. Komparic, and A. Thompson. 2020. "Deploying the Precautionary Principle to Protect Vulnerable Populations in Canadian Post-Market Drug Surveillance." *Canadian Journal of Bioethics* 3 (1): 110–8. https://doi.org/10.7202/1070232ar.

Snyder, J. 2021. "Number of COVID-19 Fines in Canada Jumped during Second Wave: Report." *National Post*, 14 May 2021. https://national post.com/news/number-of-covid-19-fines-in-canada-jumped-during-second-wave-report.

Somos, C. 2021. "Growing List of Canadian Politicians Caught Travelling Abroad despite Pandemic." CTV News, 4 January 2021. https://www.ctvnews.ca/politics/growing-list-of-canadian-politicians-caught-travelling-abroad-despite-pandemic-1.5251039.

Soumerai, S.B., D. Ross-Degnan, and J.S. Kahn. 1992. "Effects of Professional and Media Warnings about the Association between Aspirin Use in Children and Reye's Syndrome." *Millbank Quarterly* 70: 155–82.

Span, P. 2021. "For Older Adults, Home Care Has Become Harder to Find." *New York Times*, 24 July 2021. https://www.nytimes.com/2021/07/24/health/coronavirus-elderly-home-care.html.

Speer, S. 2022. "Sean Speer: In 2022, Can We Finally Be Honest about Our Health System's Failures?" The Hub, 5 January 2022. https://thehub.ca/2022-01-05/can-we-finally-be-honest-about-our-health-care-systems-failures.

Spence, R. 2020. "2/3 of Canadian Companies Offer No Paid Sick Leave." Corporate Knights, 8 October 2020. https://www.corporateknights.com/leadership/less-than-1-3-of-canadian-companies-offer-paid-sick-leave-finds-global-report.

Spencer, T. 2016. *Risk Perception: Theories and Approaches*. Psychology Research Progress Series. New York: Nova Publishers.

Sraders, A. 2021. "'The Bears Are Getting Louder': These Indicators Are Signaling a Stock Market Pullback." *Fortune*, 22 February 2021. https://fortune.com/2021/02/22/stock-market-outlook-pullback-s-andp-500-spx-decline.

Sridhar, D. 2022. "Why Can't Some Scientists Just Admit They Were Wrong about COVID?" *Guardian*, 24 March 2022. https://www.theguardian.com/commentisfree/2022/mar/24/scientists-wrong-covid-virus-experts.

Stall, N.M., K.A. Brown, A. Maltsev, A. Jones, A.P. Costa, V. Allen, and

A.D. Brown et al. 2021. "COVID-19 and Ontario's Long-Term Care Homes." Science Briefs of the Ontario COVID-19 Science Advisory Table 2 (7). https://doi.org/10.47326/ocsat.2021.02.07.1.0.

Stall, N.M., A. Jones, K.A. Brown, P.A. Rochon, and A.P. Costa. 2020. "For-Profit Long-Term Care Homes and the Risk of COVID-19 Outbreaks and Resident Deaths." Canadian Medical Association Journal 192 (33): e946–55. https://doi.org/10.1503/cmaj.201197.

Staples, D. 2020a. "The Road to Canada's COVID-19 Outbreak: Timeline of Federal Government Failure at Border to Slow the Virus." Edmonton Journal, 28 April 2020. https://edmontonjournal.com/news/national/the-road-to-canadas-covid-19-outbreak-timeline-of-federal-government-failure-at-border-to-slow-the-virus.

– 2020b. "The Road to Canada's COVID-19 Outbreak, PT. 2: Timeline of Federal Government Failure at Border to Slow the Virus." Edmonton Journal, 12 April 2020. https://edmontonjournal.com/news/politics/the-road-to-canadas-covid-19-outbreak-pt-2-timeline-of-federal-government-failure-at-border-to-slow-the-virus-2.

Starr, C. 1969. "Social Benefit versus Technological Risk." Science 165 (3899): 1232–8.

Statista. 2021. "Monthly Retail Sales of Grocery Stores in Canada from January 2015 to June 2021 (In Billion Canadian Dollars)." Modified 17 September 2021. https://www.statista.com/statistics/461774/monthly-retail-sales-of-grocery-stores-canada.

Statistics Canada. 2011. "Travel and Tourism." Chap. 31 in Canada Year Book 2011, catalogue no. 11-402-X: 448–59. https://www150.statcan.gc.ca/n1/en/pub/11-402-x/2011000/pdf/travel-voyages-eng.pdf?st=NwHdG9iz.

– 2017. "National Tourism Indicators, Fourth Quarter 2016." Daily, 30 March 2017. https://www150.statcan.gc.ca/n1/en/daily-quotidien/170330/dq170330b-eng.pdf?st=4DxAoC2j.

– 2018a. "The Evolution of Canadian Tourism, 1946 to 2015." Modified 17 May 2018. https://www150.statcan.gc.ca/n1/pub/11-630-x/11-630-x2017001-eng.htm.

– 2018b. General Social Survey, 2016. https://www23.statcan.gc.ca/imdb/p2SV.pl?Function=getSurvey&SDDS=5221.

– 2019a. "Annual Demographics Estimates: Canada, Provinces and Territories, 2019." Modified 30 September 2019. https://www150.statcan.gc.ca/n1/pub/91-215-x/91-215-x2019001-eng.htm.

– 2019b. "Population Projections for Canada (2018 to 2068), Provinces and Territories (2018 to 2043)." Catalogue no. 91-520-X. https://www150.statcan.gc.ca/n1/en/pub/91-520-x/91-520-x2019001-eng.pdf?st=aDuPet4e.

– 2020a. "Canada's Population Estimates: Age and Sex, July 1, 2020." Daily, 29 September 2020. https://www150.statcan.gc.ca/n1/en/daily-quotidien/200929/dq200929b-eng.pdf?st=hHSoukJP.

– 2020b. "Canadian Consumers Prepare for COVID-19." Modified 11 May 2020.https://www150.statcan.gc.ca/n1/pub/62f0014m/62f0014m2020004-eng.htm.

– 2020c. "Canadian Perspectives Survey Series 1: Impacts of COVID-19." Daily, 8 April 2020. https://www150.statcan.gc.ca/n1/daily-quotidien/200408/dq200408c-eng.htm.

– 2020d. "Canadians Made Fewer Trips within Canada and around the World in 2019." Daily, 9 December 2020. https://www150.statcan.gc.ca/n1/en/daily-quotidien/201209/dq201209e-eng.pdf?st=e5D9WeVd.

– 2020e. "Caregivers in Canada, 2018." Daily, 8 January 2020. https://www150.statcan.gc.ca/n1/en/daily-quotidien/200108/dq200108a-eng.pdf?st=gVh-xgb5.

– 2020f. "Care Receivers in Canada, 2018." Daily, 22 January 2020. https://www150.statcan.gc.ca/n1/en/daily-quotidien/200122/dq200122e-eng.pdf?st=j-fqvTSo.

– 2020g. COVID-19 in Canada: A Six-Month Update on Social and Economic Impacts. https://www150.statcan.gc.ca/n1/en/pub/11-631-x/11-631-x2020003-eng.pdf?st=D8in1eb6.

– 2020h. "The Impact of COVID-19 on Key Housing Markets." https://www150.statcan.gc.ca/n1/pub/11-627-m/11-627-m2020050-eng.pdf.

– 2020i. Impacts on Immigrants and People Designated as Visible Minorities. https://www150.statcan.gc.ca/n1/pub/11-631-x/2020004/s6-eng.htm.

– 2020j. "Labour Force Survey, August 2020." Daily, 4 September 2020. https://www150.statcan.gc.ca/n1/en/daily-quotidien/200904/dq200904a-eng.pdf?st=dznXEWAL.

– 2020k. "National Tourism Indicators, Fourth Quarter 2019 and First Quarter 2020." Daily, 30 June 2020. https://www150.statcan.gc.ca/n1/en/daily-quotidien/200630/dq200630b-eng.pdf?st=gRS9Toae.

– 2020l. "Provisional Data on Causes of Death, January to April 2019 and January to April 2020." https://www150.statcan.gc.ca/n1/daily-quotidien/200703/dq200703b-eng.htm.

– 2020m. "Table 36-10-0634-01: Jobs, Hours Worked and Employment Income in Tourism Industries, by Class of Worker and Work Activity." https://doi.org/10.25318/3610063401-eng.

– 2020n. "Table 36-10-0638-01: Tourism Sector's Share of Jobs and Employment Income." https://doi.org/10.25318/3610063801-eng.

– 2020o. "Three-Fifths of Total Federal, Provincial, Territorial and Local Spending Went to Social Protection, Health Care and Education in 2019." Daily, 27 November 2020. https://www150.statcan.gc.ca/n1/daily-quotidien/201127/dq201127a-eng.htm.

– 2020p. "Tourism Human Resource Module, 2019." Daily, 30 October 2020. https://www150.statcan.gc.ca/n1/en/daily-quotidien/201030/dq201030c-eng.pdf?st=8_9PA89S.

– 2020q. "Travel between Canada and Other Countries, December 2019." Daily, 21 February 2020. https://www150.statcan.gc.ca/n1/en/daily-quotidien/200221/dq200221b-eng.pdf?st=J4DHon6j.

– 2020r. "Travel between Canada and Other Countries, March 2020." Daily, 22 May 2020. https://www150.statcan.gc.ca/n1/en/daily-quotidien/200522/dq200522c-eng.pdf?st=kZeH6cYS.

– 2021a. "Alcohol and Cannabis Use during the Pandemic: Canadian Perspectives Survey Series 6." Daily, 4 March 2021. https://www150.statcan.gc.ca/n1/daily-quotidien/210304/dq210304a-eng.htm.

– 2021b. "COVID-19 in Canada: A One-Year Update on Social and Economic Impacts." 11 March 2021. https://www150.statcan.gc.ca/n1/pub/11-631-x/11-631-x2021001-eng.htm.

– 2021c. "COVID-19 Vaccine Willingness among Canadian Population Groups." StatCan COVID-19: Data to Insights for a Better Canada, catalogue no. 45280001. https://www150.statcan.gc.ca/n1/pub/45-28-0001/2021001/article/00011-eng.pdf.

– 2021d. "Household Economic Well-Being during the COVID-19 Pandemic, Experimental Estimates, First Quarter to Third Quarter of 2020." Daily, 1 March 2021. https://www150.statcan.gc.ca/n1/en/daily-quotidien/210301/dq210301b-eng.pdf?st=Pa_VWCpK.

– 2021e. "Impact of COVID-19 Pandemic on Canadian Seniors." Insights on Canadian Society, catalogue no. 75-006-X. https://www150.statcan.gc.ca/n1/en/pub/75-006-x/2021001/article/00008-eng.pdf?st=a_tLXrbr.

– 2021f. "Job Vacancies, Second Quarter 2021." Daily, 21 September 2021. https://www150.statcan.gc.ca/n1/en/daily-quotidien/210921/dq210921a-eng.pdf?st=4fMVvQya.

– 2021g. "National Tourism Indicators, First Quarter 2021." Daily, 29 June 2021. https://www150.statcan.gc.ca/n1/en/daily-quotidien/210629/dq210629a-eng.pdf?st=-48vpzle.

– 2021h. "Provisional Death Counts and Excess Mortality, January 2020 to February 2021." Daily, 14 May 2021. https://www150.statcan.gc.ca/n1/en/daily-quotidien/210514/dq210514c-eng.pdf?st=JoVoC3tZ.

– 2021i. "School Closures and COVID-19: Interactive Tool." https://www150.statcan.gc.ca/n1/pub/71-607-x/71-607-x2021009-eng.htm.

– 2021j. "Selected Police-Reported Crime and Calls for Service during the COVID-19 Pandemic, March to October 2020." Daily, 27 January 2021. https://www150.statcan.gc.ca/n1/en/daily-quotidien/210127/dq210127c-eng.pdf?st=YtFXSfTe.

– 2021k. "Statistics Canada and Contact Tracing." Modified 8 February 2023. https://www.statcan.gc.ca/eng/transparency-accountability/contact-tracing.

– 2021l. "Table 13-10-0774-01: Detailed Preliminary Information on Cases of COVID-19, 2020–2021: 6-Dimensions (Aggregated Data)." Public Health Agency of Canada, May 2021. https://www150.statcan.gc.ca/t1/tbl1/en/tv.action?pid=1310077401.

– 2021m. "Table 14-10-0377-01: Employment by Class of Worker and Industry, Annual (x 1,000)." https://doi.org/10.25318/1410037701-eng.

– 2021n. "Table 20-10-0016-01: Retail Commodity Survey, Retail Sales (x 1,000)." May 2021. https://www150.statcan.gc.ca/t1/tbl1/en/tv.action?pid=2010001601.

– 2021o. "Table 24-10-0003-01: Non-resident Travellers Entering Canada, by Country of Residence (Excluding the United States)." https://doi.org/10.25318/2410000301-eng.

– 2022a. "Canadian Tourism Activity Tracker, March 2022." Daily, 10 June 2022. https://www150.statcan.gc.ca/n1/en/daily-quotidien/220610/dq220610d-eng.pdf?st=40-A_d1s.

– 2022b. "Deaths, 2020." Daily, 24 January 2022. https://www150.statcan.gc.ca/n1/en/daily-quotidien/220124/dq220124a-eng.pdf?st=_J2Sd5oh.

– 2022c. "Disaggregated Trends in Poverty from the 2021 Census of Population." Modified 9 November 2022. https://www12.statcan.gc.ca/census-recensement/2021/as-sa/98-200-X/2021009/98-200-x2021009-eng.cfm.

– 2022d. "Energy Statistics, March 2022." 7 June 2022. https://www150.statcan.gc.ca/n1/en/daily-quotidien/220607/dq220607c-eng.pdf?st=MPdJabhu.

– 2022e. "Fewer Babies Born as Canada's Fertility Rate Hits a Record Low in 2020." StatsCan Plus, 16 May 2022. https://www.statcan.gc.ca/o1/en/plus/960-fewer-babies-born-canadas-fertility-rate-hits-record-low-2020.

– 2022f. "A Fifty-Year Look at Divorces in Canada, 1970 to 2020." Daily, 9 March 2022. https://www150.statcan.gc.ca/n1/daily-quotidien/220309/dq220309a-eng.pdf.

– 2022g. "Labour Shortage Trends in Canada." Modified 24 June 2022. https://www.statcan.gc.ca/en/subjects-start/labour_/labour-shortage-trends-canada.

– 2022h. "Pandemic Benefits Cushion Losses for Low Income Earners and Narrow Income Inequality – After Tax Income Grows across Canada except in Alberta and Newfoundland and Labrador." Daily, 13 July 2022. https://www150.statcan.gc.ca/n1/daily-quotidien/220713/dq220 713d-eng.htm.

– 2022i. "Provisional Death Counts and Excess Mortality, January 2020 to January 2022." Daily, 14 April 2022. https://www150.statcan.gc.ca/n1/ en/daily-quotidien/220414/dq220414d-eng.pdf?st=oQm28lzm.

– 2022j. "Provisional Death Counts and Excess Mortality, January 2020 to July 2022." Daily, 13 October 2022. https://www150.statcan.gc.ca/n1/ daily-quotidien/221013/dq221013b-eng.pdf.

– 2022k. "Table 12-10-0011-01: International Merchandise Trade for All Countries and by Principal Trading Partners, Monthly (x 1,000,000)." January–December 2019. https://www150.statcan.gc.ca/t1/tbl1/en/tv. action?pid=1210001101.

– 2022l. "Table 24-10-0041-01: International Travellers Entering or Returning to Canada, by Type of Transport." 23 February 2022. https:// doi.org/10.25318/2410004101-eng.

– 2022m. "Table 25-10-0063-01: Supply and Dispositions of Crude Oil and Equivalent." https://doi.org/10.25318/2510006301-eng.

– 2022n. "Table 33-10-0270-01: Experimental Estimates for Business Openings and Closures for Canada, Provinces and Territories, Census Metropolitan Areas, Seasonally Adjusted." https://doi.org/10.25318/ 3310027001-eng.

– 2022o. "Table 35-10-0169-01: Selected Police-Reported Crime and Calls for Service during the COVID-19 Pandemic." 9 August. https://doi.org/ 10.25318/3510016901-eng.

– 2022p. "Travel between Canada and Other Countries, March 2022." Daily, 24 May 2022. https://www150.statcan.gc.ca/n1/en/daily-quotidien/220524/dq220524b-eng.pdf?st=GRWCUEuP.

– 2022q. "Truck Transportation." Modified 19 July 2022. https://ic.gc.ca/ app/scr/app/cis/businesses-entreprises/484.

– 2023a. "Health Outcomes." Modified 13 October 2023. https://www150. statcan.gc.ca/n1/pub/82-570-x/2023001/section1-eng.htm#a1_1.

– 2023b. "Provisional Deaths and Excess Mortality in Canada Dashboard." Modified 9 November 2023. https://www150.statcan.gc.ca/n1/pub/71-607-x/71-607-x2021028-eng.htm.

Stecula, D., M. Pickup, and C. van der Linden. 2020. "Who Believes in COVID-19 Conspiracies and Why It Matters." Policy Options, 6 July 2020. https://policyoptions.irpp.org/magazines/july-2020/who-believes-in-covid-19-conspiracies-and-why-it-matters.

Stevens, A. 2020. "Governments Cannot Just 'Follow the Science' on COVID-19." *Natural Human Behaviour* 4 (June): 560. https://doi. org/10.1038/s41562-020-0894-x.

Stevenson, L. 2021. *Maples Personal Care Home COVID-19 Outbreak: External Review Final Report.* 15 January 2021. https://manitoba.ca/ asset_library/en/proactive/2020_2021/maples-pch-covid19-review.pdf.

Stone, L., and A. Cyr. 2021. "Provinces Diverge on COVID-19 Vaccine Passports as Some Sectors Begin Requiring Proof of Immunization." *Globe and Mail,* 14 July 2021. https://www.theglobeandmail.com/ canada/article-provinces-diverge-on-vaccine-passports-as-some-sectors-begin-requiring.

Stone, L., and K. Howlett. 2020. "Ontario Rejects Call to Take Over Operations at Long-Term Care Homes Where 54 Residents Have Died." *Globe and Mail,* 17 April 2020. https://www.theglobeandmail.com/ canada/article-ontario-rejects-call-to-take-over-operations-at-long-term-care-homes.

Stone, L., K. Howlett, and T.T. Ha. 2020. "Ontario Long-Term Care Plan Raises Concerns about Loopholes, Staff Wages amid COVID-19 Pandemic." *Globe and Mail,* 15 April 2020. https://www.theglobeand mail.com/canada/article-ontario-long-term-care-plan-raises-concerns-about-loopholes-staff.

Stone, L., and J. Keller, J. 2020. "Ontario Relying on Volunteers to Help Staffing Shortage in Long-Term Care as Feds Release New Guidelines." *Globe and Mail,* 12 April 2020. https://www.theglobeandmail.com/ canada/article-ontario-relying-on-volunteers-to-help-staffing-shortage-in-long-term.

Stone, L., and W. Leung. 2021. "Canada to Require Vaccination for Air, Rail and Marine Travellers as Well as Federal Employees." *Globe and Mail,* 13 August 2021. https://www.theglobeandmail.com/canada/ article-canada-to-require-vaccination-for-air-rail-and-marine-travellers-as.

Stoto, M.A., A. Woolverton, J. Kraemer, P. Barlow, and M. Clarke. 2022. "COVID-19 Data Are Messy: Analytic Methods for Rigorous Impact Analyses with Imperfect Data. *Global Health* 18, 2. https://doi.org/ 10.1186/s12992-021-00795-0.

STR. 2022a. "Canada Hotel RevPAR 54% Recovered in 2021." https://str. com/press-release/str-canada-hotel-revpar-54-percent-recovered-2021.

– 2022b. "Canadian Hotel Rates Exceeded 2019 Levels in March." https:// str.com/press-release/str-canada-hotel-rates-exceeded-2019-levels-march.

Subedi, R., L. Greenberg, and M. Turcotte. 2020. "COVID-19 Mortality Rates in Canada's Ethno-Cultural Neighbourhoods." Statistics Canada, 28 October 2020. https://www150.statcan.gc.ca/n1/pub/45-28-0001/ 2020001/article/00079-eng.htm.

Sun, L., G. Wang, and L. Gao. 2022. "Modelling the Impact of Tourism on Mental Health of Chinese Residents: An Empirical Study." *Discrete Dynamics in Nature and Society* 2022 (4): 1–6. https://doi. org/10.1155/2022/7108267.

Sun, Y., Y. Wu, S. Fan, T. Dal Santo, X. Jiang et al. 2023. "Comparison of Mental Health Symptoms before and during the COVID-19 Pandemic: Evidence from a Systematic Review and Meta-Analysis of 134 Cohorts." *BMJ* 380:e074224. https://www.bmj.com/content/380/bmj-2022-074224.

Sunstein, C.R. 2002a. "The Paralyzing Principle: Does the Precautionary Principle Point Us in Any Helpful Direction?" *Regulation* 25 (4): 32–7.

– 2002b. "Probability Neglect: Emotions, Worst Cases, and Law." *Yale Law Journal* 112 (61): 61–107. https://www.yalelawjournal.org/essay/probability-neglect-emotions-worst-cases-and-law.

– 2005a. *Laws of Fear: Beyond the Precautionary Principle*. Cambridge: Cambridge University Press.

– 2005b. "The Precautionary Principle as a Basis for Decision Making." *The Economists' Voice* 2 (2): 1–9. https://dash.harvard.edu/bitstream/1/29998410/1/PrecautionaryPrinciple.pdf.

– 2009. Worst-Case Scenarios. Cambridge, MA: Harvard University Press.

Sześciło, D. 2020. "Agencification Revisited: Trends in Consolidation of Central Government Administration in Europe." *International Review of Administrative Sciences* 88 (4): 995–1012. http://dx.doi.org/10.1177/0020852320976791.

Szklarski, C. 2020. "Canada's Proportion of COVID-19 Deaths in Long-Term Care Double the Average of Other Countries, Study Shows." CBC News, 25 June 2020. https://www.cbc.ca/news/health/coronavirus-canada-long-term-care-deaths-study-1.5626751.

Tait, C. 2020. "Alberta COVID-19 Testing System Overwhelmed as Infections Spike." *Globe and Mail*, 20 July 2020. https://www.theglobeandmail.com/canada/alberta/article-alberta-covid-19-testing-system-overwhelmed-as-infections-spike.

– 2021. "Alberta Health Authority Cancels All Elective Surgeries in Calgary Region as COVID-19 Hospital Admissions Soar." *Globe and Mail*, 10 September 2021. https://www.theglobeandmail.com/canada/alberta/article-alberta-health-authority-cancels-all-elective-surgeries-in-calgary.

Tait, J. 2008. "Risk Governance of Genetically Modified Crops – European and American Perspectives." In *Global Risk Governance: International Risk Governance Council*, edited by O. Renn and K.D. Walker, 133–53. Dordrecht, Netherlands: Springer. https://doi.org/10.1007/978-1-4020-6799-0.

Talbot, D., and E. Ordonez-Ponce. 2020. "Canadian Banks' Responses to COVID-19: A Strategic Positioning Analysis." *Journal of Sustainable*

Finance & Investment 12 (2): 423–30. https://www.tandfonline.com/doi/full/10.1080/20430795.2020.1771982.

Taleb, N.N. 2007. *The Black Swan: The Impact of the Highly Improbable.* New York: Random House.

Tam, S., S. Sood, and C. Johnston. 2021a. "Impact of COVID-19 on Small Businesses in Canada, First Quarter of 2021." StatCan COVID-19: Data to Insights for a Better Canada, catalogue no. 45280001. https://www150.statcan.gc.ca/n1/en/pub/45-28-0001/2021001/article/00009-eng.pdf?st=jloNIgWy.

– 2021b. "Impact of COVID-19 on the Tourism Sector, Second Quarter of 2021. StatCan COVID-19: Data to Insights for a Better Canada, catalogue no. 45-28-0001. https://www150.statcan.gc.ca/n1/en/pub/45-28-0001/2021001/article/00023-eng.pdf?st=PSk_i3pW.

Tang, B., X. Wang, Q. Li, N.L. Bragazzi, S. Tang, Y. Xiao, and J. Wu. 2020. "Estimation of the Transmission Risk of the 2019-nCov and Its Implication for Public Health Interventions." *Journal of Clinical Medicine* 9 (2): e462. https://doi.org/10.3390/jcm9020462.

Tarrow, S. 1988. "National Politics and Collective Action: Recent Theory and Research in Western Europe and the United States." *Annual Review of Sociology* 14: 421–40. https://doi.org/10.1146/annurev.so.14.080188.002225.

Tasker, J.P. 2020a. "Government Documents Reveal a Slow Start to Canada's COVID-19 Response." CBC News, 10 April 2020. https://www.cbc.ca/news/politics/covid-19-government-documents-1.5528726.

– 2020b. "Health Canada Approves Pfizer-BioNTech COVID-19 Vaccine." CBC News, 9 December 2020. https://www.cbc.ca/news/politics/vaccine-rollout-plan-phac-1.5833912.

– 2020c. "Ottawa Slow to Respond to PPE Shortages Flagged in February: Documents." CBC News, 14 August 2020. https://www.cbc.ca/news/politics/ppe-shortages-slow-response-1.5684962.

– 2021. "Federal Health Agency Wasn't Ready for Pandemic Equipment Demand, Auditor Finds." CBC News, 26 May 2021. https://www.cbc.ca/news/politics/ag-ness-ppe-1.6041158.

– 2022a. "Canada Needs to Adopt a 'More Sustainable' Approach to COVID-19, Tam Says." CBC News, 4 February 2022. https://www.cbc.ca/news/politics/canada-more-sustainable-covid-response-1.6339609.

– 2022b. "Liberal MP Joël Lightbound Says His Party's COVID Policy 'Stigmatizes and Divides People.'" CBC News, 8 February 2022. https://www.cbc.ca/news/politics/liberal-mp-politicization-pandemic-1.6343730.

Tausczik, Y., K. Faase, J.W. Pennebaker, and K.J. Petrie. 2011. "Public Anxiety and Information Seeking Following the H1N1 Outbreak: Blogs,

Newspaper Articles and Wikipedia Visits." *Health Communication* 27 (2): 179–85.

Taylor, K. 2021. "When the Music's Over: COVID-19 Decimated the Arts in Canada, and the Worst May Be Yet to Come." *Globe and Mail*, 11 March 2021. https://www.theglobeandmail.com/arts/article-when-the-musics-over-covid-19-decimated-the-arts-in-canada-and-the.

Taylor, M.G. 1960. "The Role of the Medical Profession in the Formulation and Execution of Public Policy." *Canadian Journal of Economics and Political Science* 26 (1): 108–27. https://www.jstor.org/stable/138823.

Taylor, S., L. Berthiaume, and C. Tran. 2022. "Trudeau Says He's 'Absolutely Serene' about Invoking Emergencies Act." MSN, 25 November 2022. https://www.msn.com/en-ca/news/canada/threat-of-violence-was-key-factor-in-decision-to-invoke-emergencies-act-trudeau/ar-AA14xrQD.

Taylor-Gooby, P. 2006. "The Efficiency/Trust Dilemma in Public Policy Reform." Social Contexts and Responses to Risk Network, Working Paper 9-2006. Canterbury, UK: School of Social Policy, Sociology and Social Research, University of Kent.

ter Meulen, R.H.J. 2005. "The Ethical Basis of the Precautionary Principle in Health Care Decision Making." *Toxicology and Applied Pharmacology* 207 (2): 663–7. https://doi.org/10.1016/j.taap.2004.11.032.

Theckedath, D. 2014. "Canada's Tourism Economy (In Brief)." Library of Parliament, Publication no. 2014-74-E. https://lop.parl.ca/staticfiles/PublicWebsite/Home/ResearchPublications/InBriefs/PDF/2014-74-e.pdf.

Therrien, M.C., J.M. Normandin, and J.L. Denis. 2017. "Bridging Complexity Theory and Resilience to Develop Surge Capacity in Health Systems." *Journal of Health Organization and Management* 31 (7): 96–109. https://doi.org/10.1108/jhom-04-2016-0067.

Tholl, B., J.P. Hirdes, and P. Hébert. 2020. "A Rare Window of Opportunity to Finally Fix Long-Term Care." *Policy Options*, 10 July 2020. https://policyoptions.irpp.org/magazines/july-2020/a-rare-window-of-opportunity-to-finally-fix-long-term-care.

Thompson, A., N.M. Stall, K.B. Born, J.L. Gibson, U. Allen, J. Hopkins, A. Laporte, A. Maltsev, R. McElroy, and S. Mishra. 2021. "Benefits of Paid Sick Leave during the COVID-19 Pandemic." Science Briefs of the Ontario COVID-19 Science Advisory Table 2 (25): 1–13. https://doi.org/10.47326/ocsat.2021.02.25.1.0.

Thompson, E. 2020. "Federal Government Open to New Law to Fight Pandemic Misinformation." CBC News, 16 April 2020. https://www.cbc.ca/news/politics/covid-misinformation-disinformation-law-1.5532325.

– 2022. "Security Tightened for Eight Cabinet Ministers and Theresa Tam before Convoy Protest Arrived." CBC News, 23 November 2022. https://www.cbc.ca/news/politics/convoy-protest-cabinet-security-1.6661338.

Thompson, E., R. Rocha, and A. Leung. 2022. "Hacked Convoy Data Shows More than Half of Donations Came from U.S." CBC News, 15 February 2022. https://www.cbc.ca/news/politics/convoy-protest-donations-data-1.6351292.

Thompson, N. 2021. "Reports of Domestic, Intimate Partner Violence Continue to Rise during Pandemic." CBC News, 15 February 2021. https://www.cbc.ca/news/canada/toronto/domestic-intimate-partner-violence-up-in-pandemic-1.5914344.

TIAC (Tourism Industry Association of Canada). n.d. "About TIAC." Accessed 25 November 2021. https://tiac-aitc.ca/About.html.

Tickner J.A., D. Kriebel, and S. Wright. 2003. "A Compass for Health: Rethinking Precaution and Its Role in Science and Public Health." *International Journal of Epidemiology* 32 (4): 489–92. https://doi.org/10.1093/ije/dyg186.

Tighe, D. 2021. "Monthly Retail Sales of Grocery Stores in Canada from January 2015 to June 2021." Statista, 17 September 2021. https://www.statista.com/statistics/461774/monthly-retail-sales-of-grocery-stores-canada/#statisticContainer.

Timney, M.M. 1996. "Institutionalism and Public Administration or 'I'm from the Government and I'm Here to Help.'" *Administrative Theory & Praxis* 18 (2): 101–7. https://www.jstor.org/stable/25611180.

Tinder Newsroom. 2021. "The Future of Dating Is Fluid." https://www.tinderpressroom.com/futureofdating.

Top Class Actions. 2020. "British Columbia COVID-19 Business Interruption Insurance Lawsuit." https://ca.topclassactions.com/lawsuit-settlements/coronavirus-covid-19/british-columbia-covid-19-business-interruption-insurance-lawsuit.

– 2021. "Canada's Guide to Coronavirus Outbreak Legal Issues." 11 March 2021. https://ca.topclassactions.com/coronavirus-covid-19/canadian-consumers-guide-to-coronavirus-outbreak-legal-issues.

Toronto Star. 2021. "Canada to Benefit from U.S. Rebound, Says OECD." 9 March 2021. https://www.thestar.com/business/2021/03/09/canada-to-benefit-from-us-rebound-says-oecd.html.

Tourism HR Canada. 2019. "10 Reasons Why 10% Matters: Tourism Employment Transforms Lives and Communities." 20 February 2019. https://tourismhr.ca/10-reasons-why-10-matters-tourism-employment-transforms-lives-communities.

– 2023. *Snapshot of the Tourism Sector Labour Market – National Report: Canada.* https://tourismhr.ca/wp-content/uploads/National-Report-1.pdf.

– n.d.a. "Employment by Demographic Groups – Chart 9: Employment by Age Category (Monthly)." Accessed 31 July 2022. https://tourismhr.ca/labour-market-information/tourism-employment-tracker-insights-into-covid-19s-impact/#Age-Gender.

– n.d.b. "Employment by Demographic Groups – Chart 11: Employment by Immigration Status." Accessed 31 July 2022. https://tourismhr.ca/labour-market-information/tourism-employment-tracker-insights-into-covid-19s-impact.

– n.d.c. "Tourism Business Openings and Closings – Chart 4: Tourism Business Openings and Closures." Accessed 31 July 2022. https://tour ismhr.ca/labour-market-information/tourism-employment-tracker-insights-into-covid-19s-impact.

– n.d.d. "Tourism Employment Tracker – Unemployment Rate." Accessed 31 July 2022. https://tourismhr.ca/labour-market-information/tourism-employment-tracker-insights-into-covid-19s-impact.

– n.d.e. "Tourism Facts." Accessed 31 July 2022. https://tourismhr.ca/labour-market-information/tourism-facts.

– n.d.f. "Tourism Labour Force Survey." Accessed 31 July 2022. https://tourismhr.ca/labour-market-information/tourism-labour-force-survey.

– n.d.g. "Unemployment Rate – Chart 3: Tourism Unemployment Rate." Accessed 31 July 2022. https://tourismhr.ca/labour-market-information/tourism-employment-tracker-insights-into-covid-19s-impact.

Tozer-Pennington, V. 2021. *The Aviation Industry Leaders Report 2021: Route to Recovery*. https://assets.kpmg/content/dam/kpmg/ie/pdf/2021/01/ie-aviation-industry-leaders-report-route-to-recovery.pdf.

– 2022. *The Aviation Industry Leaders Report 2022: Recovery through Resilience*. https://assets.kpmg/content/dam/kpmg/ie/pdf/2022/01/aviation-industry-leaders-report-2022.pdf.

Transport Canada. 2020a. "Minister Garneau Announces New Measures for the Use of Face Coverings in the Canadian Transportation Sector." Government of Canada, 3 June 2020. https://www.canada.ca/en transport-canada/news/2020/06/minister-garneau-announces-new-measures-for-the-use-of-face-coverings-in-the-canadian-transportation-sector.html.

– 2020b. "New Measures Introduced for Non-medical Masks or Face Coverings in the Canadian Transportation System." Government of Canada, 17 April 2020. https://www.canada.ca/en/transport-canada/news/2020/04/new-measures-introduced-for-non-medical-masks-or-face-coverings-in-the-canadian-transportation-system.html.

– 2021. "Canadian Motor Vehicle Traffic Collision Statistics: 2018." Government of Canada, modified 7 May 2021. https://tc.canada.ca/en/

road-transportation/statistics-data/canadian-motor-vehicle-traffic-collision-statistics-2018.

Treasury Board Secretariat. 2022. "Policy on Cost-Benefit Analysis." Government of Canada, modified 29 March 2022. https://www.canada.ca/en/government/system/laws/developing-improving-federal-regulations/requirements-developing-managing-reviewing-regulations/guidelines-tools/policy-cost-benefit-analysis.html.

– n.d. "Mandatory Vaccination Policy." Government of Newfoundland and Labrador. Accessed 24 February 2022. https://www.gov.nl.ca/exec/tbs/mandatory-vaccination-policy.

Trevelyan, L. 2013. "Haiti Tries to Boost Its Tourism Industry." BBC, 26 June 2013. https://www.bbc.com/news/world-latin-america-23035402.

Trichur, R. 2021. "Investors, Speak Up. Securities Regulators Need to Hear Your Grievances about Online AGMs." *Globe and Mail*, 22 November 2021. https://www.theglobeandmail.com/business/commentary/article-investors-speak-up-securities-regulators-need-to-hear-your-grievances.

Trifiletti, E., S.E. Shamloo, M. Faccini, and A. Zaka. 2021. "Psychological Predictors of Protective Behaviours during the COVID-19 Pandemic: Theory of Planned Behaviour and Risk Perception." *Journal of Community & Applied Social Psychology* 32 (3): 382–97. https://dx.doi.org/10.1002%2Fcasp.2509.

Truss, L. 2024. *Ten Years to Save the West: Lessons from the Only Conservative in the Room*. Washington, DC: Regnery. https://www.simonandschuster.ca/books/Ten-Years-to-Save-the-West/Liz-Truss/9781684515622.

Tsai, T.C., B.H. Jacobson, and A.K. Jha. 2020. "Effect of COVID-19 on Critical ICU Capacity in US Acute Care Hospitals." *medRxiv*, December 2020. https://doi.org/10.1101/2020.12.16.20248366.

Tucker, A. 2021. "North Sees 34% Drop in International Students Due to COVID-19." CBC News, 18 February 2021. https://www.cbc.ca/news/canada/north/north-sees-drop-in-international-students-due-to-covid-19-1.5917156.

Tucker, S., and A. Keefe. 2021. *2021 Report on Work Fatality and Injury Rates in Canada*. University of Regina. https://www.uregina.ca/business/assets/faculty_staff/2021-Report-on-Workplace-Fatalities-and-Injuries-2021-Oct-21.pdf.

Tumilty, R. 2020. "Are You an Essential Worker? In Canada, It Depends on Where You Live." *National Post*, 18 July 2020. https://nationalpost.com/news/canada/are-you-an-essential-worker-in-canada-it-depends-on-where-you-live.

– 2021. "Canada's COVID Models Have Been Largely Accurate, but Worst Cases Have Not Materialized." *National Post*, 26 February 2021. https://nationalpost.com/news/canada/canadas-covid-models-have-been-largely-accurate-but-worst-cases-have-not-materialized.

Tunney, C. 2021a. "Organized Crime 'Knowingly and Actively' Exploited Federal Pandemic Benefits: Intelligence Reports." CBC News, 12 November 2021. https://www.cbc.ca/news/politics/cerb-organized-crime-1.6241211.

– 2021b. "With Just 141 Tickets Issued, PHAC Says Most Travellers Are Following Quarantine Laws." CBC News, 3 February 2021. https://www.cbc.ca/news/politics/quarantine-act-enforcement-1.5897682.

– 2022a. "Court Grants Injunction to Silence Honking in Downtown Ottawa for 10 Days." CBC News, 8 February 2022. https://www.cbc.ca/news/politics/injunction-ottawa-granted-1.6342468.

– 2022b. "Federal Government Invoked Emergencies Act for First Time Ever in Response to Protests, Blockades." CBC News, 15 February 2022. https://www.cbc.ca/news/politics/trudeau-premiers-cabinet-1.6350734.

Tunney, J. 2022. "Prime Minister Justin Trudeau Took the Stand at the Emergencies Act Inquiry – Here's What We Learned." CBC News, 26 November 2022. https://www.cbc.ca/news/politics/trudeau-testifies-public-order-emergency-commission-1.6664962.

Tupper, P., and C. Colijn. 2021. "Screening with Rapid Tests to Prevent COVID-19 Transmission in Long-Term Care (LTC)." SafeCare BC, 29 January 2021. https://www.safecarebc.ca/wp-content/uploads/2021/01/ltc_modeling_tupper_colijn_final.pdf.

Turcotte, M. 2010. "Working at Home: An Update." Canadian Social Trends, catalogue no. 11-008-X. https://www150.statcan.gc.ca/n1/en/pub/11-008-x/2011001/article/11366-eng.pdf?st=gSZaJbuD.

Turcotte, M., and K. Savage. 2020. "The Contribution of Immigrants and Population Groups Designated as Visible Minorities to Nurse Aide, Orderly and Patient Service Associate Occupations." StatCan COVID-19: Data to Insights for a Better Canada, catalogue no. 45280001. https://www150.statcan.gc.ca/n1/pub/45-28-0001/2020001/article/00036-eng.pdf.

Turnbull, S. 2020. "Health Canada Looking Into Private Clinics Offering COVID-19 Tests." CTV News, 5 October 2020. https://www.ctvnews.ca/politics/health-canada-looking-into-private-clinics-offering-covid-19-tests-1.5133854.

– 2021. "After $500M of Double CERB Payments Made, Investigation Needed into Fraud: AG." CTV News, 25 March 2021. https://www.

ctvnews.ca/politics/after-500m-of-double-cerb-payments-made-investigation-needed-into-fraud-ag-1.5362115.

Turner, C. 2019. "The 'Climate Change Election' Is Over: What Happens Now?" *Globe and Mail*, 25 October 2019. https://www.theglobeandmail. com/opinion/article-the-climate-change-election-is-over-what-happens-now.

Tversky, A., and D. Kahneman. 1973. "Availability: A Heuristic for Judging Frequency and Probability." *Cognitive Psychology* 5 (1): 207–33.

– 1981. "The Framing of Decisions and the Psychology of Choice." *Science* 211 (4481): 453–8. https://doi.org/10.1126/science.7455683.

UK Health Security Agency. 2020. "Cost Utility Analysis: Health Economic Studies." Government of the United Kingdom, 13 October 2020. https:// www.gov.uk/guidance/cost-utility-analysis-health-economic-studies.

Ullah, I., K.S. Khan, M.J. Tahir, A. Ahmed, and H. Harapan. 2021. "Myths and Conspiracy Theories on Vaccines and COVID-19: Potential Effect on Global Vaccine Refusals." *Vacunas* 22 (2) (May–August): 93–7. https:// dx.doi.org/10.1016%2Fj.vacun.2021.01.001.

Ungar, L. 2022. "As 'Stealth Omicron' Advances, Scientists Are Learning More." *Globe and Mail*, 24 February 2022. https://www.theglobeand mail.com/world/article-as-stealth-omicron-advances-scientists-are-learning-more-2.

United Nations. 2010. *International Recommendations for Tourism Statistics 2008*. Department of Economic and Social Affairs, Series M no. 83, rev. 1. New York: United Nations. https://unstats.un.org/unsd/publi cation/Seriesm/SeriesM_83rev1e.pdf.

United Nations Human Rights Office of the High Commissioner. 2006. *Convention on the Rights of Persons with Disabilities*. https://www.ohchr. org/en/instruments-mechanisms/instruments/convention-rights-persons-disabilities.

United States Census Bureau. 2019. "2019 U.S. Population Estimates Continue to Show the Nation's Growth Is Slowing." United States Government, 30 December 2019. https://www.census.gov/newsroom/ press-releases/2019/popest-nation.html.

University of Toronto Joint Centre for Bioethics' Pandemic Influenza Working Group. 2005. *Stand on Guard for Thee: Ethical Considerations in Preparedness Planning for Pandemic Influenza*. https://jcb.utoronto.ca/ wp-content/uploads/2021/03/stand_on_guard.pdf.

UNWTO (United Nations World Tourism Organization). 2016. *Measuring the Sustainability of Tourism: Developing a Statistical Framework for Sustainable Tourism – Overview of the Initiative*. Statistics Department, July 2016. https://webunwto.s3.eu-west-1.amazonaws.com/s3fs-public/ 2021-06/mstoverviewinitiative_2.pdf.

– 2018. *Statistical Framework for Measuring the Sustainability of Tourism – Consultation Draft*. Draft prepared for discussion with the Working Group of Experts on Measuring the Sustainability of Tourism. https://webunwto.s3.eu-west-1.amazonaws.com/s3fs-public/2020-09/wge_mst_2nd_item_2.1_doc_o.pdf.

– 2019. "Tourism's Carbon Emissions Measured in Landmark Report Launched at COP25." 4 December 2019. https://www.unwto.org/news/tourisms-carbon-emissions-measured-in-landmark-report-launched-at-cop25.

US Department of Health and Human Services. 2005. "HHS Pandemic Influenza Plan." United States Government. https://www.cdc.gov/flu/pdf/professionals/hhspandemicinfluenzaplan.pdf.

US Department of Transportation. 2021. "Departmental Guidance on Valuation of a Statistical Life in Economic Analysis." United States Government, March 2021. https://www.transportation.gov/office-policy/transportation-policy/revised-departmental-guidance-on-valuation-of-a-statistical-life-in-economic-analysis.

van Prooijen, J.W., and K.M. Douglas. 2018. "Belief in Conspiracy Theories: Basic Principles of an Emerging Research Domain." *European Journal of Social Psychology* 48 (7): 897–908. https://dx.doi.org/10.1002%2Fejsp.2530.

Van Rosendaal, J. 2020. "Flour Mills under Pressure as New Home Bakers Take To 'COVID Baking' for Comfort." *Globe and Mail*, 1 April 2020. https://www.theglobeandmail.com/life/food-and-wine/article-flour-mills-under-pressure-as-new-home-bakers-take-to-comfort-covid.

Varadarajan, T. 2022. "How Government Spending Fuels Inflation." *Wall Street Journal*, 18 February 2022. https://www.wsj.com/articles/government-spending-fuels-inflation-covid-relief-pandemic-debt-federal-reserve-stimulus-powell-biden-stagflation-11645202057.

Varcoe, C., A.J. Browne, S. Wong, and V.L. Smye. 2009. "Harms and Benefits: Collecting Ethnicity Data in a Clinical Context." *Social Science & Medicine* 68 (9): 1659–66. https://doi.org/10.1016/j.socscimed.2009.02:034.

Varlik, N. 2021. "From Black Death to COVID-19, Pandemics Have Always Pushed People to Honor Death and Celebrate Life." The Conversation, 26 October 2021. https://theconversation.com/from-black-death-to-covid-19-pandemics-have-always-pushed-people-to-honor-death-and-celebrate-life-170517.

Vaughan, D. 1996. *The Challenger Launch Decision: Risky Technology, Culture and Deviance at NASA*. Chicago: Chicago University Press.

Väyrynen, L. 2020. "Paid Sick Leave Provision Report 2020." Corporate Knights. https://www.corporateknights.com/wp-content/uploads/2020/10/Paid-Sick-Leave-Provision-Report-2020_Final.pdf.

Victor, J. 2021. "Long Recovery Ahead for Tourism Industry in Aftermath of COVID-19 Pandemic, Report Says." Globe and Mail, 7 March 2021. https://www.theglobeandmail.com/business/article-long-recovery-ahead-for-tourism-industry-in-aftermath-of-covid-19.

Villani, M. 2020. "Frustration, Finger Pointing over Lack of Ticketing at Alberta Anti-mask Rallies." CTV News, 30 November 2020. https://calgary.ctvnews.ca/frustration-finger-pointing-over-lack-of-ticketing-at-alberta-anti-mask-rallies-1.5209944.

Vining, A.R., C. Laurin, and D. Weimer. 2015. "The Longer-Run Performance Effects of Agencification: Theory and Evidence from Québec Agencies." Journal of Public Policy 35 (2): 193–222. https://www.jstor.org/stable/43864141.

Volunteer Canada. 2020. "The Volunteering Lens of COVID-19: Fall 2020 Survey – Impacts of COVID-19 on Volunteer Engagement." Volunteer Management Professionals of Canada and spinktank, December 2020. https://volunteer.ca/vdemo/ResearchAndResources_DOCS/Vol%20Lens%202020%20Survey%20Results/VC_FallSurveyReport_2020_ENG_FINAL.pdf.

Wade, L. 2020. "From Black Death to Fatal Flu, Past Pandemics Show Why People on the Margins Suffer Most." Science, 14 May 2020. https://www.science.org/content/article/black-death-fatal-flu-past-pandemics-show-why-people-margins-suffer-most.

Wahlberg, A., and L. Sjöberg. 2000. "Risk Perception and the Media." Journal of Risk Research 3 (1): 31–50.

Wakabayashi, D., K. Weise, J. Nicas, and M. Isaac. 2020. "Big Tech Continues Its Surge Ahead of the Rest of the Economy." New York Times, 29 October 2020. https://www.nytimes.com/2020/10/29/technology/apple-alphabet-facebook-amazon-google-earnings.html.

Walker, P., and N. Davis. 2021. "To Vaccinate Children or Not? Getting Decision Right Is Far from Child's Play." Guardian, 27 August 2021. https://www.theguardian.com/society/2021/aug/27/to-vaccinate-children-or-not-getting-decision-right-is-far-from-childs-play.

Wall, G. 2006. "Recovering from SARS: The Case of Toronto Tourism." Chap. 7 in Tourism, Security and Safety: From Theory to Practice, edited by Y. Mansfeld and A. Pizam, 143–52. Burlington, ON: Elsevier.

Walsh, B. 2009. "Why Border Controls Can't Keep Out the Flu Virus." Time, 30 April 2009. http://content.time.com/time/health/article/0,8599,1894786,00.html.

Walsh, M. 2020. "National Emergency Stockpile Had $3-Million Baseline Budget, Lower than a Decade Ago." *Globe and Mail*, 24 April 2020. https://www.theglobeandmail.com/politics/article-national-emergency-stockpile-had-3-million-baseline-budget-lower.

Walsh, M., G. Robertson, and K. Tomlinson. 2020. "Federal Emergency Stockpile of PPE Was Ill-Prepared for Pandemic." *Globe and Mail*, 30 April 2020. https://www.theglobeandmail.com/politics/article-federal-emergency-stockpile-of-ppe-was-not-properly-maintained.

Walsh, M., and N. Vanderklippe. 2020. "Ottawa and the Provinces Are Navigating a 'Wild West' in the Medical Supply Market." *Globe and Mail*, 6 April 2020. https://www.theglobeandmail.com/politics/article-ottawa-and-the-provinces-are-navigating-a-wild-west-in-the-medical.

Walsh, M., and G. York. 2021. "Canada May Defer Vaccine Deliveries Rather than Launch Early Global Sharing." *Globe and Mail*, 4 May 2021. https://www.theglobeandmail.com/world/article-canada-may-defer-vaccine-deliveries-rather-than-launch-early-global.

Walters, G., J. Mair, and J. Lim. 2016. "Sensationalist Media Reporting of Disastrous Events: Implications for Tourism." *Journal of Hospitality and Tourism Management* 28 (September): 3–10. http://dx.doi.org/10.1016/j.jhtm.2016.04.008.

Warick, J. 2020. "'Without Enforcement, There Is No Law': Sask. Police, Government Urged to Sanction COVID-19 Protesters." CBC News, 11 December 2020. https://www.cbc.ca/news/canada/saskatoon/without-enforcement-there-is-no-law-sask-police-government-urged-to-sanction-covid-19-protesters-1.5836847.

Warmington, J. 2022. "Warmington: 'Freedom' Truckers May Form World's Longest Convoy." *Toronto Sun*, 29 January 2022. https://torontosun.com/news/local-news/warmington-freedom-truckers-may-form-worlds-longest-convoy.

Warnica, R., and A. Bailey. 2021. "Several of Doug Ford's Key Pandemic Decisions Were Swayed by Business Interests, Star Analysis Suggests." *Toronto Star*, 16 July 2021. https://www.thestar.com/business/2021/07/15/several-of-doug-fords-key-pandemic-decisions-were-swayed-by-business-interests-star-analysis-suggests.html.

Wason, P.C. 1960. "On the Failure to Eliminate Hypotheses in a Conceptual Task." *Quarterly Journal of Experimental Psychology* 12 (3): 129–40.

Watters, H. 2019. "How Do the Main Parties Compare on These Issues?" CBC News. https://newsinteractives.cbc.ca/elections/federal/2019/party-platforms.

– 2022. "2 Years On, There Are Calls for a Real Look at What Went Wrong in Canada during COVID-19." CBC News, 14 March 2022. https://www.

cbc.ca/news/canada/hamilton/covid-19-public-inquiry-commission-1.
6380698.

Watts, J.J., and L. Segal. 2009. "Market Failure, Policy Failure and Other
Distortions in Chronic Disease Markets." BMC *Health Services Research*
9:102. doi.org/10.1186/1472-6963-9-102.

Waxman, O., and C. Wilson. 2021. "How the Coronavirus Death Toll
Compares to Other Deadly Events from American History." *Time*, 1
September 2021. https://time.com/5815367/coronavirus-deaths-
comparison.

Wazer, C. 2016. "The Plagues That Might Have Brought Down the Roman
Empire." *The Atlantic*, 16 March 2016. https://www.theatlantic.com/
science/archive/2016/03/plagues-roman-empire/473862.

Weaver, J. 2020. "How the 'Bureaucratic' World Health Organization
Ended Up on the Hot Seat over Its COVID Response." CBC News, 10 July
2020. https://www.cbc.ca/news/world/world-health-organization-who-
covid-1.5641966.

Weber, B. 2020. "Scientists Cut Peer-Review Corners under Pressure of COVID-
19 Pandemic." CBC News, 21 April 2020. https://www.cbc.ca/news/canada/
edmonton/scientists-covid-pandemic-research-misinformation-1.5539997.

Webster, D. 2020. "Risk Management and Legal Liability." Chap. 11 in
Introduction to Tourism and Hospitality in B.C., 2nd ed., edited by M.
Westcott. Victoria, BC: BCcampus. https://opentextbc.ca/introtourism/
chapter/chapter-11-risk-management-and-legal-liability.

Weeks, C. 2022. "Fewer than One in Five Canadians Have Received a
COVID-19 Booster Shot." *Globe and Mail*, 28 October 2022. https://
www.theglobeandmail.com/canada/article-covid-19-bivalent-vaccine-
canada.

Weichel, A. 2021. "Will BC's Vaccine Mandate Cause Hospital Staffing
Shortages? Officials Preparing for Possibility." CTV News, 15 September
2021. https://bc.ctvnews.ca/will-b-c-s-vaccine-mandate-cause-hospital-
staffing-shortages-officials-preparing-for-possibility-1.5585653.

Weick, K.E., and K.H. Roberts. 1993. "Collective Mind in Organizations:
Heedful Interrelating on Flight Decks." *Administrative Science Quarterly*
12 (3): 357–81.

Weick, K.E., and K.M. Sutcliffe. 2001. *Managing the Unexpected: Assuring
High Performance in an Age of Complexity*. San Francisco, CA:
Jossey-Bass.

Welsh, M. 2020. "The Star Published an Investigation into Long-Term Care
in 2003. What's Changed since Then?" *Toronto Star*, 27 May 2020.
https://www.thestar.com/news/canada/2020/05/27/the-star-published-an-
investigation-into-long-term-care-in-2003-whats-changed-since-then.html.

Wheat, C., J. Duguid, L. Relihan, and B. Kim. 2023. "Downtown Downturn: The COVID Shock to Brick-and-Mortar Retail." JPMorgan Chase Institute. https://www.jpmorganchase.com/institute/research/cities-local-communities/downtown-downturn-covid-shock-to-brick-and-mortar.

Wherry, A. 2020. "'We Are All in This Together': Will Trudeau's Actions Match His Words?" CBC News, 1 April 2020. https://www.cbc.ca/news/politics/trudeau-pandemic-covid-coronavirus-media-1.5516383.

– 2022. "Ready or Not, a New Debate about the Future of Health Care Has Begun." CBC News, 9 January 2022. https://www.cbc.ca/news/politics/health-care-pandemic-transfers-1.6307798.

The White House. 2021. "Statement by President Joe Biden on the Investigation into the Origins of COVID-19." 27 August 2021. https://www.whitehouse.gov/briefing-room/statements-releases/2021/08/27/statement-by-president-joe-biden-on-the-investigation-into-the-origins-of-covid-%E2%81%A019.

WHO (World Health Organization). 1986. *The Ottawa Charter for Health Promotion.* https://www.who.int/teams/health-promotion/enhanced-wellbeing/first-global-conference.

– 2014. *The Case for Investing in Public Health.* Regional Office for Europe. http://apps.who.int/iris/bitstream/handle/10665/170471/Case-Investing-Public-Health.pdf.

– 2020a. "Mission Summary: WHO Field Visit to Wuhan, China 20–21 January 2020." 22 January 2020. https://www.who.int/china/news/detail/22-01-2020-field-visit-wuhan-china-jan-2020.

– 2020b. "Naming the Coronavirus Disease (COVID-19) and the Virus That Causes It." https://www.who.int/emergencies/diseases/novel-coronavirus-2019/technical-guidance/naming-the-coronavirus-disease-(covid-2019)-and-the-virus-that-causes-it.

– 2020c. *Novel Coronavirus (2019-nCOV) Situation Report – 1.* 21 January 2020. https://www.who.int/emergencies/diseases/novel-coronavirus-2019/situation-reports.

– 2020d. *Novel Coronavirus (2019-nCOV) Situation Report – 5.* 25 January 2020. https://www.who.int/emergencies/diseases/novel-coronavirus-2019/situation-reports.

– 2020e. *Novel Coronavirus (2019-nCOV) Situation Report – 8.* 28 January 2020. https://www.who.int/emergencies/diseases/novel-coronavirus-2019/situation-reports.

– 2020f. *Novel Coronavirus (2019-nCOV) Situation Report – 11.* 31 January 2020. https://www.who.int/emergencies/diseases/novel-coronavirus-2019/situation-reports.

- 2020g. *Novel Coronavirus (2019-nCOV) Situation Report – 14.* 3 February 2020. https://www.who.int/emergencies/diseases/novel-corona virus-2019/situation-reports.
- 2020h. *Novel Coronavirus (2019-nCOV) Situation Report – 40.* 29 February 2020. https://www.who.int/emergencies/diseases/novel-corona virus-2019/situation-reports.
- 2020i. "Rolling Updates on Coronavirus Disease (COVID-19)." Updated 31 July 2020. https://www.who.int/emergencies/diseases/novel-corona virus-2019/events-as-they-happen.
- 2020j. "The Top 10 Causes of Death." 9 December 2020. https://www. who.int/news-room/fact-sheets/detail/the-top-10-causes-of-death.
- 2020k. "Transmission of SARS-COV-2: Implications for Infection Prevention Precautions." 9 June 2020. https://www.who.int/news-room/ commentaries/detail/transmission-of-sars-cov-2-implications-for-infection-prevention-precautions.
- 2020l. "Virtual Press Conference 8 June 2020." https://www.who.int/docs/ default-source/coronaviruse/transcripts/who-audio-emergencies-corona virus-press-conference-08jun2020.pdf.
- 2021a. "About Us." World Health Organization Regional Office for the Eastern Mediterranean. http://www.emro.who.int/about-who/ public-health-functions/health-promotion-disease-prevention.html.
- 2021b. "Cancer." 3 March 2021. https://www.who.int/news-room/fact-sheets/detail/cancer.
- 2021c. "Contact Tracing in the Context of COVID-19." February 2021. https://www.who.int/publications/i/item/contact-tracing-in-the-context-of-covid-19.
- 2021d. "Statement – Catastrophic Impact of COVID-19 on Cancer Care." Regional Office for Europe, 4 February 2021. https://www.euro.who.int/ en/media-centre/sections/statements/2021/statement-catastrophic-impact-of-covid-19-on-cancer-care.
- 2021e. "Timeline: WHO's COVID-19 Response." Updated 25 January 2021. https://www.who.int/emergencies/diseases/novel-coronavirus-2019/ interactive-timeline.
- 2023. "China: WHO Coronavirus (COVID-19) Dashboard." Updated 20 September 2023. https://covid19.who.int/region/wpro/country/cn.
Wiafe, S., and S. Smith. 2021. "We Must Reckon with the History of Medical Racism and Violence in Order to Address Vaccine Hesitancy in African, Caribbean, Black and Indigenous Communities." Institute for Science, Society and Policy, 23 February 2021. https://issp.uottawa.ca/en/ news/we-must-reckon-history-medical-racism-and-violence-order-address-vaccine-hesitancy-african.

Williams, N., and A.M. Paperny. 2022. "Insight: In Protests and Politics, Canada's 'Freedom Convoy' Reverberates." Reuters, 4 August 2022. https://www.reuters.com/world/americas/protests-politics-canadas-freedom-convoy-reverberates-2022-08-04.

Willick, F. 2021. "Vaccines Intended for N.S., N.B. to Be Delivered to Northern Canada." CBC News, 16 February 2021. https://www.cbc.ca/news/canada/nova-scotia/covid-briefing-feb-12-1.5911954.

Willman, D. 2020. "The CDC's Failed Race against COVID-19: A Threat Underestimated and a Test Overcomplicated." Washington Post, 26 December 2020. https://www.washingtonpost.com/investigations/cdc-covid/2020/12/25/c2b418ae-4206-11eb-8db8-395dedaaa036_story.html.

Wilson, J. 2021. "Yukon, Nova Scotia Roll Out Vaccine Mandate for Employees." HR Reporter, 18 October 2021. https://www.hrreporter.com/focus-areas/legislation/yukon-nova-scotia-roll-out-vaccine-mandate-for-employees/360818.

Wilson, J.Q. 1980. The Politics of Regulation. New York: Basic Books.

Wong, J. 2021. "Hundreds Have Tried to Enter Canada with Fake COVID-19 Test Results, Proof-of-Vaccine Documents: CBSA." CBC News, 30 November 2021. https://www.cbc.ca/news/canada/edmonton/falsified-covid19-documents-cbsa-1.6266686.

Woo, A. 2021a. "COVID-19 Pandemic Has Delayed Treatment, Exacerbated Existing Health Conditions: Heart & Stroke Survey." Globe and Mail, 19 October 2021. https://www.theglobeandmail.com/canada/article-covid-19-pandemic-has-delayed-treatment-exacerbated-existing-health.

– 2021b. "Hospitals Faced with New Capacity Crisis as Unvaccinated Canadians, Reduced Public Health Measures Drive Covid-19's Fourth Wave." Globe and Mail, 7 September 2021. https://www.theglobeandmail.com/canada/article-as-covid-19s-fourth-wave-surges-hospitals-face-new-capacity-crisis-and.

– 2022. "Transmissibility of Omicron Led to Much Higher Death Totals than past Wave, Research Shows." Globe and Mail, 8 February 2021. https://www.theglobeandmail.com/canada/article-transmissibility-of-omicron-led-to-much-higher-death-totals-than-past.

Woods, M. 2021. "Paid Sick Days in Canada: What You Need to Know." Huffington Post, 13 January 2021. https://www.huffingtonpost.ca/entry/paid-sick-days-covid-ontario_ca_5ffe28f6c5b656719889e8cb.

Woolf, M. 2021. "Tories to Oppose Hybrid Parliament Proposal, Say It Weakens Government Scrutiny." Global News, 24 November 2021. https://globalnews.ca/news/8397965/tories-oppose-hybrid-parliament-proposal.

World Bank. 2018. "International L – Global Rankings 2PIO18." https://lpi.worldbank.org/international/global.

– 2020a. "Population, Total – Brazil." https://data.worldbank.org/indicator/SP.POP.TOTL?locations=BR.

– 2020b. "Population, Total – China." https://data.worldbank.org/indicator/SP.POP.TOTL?locations=CN.

– 2020c. "Population, Total – Germany." https://data.worldbank.org/indicator/SP.POP.TOTL?locations=DE.

– 2020d. "Population, Total – India." https://data.worldbank.org/indicator/SP.POP.TOTL?locations=IN.

– 2020e. "Population, Total – Italy." https://data.worldbank.org/indicator/SP.POP.TOTL?locations=IT.

– 2020f. "Population, Total – Japan." https://data.worldbank.org/indicator/SP.POP.TOTL?locations=JP.

– 2020g. "Population, Total – Mexico." https://data.worldbank.org/indicator/SP.POP.TOTL?locations=MX.

– 2020h. "Population, Total – New Zealand." https://data.worldbank.org/indicator/SP.POP.TOTL?locations=NZ.

– 2020i. "Population Total – South Africa." https://data.worldbank.org/indicator/SP.POP.TOTL?locations=ZA.

– 2022. "Current Health Expenditure (% of GDP)." https://data.worldbank.org/indicator/SH.XPD.CHEX.GD.ZS.

– n.d.a. "Inflation, Consumer Prices (Annual %) – Canada." Accessed 22 February 2022. https://data.worldbank.org/indicator/FP.CPI.TOTL.ZG?contextual=default&end=2020&locations=CA&start=2016&view=chart.

– n.d.b. "Rural Population (% of Total Population) – Canada." Accessed 22 July 2021. https://data.worldbank.org/indicator/SP.RUR.TOTL.ZS?end=2019&locations=CA&start=1960&view=chart.

World Vision. 2021. "Covid-19's Impact on the Charity Sector." *Maclean's*, 9 August 2021. https://www.macleans.ca/longforms/covid-19-impact-on-charities.

Wozniak, R. 2020. "Safety Considerations in the New Normal." *Canadian HR Reporter* 33 (7): 18–19. http://digital.hrreporter.com/i/1268696-august-2020-can/17.

WTTC (World Travel & Tourism Council). 2019. *Travel & Tourism: Generating Jobs for Youth*. https://wttc.org/Portals/0/Documents/Reports/2019/Social%20Impact-Generating%20Jobs%20for%20Youth-Jan%202019.pdf.

– 2020. *Travel & Tourism: Global Economic Impact & Trends 2020*. https://wttc.org/Portals/0/Documents/Reports/2020/Global%20Economic%20Impact%20Trends%202020.pdf.

– n.d.a. "Economic Impact Reports." Accessed 22 July 2021. https://wttc. org/Research/Economic-Impact.

– n.d.b. "'Safe Travels': Global Protocols & Stamp for the New Normal." Accessed 17 December 2021. https://wttc.org/COVID-19/SafeTravels- Global-Protocols-Stamp.

Xia, Y., H. Ma, G. Moloney, H.A. Velásquez García, M. Sirski, N.Z. Janjua, D. Vickers et al. 2022. "Geographic Concentration of SARS-COV-2 Cases by Social Determinants of Health in Metropolitan Areas in Canada: A Cross-Sectional Study." *Canadian Medical Association Journal* 194 (6): e195–204. https://doi.org/10.1503/cmaj.211249.

Xiao, M., I. Qian, T.W. Liu, and C. Buckley. 2022. "How a Chinese Doctor Who Warned of COVID-19 Spent His Final Days." *New York Times*, 6 October 2022. https://www.nytimes.com/2022/10/06/world/asia/ covid-china-doctor-li-wenliang.html.

Xu, L. 2021. "International Student Told to Be Thankful While Being Forced to Quarantine at Hotel." *Star*, 22 January 2021. https://www. thestar.com/news/canada/2021/01/22/international-student-told-to-be- thankful-while-being-forced-to-quarantine-at-hotel.html.

Yahoo Finance. 2020a. "Air Canada (AC.TO)." https://ca.finance.yahoo. com/quote/AC.TO.

– 2020b. "Amazon.com, Inc. (AMZN)." https://ca.finance.yahoo.com/quote/ AMZN.

– 2020c. "Cineplex Inc. (CGX.TO)." https://ca.finance.yahoo.com/quote/ CGX.TO.

– 2020d. "Empire Company Limited (EMP-A.TO)." https://ca.finance. yahoo.com/quote/EMP-A.TO.

– 2020e. "The Home Depot, Inc. (HD)." https://ca.finance.yahoo.com/ quote/HD.

– 2020f. "London Stock Exchange Group PLC (LSEG.L)." https://finance. yahoo.com/quote/LSEG.L.

– 2020g. "Moderna, Inc. (MRNA)." https://ca.finance.yahoo.com/quote/ MRNA.

– 2020h. "Netflix, Inc. (NFLX.NE)." https://ca.finance.yahoo.com/quote/ NFLX.NE.

– 2020i. "Novavax, Inc. (NVAX)." https://ca.finance.yahoo.com/quote/ NVAX.

– 2020j. "NYSE Composite (DJ) (^NYA)." https://finance.yahoo.com/ quote/%5ENYA.

– 2020k. "S&P/TSX Composite index (^GSPTSE)." https://ca.finance.yahoo. com/quote/%5EGSPTSE.

– 2020l. "Walmart Inc. (WMT)." https://ca.finance.yahoo.com/quote/WMT.

– 2020m. "Zoom Video Communications, Inc. (ZM)." https://ca.finance.
yahoo.com/quote/ZM.

– 2021a. "Best Buy Co., Inc. (BBY)." https://finance.yahoo.com/quote/BBY/
history.

– 2021b. "Costco Wholesale Corporation (COST)." https://finance.yahoo.
com/quote/COST/history.

– 2021c. "The Home Depot, Inc. (HD)." https://ca.finance.yahoo.com/
quote/HD.

– 2021d. "Walmart Inc. (WMT)." https://ca.finance.yahoo.com/quote/
WMT.

– 2022a. "Hilton Worldwide Holdings Inc. (HLT)." https://ca.finance.yahoo.
com/quote/HLT/history.

– 2022b. "InterContinental Hotels Group PLC (IHG)." https://ca.finance.
yahoo.com/quote/IHG/history.

– 2022c. "Marriott International, Inc. (MAR)." https://ca.finance.yahoo.
com/quote/MAR/history.

– 2022d. "Wyndham Hotels & Resorts, Inc. (WH)." https://ca.finance.
yahoo.com/quote/WH/history.

Yarr, K. 2020. "How P.E.I. Went from Zero to 2,000 Local COVID-19 Tests
a Week." CBC News, 28 April 2020. https://www.cbc.ca/news/canada/
prince-edward-island/pei-covid-19-tests-german-1.5547455.

Yeginsu, C., and N. Chokshi. 2021. "The Cruise Industry Stages a
Comeback." *New York Times*, 28 July 2021. https://www.nytimes.
com/2021/07/28/travel/cruise-industry-comeback.html.

York, G. 2021a. "Canada Donates Soon-to-Expire COVID-19 Vaccines to
Africa as Global Shortage Worsens." *Globe and Mail*, 9 September 2021.
https://www.theglobeandmail.com/world/article-canada-donates-soon-to-
expire-vaccines-to-africa-as-global-shortage.

– 2021b. "Canada Reluctant to Join International COVID-19 Vaccine-
Sharing Campaign." *Globe and Mail*, 3 June 2021. https://www.theglobe
andmail.com/world/article-canada-not-ready-to-join-international-covid-
19-vaccine-sharing.

– 2023. "Secret Vaccine Contracts in South Africa Authorized High Prices
and Huge Advance Payments." *Globe and Mail*, 5 September 2023.
https://www.theglobeandmail.com/world/article-south-africa-secret-
vaccine-contracts.

Young, M.E., N. King, S. Harper, and K.R. Humphreys. 2013. "The
Influence of Popular Media on Perceptions of Personal and Population
Risk in Possible Disease Outbreaks." *Health, Risk & Society* 15 (1):
103–14. https://doi.org/10.1080/13698575.2012.748884.

Young, M.E., G.R. Norman, and K.R. Humphreys. 2008. "Medicine in the Popular Press: The Influence of the Media on Perceptions of Disease." *PLOS ONE* 3 (10): E3552. https://doi.org/10.1371/journal.pone.000 3552.

Younglai, R. 2022. "Canadian Home Prices Jumped by Record 26.6 per cent in 2021." *Globe and Mail*, 17 January 2022. https://www.theglobe andmail.com/business/article-canadian-home-prices-jumped-by-record-266-per-cent-in-2021.

Yousif, N. 2020. "4 Million Cries for Help: Calls to Kids Help Phone Soar amid Pandemic." *Toronto Star*, 13 December 2020. https://www.thestar. com/news/gta/2020/12/13/4-million-cries-for-help-calls-to-kids-help-phone-soar-amid-pandemic.html.

Yu, A., S. Prasad, A. Akande, A. Murariu, S. Yuan, S. Kathirkamanathan, M. Ma, and S. Ladha. 2020. "COVID-19 in Canada: A Self-Assessment and Review of Preparedness and Response." *Journal of Global Health* 10 (2): 0203104. https://dx.doi.org/10.7189%2Fjogh.10.0203104.

Yu, G., P. Yanfeng, Y. Rui, F. Yuding, M. Danmeng, F. Murphy, H. Wei, and T. Shen. 2020. "How Early Signs of the Coronavirus Were Spotted, Spread and Throttled in China." *Straits Times*, 28 February 2020. https:// www.straitstimes.com/asia/east-asia/how-early-signs-of-the-coronavirus-were-spotted-spread-and-throttled-in-china.

Yukon Legislative Assembly. 2021. "Calendar." Government of Yukon. https://yukonassembly.ca/house-business/calendar.

Zahar, M.J., and M. Sondarjee. 2021. "Vaccine Nationalism and COVID-19." Open Canada, 25 January 2021. https://opencanada.org/vaccine-nationalism-and-covid-19.

Zahariadis, N., ed. 2016. *Handbook of Public Policy Agenda Setting.* Cheltenham, UK: Edward Elgar.

Zaidi, D. 2022. "Labour Shortage: Food, Hotel Industries Continue to Be Hardest Hit by Lack of Workers." CTV News, 23 June 2022. https:// www.ctvnews.ca/business/labour-shortage-food-hotel-industries-continue-to-be-hardest-hit-by-lack-of-workers-1.5960328.

Zajacova, A., A. Jehn, M. Stackhouse, P. Denice, and H. Ramos. 2020. "Changes in Health Behaviours during Early COVID-19 and Socio-demographic Disparities: A Cross-Sectional Analysis." *Canadian Journal of Public Health* 111: 953–62. https://doi.org/10.17269/s41997-020-00434-y.

Zanoni, K. 2020. "Ontario Long-Term Care Homes Hit with $600M Class Action Lawsuit Alleging Negligence." Top Class Actions, 6 August 2020. https://ca.topclassactions.com/lawsuit-settlements/coronavirus-covid-19/

ontario-long-term-care-homes-hit-with-600m-class-action-lawsuit-alleging-negligence.

Zeng, B., and R. Gerritsen. 2014. "What Do We Know about Social Media in Tourism? A Review." *Tourism Management Perspectives* 10 (April): 27–36. http://dx.doi.org/10.1016/j.tmp.2014.01.001.

Zhang, J.J. 2023. "Leisure Travel as Process: Understanding the Relationship between Leisure Travel and Subjective Well-Being among Older Adults." *Current Issues in Tourism* 26 (20): 3306–17. https://doi.org/10.1080/13683500.2023.2201418.

Zhang, R., Y. Li, A.L. Zhang, Y. Wang, and M.J. Molina. 2020. "Identifying Airborne Transmission as the Dominant Route for the Spread of COVID-19." *Earth, Atmospheric, and Planetary Sciences* 117 (26): 14857–63. https://doi.org/10.1073/pnas.2009637117.

Zheng, S. 2020. "An Open Letter from Canadian Doctors to the Chinese Community on Self-Isolation." 25 February 2020. https://n2nhelp.blog spot.com/2020/02/blog-post_7.html.

Zins, A.H., and I. Ponocny. 2022. "On the Importance of Leisure Travel for Psychosocial Wellbeing." *Annals of Tourism Research* 93 (March): 103378. https://doi.org/10.1016/j.annals.2022.103378.

Zoutman, D.E., B.D. Ford, and J. Gauthier. 2009. "A Cross-Canada Survey of Infection Prevention and Control in Long-Term Care Facilities." *American Journal of Infection Control* 37 (5): 358–63. https://doi.org/10.1016/j.ajic.2008.10.029.

Zucker, J. 2020. "Timeline of Coronavirus' Impact on Sports." Bleacher Report, March 2020. https://bleacherreport.com/articles/2880569-timeline-of-coronavirus-impact-on-sports.

Zussman, R. 2020. "Coronavirus: C.C. to Cancel All Non-urgent Surgeries to Free Up Beds for Possible Patients." Global News, 16 March 2020. https://globalnews.ca/news/6684870/government-canceling-non-urgent-surgeries-beds-covid-19.

Index

Page numbers in italics indicate references to tables or figures.